MW00721251

MANUAL OF EQUINE DERMATOLOGY

MANUAL OF EQUINE DERMATOLOGY

Reginald R.R. Pascoe AM, DVSc, FRCVS, FACVSc
Director, Oakey Veterinary Hospital, Oakey, Queensland , Australia

Derek C. Knottenbelt BVM&S, DVM&S, MRCVS
Senior Lecturer, Department of Veterinary Clinical Science and Animal Husbandry
University of Liverpool, Liverpool, United Kingdom

W B Saunders
London Edinburgh New York Philadelphia Sydney Toronto

WB SAUNDERS
An imprint of Harcourt Publishers Limited

First published 1999
Reprinted 1999

ISBN 0-7020-1968-2

British Library Cataloguing in Publication Data
A catalogue record for this book is available from the British Library

Library of Congress Cataloging in Publication Data
A catalog record for this book is available from the Library of Congress

Commissioning Editor: Catriona Byers
Project Supervisor: Mark Sanderson
Senior Project Editor: Carol Parr
Design: Eric Drewery

Typeset by Phoenix Photosetting, Chatham, Kent
Printed in Hong Kong
SWTC/02

The Publisher's policy is to use **paper manufactured from sustainable forests**

This book is dedicated to the memory of
our friend Tony Stannard who as one of the world's
great dermatopathologists provided us with so much friendship
and academic stimulation over so many years.
His death in 1997 was untimely and we shall miss
his wise and friendly counsel.

CONTENTS

Preface ix
Acknowledgements xi

PART I
PRINCIPLES AND TECHNIQUES 1

chapter 1
Introduction to clinical equine dermatology 3

chapter 2
The approach to the equine dermatological case 11

chapter 3
Diagnostic/investigative tests 21

chapter 4
Principles of dermatological therapeutics 35

PART II
SYNDROMES IN EQUINE DERMATOLOGY 63

chapter 5
Syndromes in equine dermatology 65

PART III
DISEASE PROFILES 89

Section A
Infectious Diseases 91

chapter 6
Viral diseases 91

chapter 7
Bacterial diseases 97

chapter 8
Fungal diseases 111

chapter 9
Protozoal diseases 121

chapter 10
Metazoan/parasitic diseases 123

Section B
Noninfectious Diseases 145

chapter 11
Congenital/developmental diseases 145

chapter 12
Immune-mediated/allergic diseases 155

chapter 13
Chemical and toxic dermatoses 183

chapter 14
Endocrine disorders 189

chapter 15
Nutritional disorders 191

chapter 16
Iatrogenic and idiopathic disorders 195

chapter 17
Physical and traumatic disorders 205

chapter 18
Injuries and diseases of the hoof 227

chapter 19
Neoplastic conditions 241

References 273

Index 281

PREFACE

The continuing popularity of the horse for both sport and pleasure has led to an ever-increasing need for veterinarians to update and upgrade their knowledge of equine diseases. Although the skin is the most visible and one of the largest organs of the body, its state of health is often overlooked. Skin disease in horses can be singularly distressing to many owners and so it is not surprising that if we, as animal health professionals, fail to solve problems, owners resort to often unproved and even harmful remedies to treat their horses. This frequently leads to a clinical deterioration and often an alteration in the clinical appearance of the condition. It can become increasingly difficult to reach either a definitive diagnosis or a successful outcome. We hope this book will address at least some of the simple problems of diagnosis and treatment.

The layout of this book is designed to help students and veterinary surgeons with an interest in equine dermatology to improve their diagnostic and treatment skills. Chapters covering the general clinical examination of the horse, which is very important in dermatological cases, diagnostic tests (which are an almost inevitable event in most skin diseases) and the general principles of dermatological therapy provide the basis for the following sections. The 'syndrome' chapter includes flow charts which we hope will encourage clinicians to explore the differential diagnosis of the common broad categories of disease. These are intended to facilitate the recognition of unusual manifestations of common conditions as well as the rarer diseases which can easily be overlooked. They are inevitably oversimplified and contain diseases which individual veterinary surgeons might never encounter and they should therefore be interpreted with care and clinical understanding.

The specific diseases are covered individually to provide a broad clinical understanding of each of the more common skin conditions. We have attempted to place greater emphasis on the commoner disorders while at the same time recognizing that the rarer ones are often more difficult to diagnose and treat. We hope that the reader will understand this relative emphasis and that we need to include the rarer disorders and those with limited geographical distributions. We consider that the foot is an extension of the skin and so we feel that it is justified to include a special section on disorders of the foot (excluding the orthopaedic and other internal disorders).

Skin tumours in general are relatively common in the horse, although many of the specific neoplastic disorders are very rare. Accordingly, a separate chapter has been included with detailed diagnostic, treatment and prognostic information.

Our great friend and colleague Tony Stannard persistently made the point that some equine diseases are given names which are derived from 'similar' diseases in other species but that there are often significant differences in the pathogenesis, pathology and clinical features. In many cases, for example sarcoidosis, systemic lupus erythematosus and eosinophilic granuloma, the differences are really sufficient to warrant separate names and so it has become common practice to prefix the diseases with 'equine'. It is probably unwise to therefore interpret the name of a disease as an indication of an identical pathological and clinical syndrome in other species. Consequent extrapolation of diagnostic or treatment protocols could be very disappointing.

Equine dermatology is considerably aided by visual appraisal but this can be a trap for the unwary, often leading to the diagnosis of rare conditions when, in fact, the horse may have a modified form of a common disease. Photographic material significantly enhances the value of a text book on dermatology and we have attempted to illustrate as many of the disorders as possible with high-quality colour illustrations. It is not possible to show every variation of every disease and so clinicians should interpret the illustrations as an indication of one form of the condition.

The wide variety of disease conditions means inevitably that there is some difficulty in trying to indicate which are common and which are rare. We have attempted to indicate the more common conditions but there is marked geographical variation in the prevalence of dermatological diseases. Furthermore, the breed, colour and type of horse as well as the specific husbandry practices have a significant effect on the incidence of disease. Veterinary surgeons will inevitably become aware of the more common diagnostic options in their own localities.

Air transportation and faster and more frequent movement of horses between countries mean that a wider range of disease conditions can be expected to be presented for diagnosis and treatment. It is particularly important to be aware of the possibility of spread of serious epidemic disease from this source. We have tried to include these wherever possible while recognizing that many veterinary surgeons may never encounter them. Furthermore, we recognize that hitherto geographically restricted diseases may appear almost anywhere. A geographical code has been inserted above those diseases which are currently regarded as restricted to limited areas of the world. Readers should interpret these with care and recognition that they are for the most part reliant upon literature reports alone.

Initially, readers might like to use the first section of the book as revision of the basic aspects of dermatological diagnosis and treatment. When faced with a dermatological case, reference could then be made directly to the chapter on syndromes. Having considered the most likely diagnosis from this, specific details regarding the confirmation of diagnosis and the suggested treatment can be obtained from the next section which is divided initially into the infectious and noninfectious diseases.

Reg Pascoe
Derek Knottenbelt

ACKNOWLEDGEMENTS

Joy Pascoe and Morna Knottenbelt have shown patience beyond the call of duty yet again and we thank them for this!

We are extremely grateful to Denis Duret, the IT Officer of the Faculty of Veterinary Science, University of Liverpool for his continued help with the figures and flow charts and other help throughout this project. Rebecca Magnussen and Barrie Edwards prepared some of the graphic drawings and we are very grateful for this help. Vicki Martin prepared the drawing on wound healing on p. 206. We gratefully acknowledge the contributions from the following colleagues.

Dr J. Gibson, Department of Primary Industries, Toowoomba, Australia
Dr S.G. Knott, Brisbane, Australia
Dr R. Miller, Brisbane, Australia
Professor J.R. Pascoe, Veterinary Medical Teaching Hospital, Davis, California, USA
Dr C. Pollitt, Department Veterinary Medicine, University of Queensland, Brisbane, Australia
Professor D.W. Scott, Department Clinical Sciences, Cornell University, New York, USA
Professor A.A. Stannard, Department of Veterinary Medicine, Veterinary Medical Teaching Hospital, Davis, California, USA
K. Swan, Ipswich, Queensland, Australia
Dr J.R. Vasey, Goulbourn Valley Veterinary Hospital, Shepparton, Australia
Dr Morna Knottenbelt, Heswall, UK
Dr K. van der Bergh, University of Pretoria, South Africa
Professor Marianne Sloet-von Oldruitenborg-Osterbaan, University of Utrecht, The Netherlands
Dr Ellen Singer, University of Liverpool, Liverpool, UK
Professor Barrie Edwards, University of Liverpool, Liverpool, UK
Dr Joan Rest, Rest Associates, Cambridge, UK
Dr John McGarry, University of Liverpool, Liverpool, UK
Dr Ian Nanjiani, Pfizer Ltd, Sandwich, UK
Dr Bruce McGorum, University of Edinburgh, UK

PART I

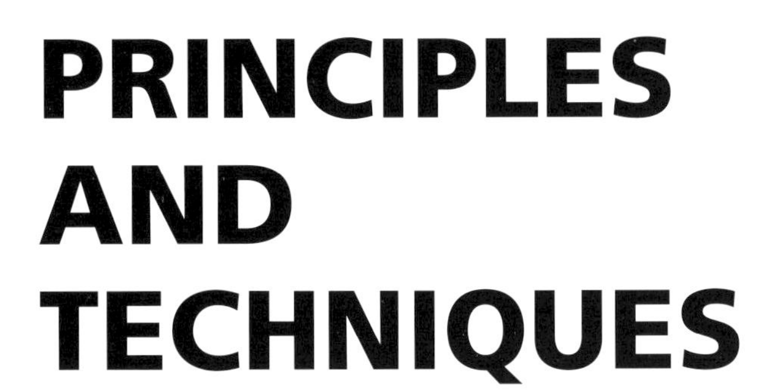

PRINCIPLES AND TECHNIQUES

chapter 1

INTRODUCTION TO CLINICAL EQUINE DERMATOLOGY

The skin is the body's largest organ and among its more important tasks are protection against the environment, thermoregulation (sweating and heat conservation), sensory perception, secretory function and pigmentation. It is conveniently examined both visually and by palpation. Deviations from normal may reflect primary skin disease and/or secondary manifestations of primary systemic disease. The latter are relatively common and the skin then may act as a significant indicator of other systemic disease and may reflect the horse's general health status.

The basis of clinical disease diagnosis must, by necessity, be guided by a thorough knowledge of what may be regarded as normal. Familiarity with dermatological terms allows a rational scientific dialogue between practitioners and dermatopathologists, reducing confusion and materially improving diagnostic accuracy. Although specific descriptive terms can be open to misinterpretation, regular usage will minimize this risk.

A careful and critical assessment of presenting clinical signs and an understanding of their significance in relation to a disease process, combined with a basic understanding of skin morphology and function, allow the clinician to categorize skin disease into broad groups. This grouping allows a clinician to reach an accurate diagnosis more easily and accurately than if attempts are made to guess a diagnosis without knowing all the facts.

The written description of various skin lesions can be both poorly understood and poorly used, and the specialized vocabulary of the dermatologist may be daunting. However, a short glossary of terms commonly used is shown at the end of this chapter (p 8). These terms make the description of well-recognized lesions more universally understood by both dermatopathologists and clinicians. Their use serves to reduce confusion in terms of recording, reporting and understanding of skin conditions but can be an oversimplification.

The normal anatomical structure of equine skin broadly follows the classical descriptions shown in many textbooks of anatomy. There are some significant differences, however, in the horse. For example, the skin is particularly well endowed with sweat glands and the horse sweats more easily and in different patterns from most other species. The growth patterns of the hair coat have a seasonal relationship which is strongly and predictably dependent upon the daylight hours and are not significantly affected by other factors such as temperature. Seasonality of coat character is an area which has been largely ignored in the horse, but the changes are very predictable both in extent and type.

The response the skin shows to insult or disease is reflected in changes in its physical appearance or texture. Alterations in the hair density or colour are also common signs of skin disease, but in some cases these occur in the absence of any apparent local disease process. Changes in physical appearance might be very significant to the dermatologist but taken alone may serve to confuse the possible diagnosis and treatment. The skin can also be seriously affected by systemic disease and so skin disorders may be secondary to an apparently unrelated condition.

INFLAMMATION

One of the most important aspects of skin disease is the inflammatory response. It can be defined as the response of living tissue to injury.[1] The response can only occur in vascularized tissues and is essential for protection against invading pathogens and for instigating the repair processes. It is also an essential defence mechanism and an important pathological process with both desirable and undesirable consequences. Inflammation is a highly complex process which proceeds in a co-ordinated fashion to produce the response in the injured tissue. Failure of the normal defence mechanisms to respond adequately to an insult can result in infection and progressive tissue damage while an inappropriate, overactive response can also result in tissue damage as a result of (auto-immune) self-damage. One of the main values of inflammation is the repair of injured tissues after foreign matter and infection have been eliminated. A detailed knowledge of the particular inflammatory responses in an organ and the cells involved in the process provides the clinician with the means to manipulate the response and to develop new and more effective therapeutic regimens.

In some types of injury, such as simple lacerated/incisional wounds, inflammation leads specifically and directly to repair. In infected tissues the response leads first to the removal of necrotic tissues, infectious organisms and foreign matter and then to repair. However, in some infections the process of elimination of bacteria may lead to the release of enzymes which have tissue-destructive properties. This process, which may also involve other causes of tissue destruction, can result in disruption of the normally beneficial inflammatory response.

The inflammatory process is largely similar for a wide range of applied insults – it can be regarded as the end point of damage however it is caused. The responses seen in the skin are generally, therefore, not pathognomonic for a particular cause. However, there are some responses which show significant and identifiable differences that make diagnosis simpler. These conditions are often easily recognized.

There are several distinct ways in which the skin can respond to an applied insult. The first of these is the inflammatory response and the others largely fall into the categories of injury or hypersensitivity. However, it is important to realize that a skin laceration, for example, will be accompanied by inflammation and, indeed, its resolution (healing and repair) depends upon the existence and efficiency of the inflammatory response. Similarly, a hypersensitivity response, to an insect bite for example, will inevitably result in an acute inflammatory response. The intensity and duration of the response will depend in large part on the nature and severity of the insult and any complicating factors which develop. Even self-inflicted trauma (such as might arise from pruritus) and mild infections will have a profound influence on the overall response. It is therefore often difficult to establish the primary problem when such complicating factors exist.

Typical of all aspects of physiological response, the processes are linked seamlessly and undue reliance upon categories of response is likely to lead to errors of interpretation. Inflammation can conveniently be divided into acute and chronic forms, although this division is arbitrary and elements of both are almost always present at some point in the healing/repair process. The balance between the two is probably not clinically definable, but acute inflammation usually evolves into chronic inflammation with or without a repair phase. In some cases there is no detectable acute phase and the injury appears to pass directly into a chronic response. Chronic inflammation is usually of longer duration than acute inflammation and is characterized by the presence of mononuclear cells (macrophages, lymphocytes and plasma cells) and marked fibroblastosis.

THE ACUTE INFLAMMATORY RESPONSE

Following an insult to the skin (which may include physical injury, insect bite or a response from interactions within the body itself, etc.) that involves a vascular response to injury, a transient period of vasoconstriction develops. This is followed by vasodilatation and an increase in arteriolar permeability both to cells and to bioactive proteins. This results in the extravasation of fluid and proteins (and blood cells if the damage is sufficiently severe). There is a resultant relative haemoconcentration and increased viscosity of the blood which slows the circulation down. This allows stasis of erythrocytes and platelets and margination of leukocytes to occur. Once attached to the vascular endothelium they migrate into the extravascular space.

Neutrophils and monocytes identify and attack noxious particles such as foreign matter and bacteria, removing them by phagocytosis. However, most bacteria must first be coated with serum proteins (opsonins) (which have also leaked into the tissue fluid as a result of the vascular damage). Opsonins include IgG (antibodies to antigens encountered previously), and complement. Once phagocytosed, the bacteria are destroyed in the cell itself, but some of the products of this breakdown and the lysis of cells can escape into the region of the injury and here they may exacerbate the tissue destruction. A cascade of biophysiological responses is instigated which culminates in the development of one or more of the cardinal signs of inflammation. These are heat, pain (or pruritus), swelling and (less obviously in the skin of horses) redness.

The cells involved in the acute inflammatory process are largely delivered to the site via the circulation. They include the granulocytes (neutrophils, eosinophils and basophils), mast cells, monocytes and lymphocytes. The neutrophil is the predominate cell in acute inflammation particularly when bacterial infection is present.

The neutrophil These contain two major types of granules which are involved in the process. While they have a predominately beneficial effect on acutely inflamed tissue, disruption of the cells can cause the release of destructive enzymes which can lead to further cell death. Furthermore, they can elicit the production of free radicals, hydrogen peroxide and hypochlorous acid which are all harmful to the tissues.

Other granulocytes Eosinophils, basophils and mast cells release a variety of lipid and peptide mediators which instigate aspects of the inflammatory response. The eosinophil seems to be particularly involved in the defence mechanisms for parasitic infections/insults while the basophil and mast cell are probably involved in allergic or immediate hypersensitivity responses.

Macrophages These are probably the most important cell type in the inflammatory responses. They are especially important in chronic inflammation in all organs and structures. They are produced by monocytes in the bone marrow and are delivered to the damaged tissues by the circulation. The monocytes are long-lived tissue cells which can differentiate under suitable stimulus into macrophages with secretory and phagocytic properties. They have a highly active phagocytic function and their role in the process of defence inflammation involves many bioactive substances (including plasminogen activation factor, collagenase, interleukin-1, tumour necrosis factor and complement).

Activated macrophages also produce oxygen molecules (including free radicals) and eicosanoids (including prostaglandins and thromboxane). The majority of the products from macrophage metabolism and destruction augment inflammation, and while this may result in significant defence against microorganisms it may also cause further tissue destruction.

A further role for macrophages is as an intermediary in the development of humoral response/antibody production. They serve to carry and present antigens to T lymphocytes.

Lymphocytes These cells are important for identification of foreign and autoantigens. B cells recognize the antigens and will produce antibody-forming T cells. T cells also recognize antigens and will proliferate in response to specific antigens.

CHRONIC INFLAMMATION

Coordination of the vascular and cellular responses is important in the inflammatory process. This is provided by a series of mediators which are derived from the circulation (complement, albumin, fibrinogen and kinins) and from cells in the tissue (either migratory cells or cells comprising the local vasculature or other tissues). Cyclooxygenases catalyse the breakdown of arachidonic acid and this culminates in the production of prostaglandins or thromboxane. The prostaglandins are mediators of the vascular phases of inflammation causing profound vasodilatation, and with histamine and kinins cause increased vascular permeability. In addition to the pro-inflammatory effects, these also have significant suppressive effects on B and T lymphocytes as well as interleukin-2. Lipoxygenase proteins also support the bonding of oxygen, but in this case to fatty acids (and arachidonic acid in particular). This reaction proceeds to the production of leukotrienes, which are important chemoattractants for leukocytes. The interrelationships of these chemical processes is very complex.

A large number of factors are capable of influencing the inflammatory process including the nonsteroidal anti-inflammatory drugs (such as aspirin, phenylbutazone, ketoprophen and flunixin meglumine). These drugs act by inhibiting cyclooxygenase and individual drugs have greater or lesser effect in this direction. Corticosteroids also have a profound effect on the process by inhibiting the synthesis of prostaglandins and leukotrienes. They have an important difference from the nonsteroidal drugs in that they affect both cyclooxygenase and lipoxygenase production. Thus, the two classes of drugs can be used to disrupt different aspects of the process and are particularly useful when one side or the other of the process is having a deleterious or harmful effect on the tissue.

Growth factors and cytokines are complex bioactive proteins which influence the behaviour of cell types, through either stimulation or inhibition. The relative proportions of these are vital in the coordination of the repair processes which follow inflammation. Uncoordinated production with consequent alterations in cell behaviour are blamed for many abnormal or idiosyncratic responses in the skin including the failure of some skin wounds to heal.

Proteinases (including the metalloproteinases which rely upon zinc in particular) are some of the most significant mediators of injury and tissue

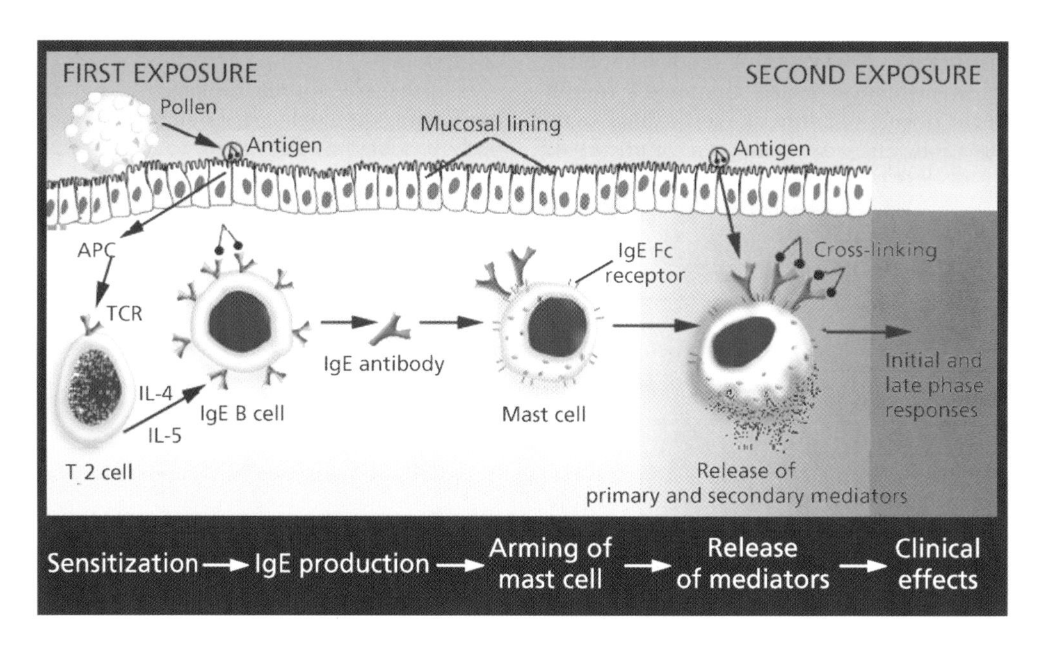

Figure 1.1 Type 1 Hypersensitivity (Immediate/anaphylactic response). These responses are primarily the result of dramatic mast cell degranulation. The IgE binds to the surface of mast cells or basophils and on subsequent exposure to the same antigen, degranulation occurs with release of inflammatory mediators. The release of inflammatory mediators results in a dramatic and immediate local damage and sometimes systemic signs. The response is usually immediate (within minutes) and may be severe, resulting in an acute systemic anaphylaxis. The response can, however, be delayed for several hours and indeed there may be a biphasic response (an immediate response with a second response in 1–2 hours).

Typical examples of this response include anaphylaxis, atopy and food hypersensitivity.

destruction. In some cases they are responsible for bacterial and cell debris degradation but they have a significant and desirable role in collagenolysis and natural disruption of the extracellular matrix in healthy, healing tissue. The role of these proteins in skin diseases of the horse has not yet been established but their study is currently one of the most exciting areas of research.

It is probable that all aspects of the inflammatory process have both advantages and disadvantages. The balance and coordination of the process appears to be the most significant aspect in promoting the beneficial while suppressing the harmful effects. All therapeutic measures applied to the repair of skin injuries and the curing of skin disease have to take account of these processes and drugs or manipulations which sacrifice the beneficial aspects must be viewed with some caution.

SKIN REACTIONS – COOMBS' SENSITIVITY REACTIONS

The extent of the inflammatory response outlined above is also influenced by various other types of responses which precede inflammation. These are usefully categorized into four types of reaction which depend variously on the type of insult that is applied. An in-depth description of these responses can be found in most texts on immunology and pathology. Although some skin diseases can be attributed to a single one of these responses, most have aspects of several and so the

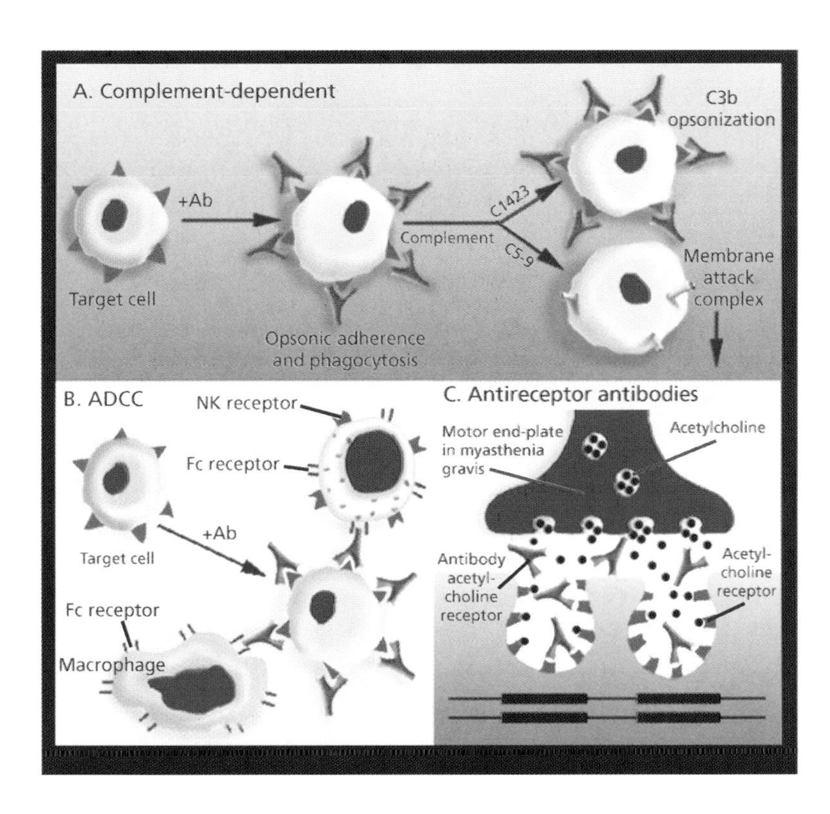

Figure 1.2 Type 2 Hypersensitivity (Cytotoxic response). Antibodies and complement bind onto complete antigens on or in body tissues and result in antibody-dependent cytotoxicity with resultant cell damage or disruption. This response also arises from antibody binding to exogenous antigen which has become associated with a cell-surface or with a basement membrane.

Examples include haemolytic disease of foals (neonatal isoerythrolysis), pemphigus complex of diseases and immune-mediated thrombocytopenia. Drug eruptions may also be associated with this type of reaction.

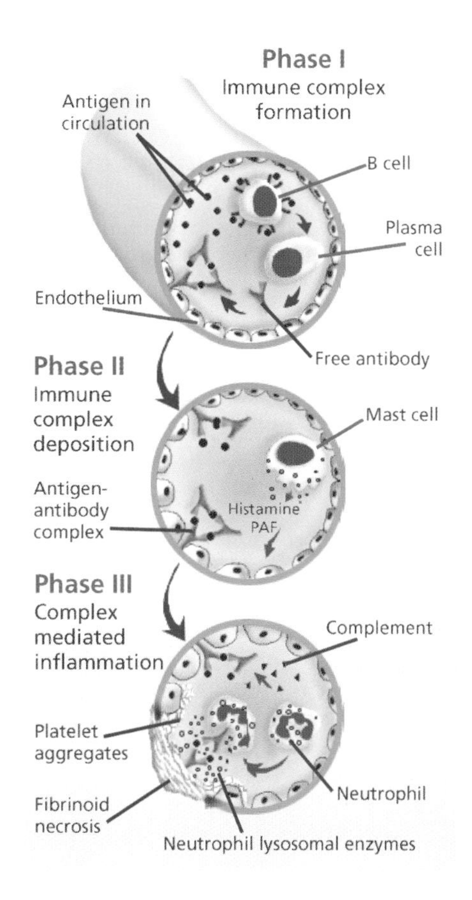

Figure 1.3 Type 3 Hypersensitivity (Immune-complex hypersensitivity reactions). Antigen–antibody complexes (immune complexes) are formed which can exist freely in the circulation or can be deposited in capillary beds, basement membranes or other tissues. These antigen–antibody complexes are deposited on circulating cells (e.g. red cells or platelets) or the cells of major organs. Deposition onto vascular endothelial cells is particularly frequent. Their deposition at these sites is strongly attractive to neutrophils, and when these are disrupted they release tissue destructive hydrolytic and proteolytic enzymes which induce tissue damage. The consequent damage to blood vessel walls causes small haemorrhages (petechial and ecchymotic haemorrhages) and leakage of protein which results in localized oedema. Serious secondary systemic effects can arise. Cell damage can therefore occur without specific antibody to the cells themselves. This is the presumed mechanism for the autoimmune haemolytic anaemia which accompanies internal infections or neoplasia. Pastern leukocytoclastic vasculitis, purpura haemorrhagica and systemic lupus erythematosus-like syndrome are cutaneous examples of this response.

categorization is arbitrary. It is however, helpful at a basic level.

CLINICAL DESCRIPTIONS OF SPECIFIC TYPES OF LESIONS SEEN IN THE HORSE

It is important to describe lesions accurately even if a definitive diagnosis cannot be attained. These definitions are useful when describing a clinical condition but typically many lesions have some characteristics of several single lesions. The correct use of the terms below facilitate the understanding between clinicians and dermatopathologists but can be oversimplified and therefore misleading. Examples of each type of lesion are shown in other chapters of this book.

Primary lesions

Macule A small (< 1 cm diameter) circumscribed, flat, impalpable area of colour change in the skin (hypo- or hyperpigmentation). (See Figure 6.3.)

Patch A macule > 1 cm diameter. (See Figure 12.21.)

Papule Small (< 1 cm diameter), circumscribed, solid, slightly raised mass in skin. A papule is always palpable as an abnormality of the normal skin texture/structure. Papules may be discoloured (pink or red). They are often associated with insect bites etc. and may be pruritic. (See Figure 6.2.)

Plaque Solid elevated, flat-topped, regular or irregular thickening > 1 cm diameter arising as result of coalescence of papules. (Usually allergic in origin, e.g. urticarial lesions.) A plaque which has a closely packed irregular projecting surface is termed a *vegetation*. (See Figure 12.5.)

Vesicle These are sharply demarcated, raised lesions filled with a clear watery fluid. Very large vesicles are called 'bullae'. They can be epidermal or subepidermal. It is easy to appreciate that the thin overlying epidermis makes them very fragile and liable to rupture from even minor trauma – these are therefore rarely seen intact (e.g. early equine coital exanthema, blistering etc.). (See Figure 12.13.)

Pustule A small well-defined and circumscribed mass in the skin which is filled with purulent material and inflammatory debris. They are usually yellow in colour but may have a green or dark brown hue. (See Figure 6.8.)

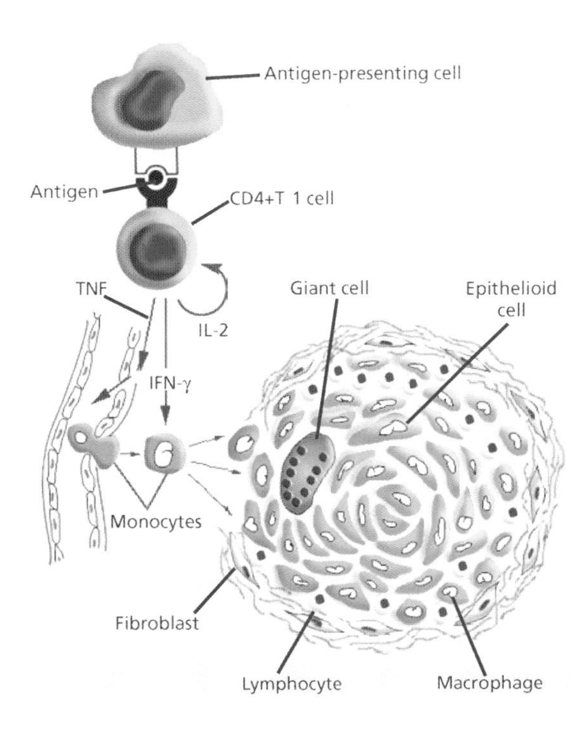

Figure 1.4 Type 4 Hypersensitivity (Cell-mediated responses). These responses arise when an antigen reacts with a tissue protein to form a recognizable antigen against which the body's cellular responses are marshalled. The monocyte/macrophage (or Langerhans') cells then present the antigen to the lymphoreticular tissue where T lymphocytes respond by releasing mediators which cause tissue damage and generalized systemic effects such as extensive pruritus. The hypersensitivity reaction/response is therefore delayed for up to 48–72 hours (or sometimes longer). This reaction is typified by the intradermal tuberculin test in cattle and humans and the intradermopalpebral Mallein test for glanders in horses.

Drug eruptions and culicoides hypersensitivity (sweet itch) are examples of this response.

An **abscess** is a localized collection of pus in a cavity formed by disintegration of tissue. (See Figure 3.5.)

Wheal A well-defined, circular, flat-topped, oedematous lesion of variable size which usually causes no changes in the overlying skin or hair coat. They usually appear and disappear rapidly (e.g. urticarial reactions). (See Figure 12.2.)

Nodule Raised, circumscribed (round) solid lump > 1 cm diameter which usually extends into the deeper layers of the skin (e.g. sarcoid, melanoma, neurofibroma, eosinophilic granuloma, some allergic responses). (See Figure 19.5.)

Cyst A smooth, well-defined, circumscribed structure lined with epithelium and containing solid or liquid matter secreted by cells in the lining. (See Figure 11.12.)

Tumour Mass of (usually) neoplastic origin (benign or malignant) (e.g. sarcoid, melanoma, papilloma, etc.). (See Figure 19.12.)

Secondary lesions

Alopecia Partial or complete loss of hair from whatever cause. Most alopecia is secondary but it can be primary. (See Figure 12.21.)

Scales Accumulation of loose epidermal debris (usually white or discoloured yellowish/brown by sebum, serum or blood). (See Figure 14.1.)

Crust Solid, dry, adherent accumulation of dried serum, blood, pus or scales. (See Figure 8.2.)

Scar/cheloid Fibrous tissue of healed lesion in skin

(see Figure 17.13.) Abnormal or inappropriate scarring may be hypertrophic (see Figure 17.5) or cheloid (see Figure 17.14.)

Erosion Shallow skin defects not penetrating the basement membrane (these do not result in scarring). (see Figure 10.14.)

Ulcers Erosion which penetrates the full depth of the skin (scar formation is invariable when healing has taken place). (See Figure 10.4.)

Lichenification Thick, hard skin which is often hyperpigmented and alopecic. Marked folding and thickening is often present. (See Figure 12.28.)

Fissure Splitting of skin (often with bleeding) and loss of natural elasticity. (see Figure 7.10.)

Hypo-/hyperpigmentation Damaged skin resulting in changes in natural pigment distribution in the immediate vicinity. This can be either white (leukoderma/leukotrichia) or black (melanoderma/melanotrichia). (See Figure 11.9.)

chapter 2

THE APPROACH TO THE EQUINE DERMATOLOGICAL CASE

Owners of horses commonly become distressed when skin problems fail to resolve, or even to follow a predicted course. This may happen because of misinformation, misdiagnosis or improper treatment. Without an accurate diagnosis, any treatment becomes little better than an educated guess. Without a logical and systematic approach, there are few more frustrating situations than the diagnosis and treatment of skin disease in horses.

A problem-orientated approach, in which the diagnostic process is directed towards the identification of the recognizable problems which the horse has, is an effective way of exploring a dermatological case. An accurate diagnosis can often be made then and effective and economic treatment instituted. The problems may be primarily dermal, but it is important to realize that significant skin disease can arise as a secondary manifestation of a primary systemic disease.

The initial clinical objective should be to identify the predominant clinical sign. The most common components of equine skin disease are

- Pruritus (itching dermatoses)
- Hair loss (alopecic dermatoses)
- Scaling and crusting (dry/flaking dermatoses)
- Weeping and seeping (moist dermatoses)
- Alterations in pigmentation
- Nodular lesions (skin-thickening dermatoses)

Before performing any clinical examination or other investigation the clinician should always obtain an accurate historical account of the case. A clinical examination might then allow the disease to be categorized into one or more of the above major disease patterns. While it may be more correct scientifically to make an approach based on the causal agent or agents, these are commonly not obvious and often require further tests.

EXAMPLE OF A DERMATOLOGICAL EXAMINATION FORM

This form is included to illustrate the type of form which might prove useful in investigation of dermatological problems in horses. A suitable abbreviated form can be prepared to cover re-examinations at subsequent dates. Clinicians are invited to copy or modify this to suit their own needs.

Equine Dermatology Diagnostic Form

Date: Name of horse: CASE NUMBER:

(Referring) Veterinarian: Owner:
Address:

Tel:
INSURANCE: YES/NO
Type: Company: Tel:

Breed/Type: Age: Sex:

Colour: Height: ID MARK:

Clinical Problem

HISTORY
Duration of ownership: Prepurchase exam: YES/NO

Use of horse:

Deworming: Vaccination:

Management:

Diet:

Environment: inside:

outside:

Contagion/Contact : contact with other horses? YES/NO
do they have skin problems? YES/NO
are the lesions the same? YES/NO
with other species? YES/NO
any skin lesions on the owners? YES/NO

History of skin problem

Date of onset:

Initial signs:

How has it progressed?

Pruritus present: YES/NO

Which parts of the horse are affected?

Feet	Legs	Head
Body	Mane	Tail

Fly control measures taken:

Previous treatment for the problem?

Did it help?:

General health:

date of start: finish:

other diseases or illness:

other treatments administered:

drug:
frequency:
period:
effect:

Summing-up from history:

Physical examination:

Vital signs

Rectal temperature: °C Pulse: b/m Respiration: b/m

Capillary refill time: sec Mucous membrane colour:

Body condition: (0–10) Weight: kg (estimate/band/scale)

Body Systems

(Record abnormalities only; N/A = no abnormalities detected)

Alimentary system:

Cardiovascular system:

Respiratory system:

Nervous system:

Special senses (eye/ear):

Hepatic and endocrine systems:

Urinary system:

Reproductive system:

Endocrine system:

Musculoskeletal system:

Dermatological examination

Pruritus:	Present/Absent	Mild	Moderate	Severe

Primary lesions: (circle)	macule	papule	patch
	pustule	vesicle	bulla
	wheal	nodule	tumour
Secondary lesions:	erythema	scale	crust
	fissure	alopecia	comedone
	ulcer	erosion	excoriation
	hyperpigmentation		lichenification
Hair – Colour change?:	Easily epilated?:		Greasy/Dry?
Skin – Normal	Thickened		Thin

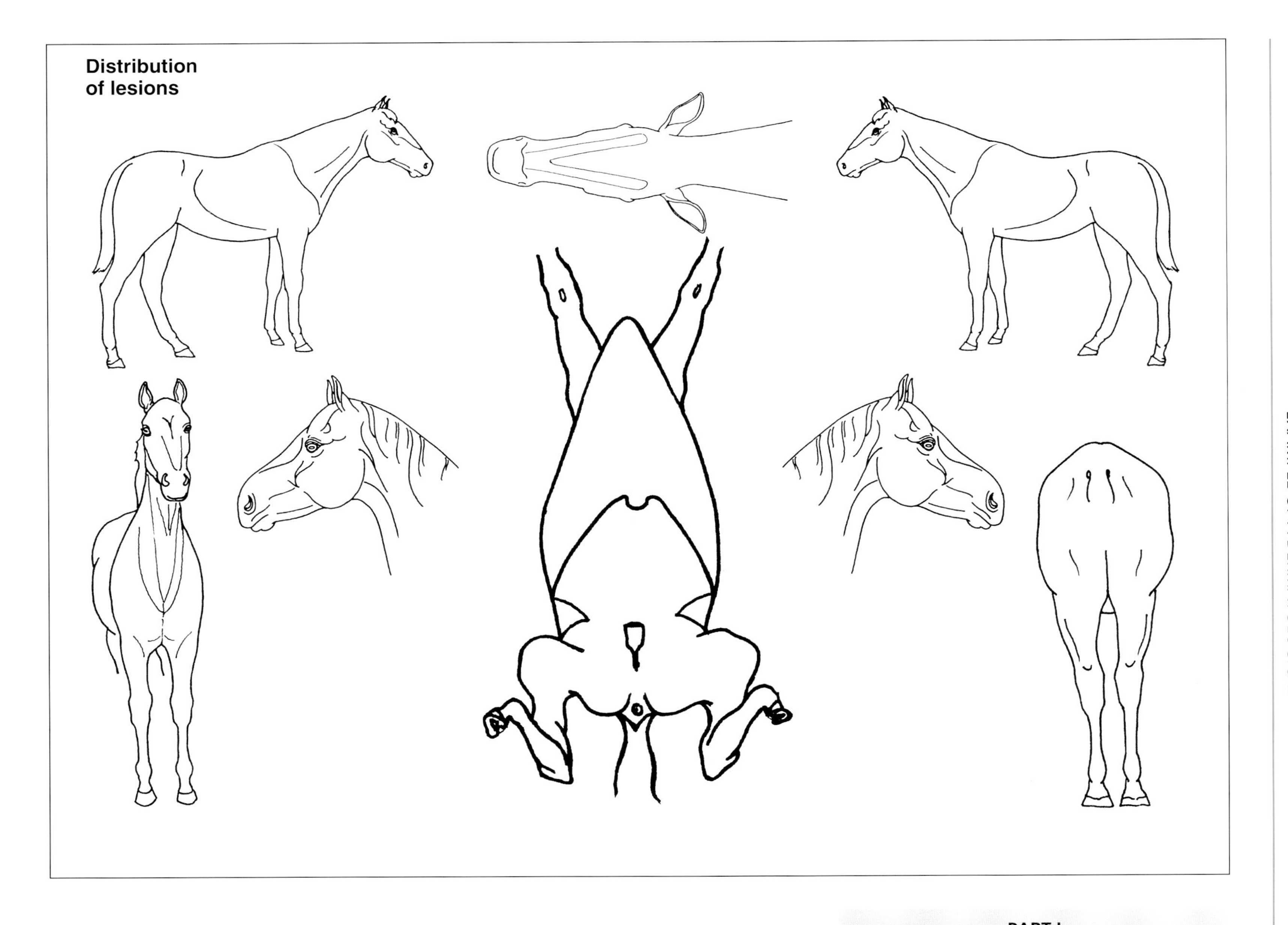
Distribution
of lesions

Problem List:

Differential diagnosis (in order of likelihood):

Diagnostic tests and results
(ring tests performed and * if test performed 'in house')
Name of laboratory: Report number:
Date of dispatch: Date of result/report:
phone:
written:

1. Skin scrapings:
2. Sellotape preparation:
3. Groomings:
4. Culture/sensitivity
   - Viral culture/ID
   - Fungal swab/culture:
   - Yeast prep/culture:
   - Bacterial swab:
   - *Dermatophilus* prep/culture:
5. Needle aspirate:
6. Biopsy: bacterial culture:
   histopathology:
   immunofluorescence:
7. Serology:
8. Other:

Diagnosis:

Treatment prescribed (in detail):

Photographs (number/location/type):

Revisits: YES/NO

Date: **Sheet number:** **Case number:**

History taking (anamnesis)

The history of both the animal and the presenting problem are important parts of all clinical procedures. These should preferably be established and recorded before any clinical assessment or judgement is made. Failure to obtain an adequate history often leads to gross errors of interpretation and diagnosis. For example, if the clinician is not aware that the owner has already attempted treatment with antiparasitic medication, he or she might be misled by the failure to find ectoparasites during subsequent clinical and laboratory investigations. Diseases which have been subjected to repeated (and sometimes ill-conceived) treatment attempts are particularly common in equine practice and a truthful, long-term history of the animal is very helpful. Careful, exhaustive inquiry of the client is a time-consuming exercise but is clearly essential.

The history should establish relevant long-term information about the animal such as previous disease or illness, surgery, medication and the vaccination and worming status. Work and management details (including bedding types and feed regimens) provide useful information, particularly when considered with the time of onset of the condition. Careful reviews of in-contact horses (or other species) and the environment are useful additions.

The clinical problem as perceived by the owner (usually called the 'owner's complaint') is often a useful starting point for the process of obtaining the history of the specific complaint. The value of an individually formulated examination sheet (such as is shown), cannot be understated – it allows a structured, thorough questioning without omissions. However, even this may not always be totally comprehensive. No information is too trivial – subtle facts may ultimately be the most significant. It is important to avoid undue repetitions but it may be necessary to ask questions in different ways to obtain the most helpful and reliable answers.

Particular attention should be paid to previous diagnostic tests, diagnoses and attempts at treatment (by owners, well-meaning lay people and previous veterinary surgeons). The nature of practice sometimes makes this difficult to establish, but it is important to determine whether any measures have had significant effects on the course of the condition (for better or worse). It is often helpful in long-standing cases to ask the client to provide a chronological list of the disease's progress, variation of feed or environment or of rider tack or harness which has been used. Management changes such as feed, water, bedding, pasture and transport, or unusual circumstances such as access to toxic waste or preservative-treated fence posts, should be established early.

Including the historical information on a 'Dermatological Examination Form' provides a record of these events. It is often possible to come to a broad conclusion as to the nature of the case based upon the history alone. For example, contact with other horses known to be affected by dermatophytosis ('ringworm') might be suggestive of the problem, but failure to continue the investigation by clinical assessment is potentially dangerous.

The clinical examination of the horse

Failure to perform a full clinical examination of all the body systems can lead to errors of diagnosis. For example, a horse showing evidence of photosensitization might also exhibit icterus (jaundice) and ventral oedema and the underlying primary problem may be hepatic failure. Subsequent treatment of the dermatological problem alone may be disappointing without the primary disease being addressed. In practice, exhaustive clinical examinations are not always performed.

Many of the common skin diseases are primary and present with sufficient clinical signs and history to justify an abbreviated clinical examination. However, there is then a significant danger with problem skin diseases, and especially those which do not fall neatly into recognizable patterns, that important aspects of the general health of the patient might be missed.

The clinical examination should begin with the assessment of the general health, demeanour and bodily condition of the horse. An early overall view of the horse in good light is useful and might help to establish the distribution of skin abnormalities. The condition may be very localized or more generalized. This in itself aids the diagnosis, as some conditions are never (or very rarely) generalized and some others are not usually localized.

The physical examination should include the recording of the vital signs and the assessment of each body system in turn. Clearly, there are justifiable short-cuts which are acceptable after experience has been gained, but clinicians should be particularly wary of jumping to conclusions in dermatological disease. Thus, an examination of the musculoskeletal system and a lameness work-up should not be needed in most cases. An assessment of the neurological system may be specifically helpful in some cases such as photosensitization when hepatic encephalopathy may be present.

Following a broad physical examination, there may be indications for organ function tests. These might include haematological analysis, serum biochemistry, abdominocentesis, faecal and urine analyses, rectal examination, ultrasonography and gastrointestinal absorption tests. The dermatologist should be particularly wary of the trap of a 'haematological diagnosis'. There are very few primary skin diseases which exhibit significant haematological findings, but some diseases with secondary dermatological changes have important haematological changes (e.g. Cushing's disease and photosensitization arising from hepatic disease).

The physical examination may require to be repeated at a later stage, particularly when an apparently simple skin disease fails to respond to treatment, and it is important to record all the findings of the initial and subsequent examinations. Where skin disease appears as a consequence of internal disease, local skin treatment is likely to be ineffective (or palliative) unless the underlying disease is resolved. Furthermore, successful treatment of the underlying disease may result in rapid resolution of the skin disease without the need for extensive local treatment beyond obvious supportive measures. In dermatological cases a thorough clinical examination may therefore be particularly rewarding.

The specific dermatological examination is obviously a major part of the clinical process of investigation of skin disease and again the method for this can be laid out on a prepared form so that little is omitted or ignored. The form can be used again for reference if the problem fails to resolve. Reference to the type and size of lesions is based upon the accepted lesion descriptions (see Chapter 1), which should be readily recognized by the clinician. The nature, number, size and distribution of the lesions should be recorded. It is often useful to refer to these recognized lesion types when discussing the case with colleagues or with a pathologist who might become involved in the case.

Furthermore, reference to previous records provides information on the extent and type of changes since the last examination. The owner (and veterinarian) might be under the impression that the condition has deteriorated whereas in fact it might have improved or new lesions might have developed with a different distribution. A chronological record is particularly useful to pathologists in identifying the likely age of a lesion or change in the skin.

A photographic record is a very useful and underutilized asset in dermatology. Skin diseases are often very photogenic and photographs provide an exact description which cannot always be effectively provided by a written account.

The problem list

Following the history taking, clinical examination and recording of the 'owner's complaint', a problem list should be compiled. This provides a concise summary of the salient features of the case as well as the findings of clinical and historical examinations. The list can be as detailed as the clinician feels is useful. It serves to focus attention on the defined problem(s) which have been identified. It is often possible at this stage to detect the presence or absence of systemic disease involvement (whether related to the dermatological problem or not). Although this may in some cases be misleading, it may still have profound influences on treatment options. Thus, a pony with laminitis may be precipitated into a life-threatening acute episode following a single corticosteroid dose administered to treat a mild skin disease. Similarly, a horse with liver failure may show no skin disease until it is subjected to high levels of ultraviolet light/sunlight and may then not benefit from being turned out into sunlight as part of an attempt to treat a suspected or confirmed dermatophytosis (ringworm).

The term *syndrome* is defined as an aggregate of clinical features, signs or symptoms which form the picture of a disease entity. This is therefore not a term which is theoretically applicable to the features of dermatological disease. In the horse the range of clinical signs is limited for a wide range of disparate disorders and so for the purposes of this text they will be termed syndromes. Further breakdown of these can be found in Chapter 5 in which a number of possible diagnoses can be found for each syndrome. The clinical problem can usually be classified into one or more of the major classes outlined below.

1. **Pruritus** Itching or irritation of the skin which encourages behavioural changes such as self-inflicted trauma.
2. **Alopecia and alteration of hair quantity or quality** Complete or partial baldness (loss of hair) or alteration in hair density or quality or over a variable area.

3. **Nodule** A circumscribed thickening of the skin of variable size and extent.
4. **Dry dermatosis (scaling and crusting)** An accumulation of dry scales and crusts arising from excessive flaking of the skin or from accumulation of dried exudate on the surface of the skin.
5. **Moist dermatosis (weeping and seeping)** An accumulation of fluid exudate on the skin surface arising directly from skin damage/inflammation or another pathological process.
6. **Pigmentary alterations** Changes in the normal pigmentary pattern of the hair coat and/or the skin.

It is entirely possible that the problem list will include more than one of the major problem categories (syndromes), but this should not distort or bias the diagnostic process. Each condition should be initially considered in its own right and the combined lists examined to see whether there are common diagnostic possibilities.

One or more of the major forms of skin disease may be presented and this should be considered with other clinical features such as the anatomical location of the problem. This will inevitably form a major part of the problem list. For example, scaling and crusting over the fetlock region and facial and limb pruritus might be recognized. Although these specific points serve to identify the character of the problem, in themselves they provide little information on the aetiology, diagnosis or treatment options.

A specific diagnosis must then be the objective of the clinician but may be difficult to achieve directly from the problem list in many cases. It is made even more difficult when a logical diagnostic process is not applied. The next stage in the process is to establish a list of differential diagnoses, i.e. specific diseases which may be present or which have the features identified.

Differential diagnosis

After completion of the problem list, a differential diagnosis list consisting of probable and possible diseases can be assembled. Flow charts (algorithms) can be useful for both inexperienced and experienced clinicians to develop the differential diagnosis (see Chapter 5). Serious errors can be made by attempting to make a disease fit a single or few clinical features. Very few diseases are predictably identical in all cases. Subtle and more obvious variations are usually present to trap the unwary clinician. The most likely conditions (probably being placed at the top of the differential diagnosis list) will vary widely in different geographical areas, at different times in the year and under different management conditions. Thus, some diseases are common in some areas and almost never encountered in others. Some conditions are strictly limited geographically and these can justifiably be left out of the consideration in the rest of the world. For example, glanders is currently very restricted and could possibly justifiably be ignored in the United Kingdom – however the dangers of such an approach are obvious! Deep mycosis such as Florida leech disease occurs in a restricted area in the Gulf states of the United States, South America and Australia and has not been recorded elsewhere. There are other areas where it is theoretically possible and it may then be placed low on the list. Geographical restriction of diseases is becoming much less significant as rapid, worldwide transport of horses has become commonplace. Unusual diseases may appear and epidemics of highly contagious diseases can also occur more readily. It is, of course, impossible in a book of this type to list every variation in every disease.

It may of course be possible to identify at this point a specific and definitive diagnosis and take appropriate therapeutic measures. More likely, a short-list of possible diagnoses whose clinical features are basically similar and which are not separable on clinical grounds alone will be considered. These may then require special tests for confirmation of a definitive diagnosis or elimination of some of the alternatives.

Diagnostic confirmation/ investigative tests

The diagnosis is that part of the investigation which leads to the establishment of a specific disease process. From the differential diagnosis list, a number of further investigative methods can be identified either to confirm or to eliminate specific conditions. Supportive diagnostic tests are often used in dermatological cases because of the outward clinical similarity of many conditions and the limited range of clinical signs detectable through clinical examination alone. There is a significant danger in proceeding straight to this stage without any previous clinical examination or historical information, thus relying totally on the services of a bacteriologist, pathologist or clinical pathologist. This is not an acceptable practice in dermatological cases and the specialist concerned carries an unfair and unjustifiable responsibility for diagnosis.

If a diagnosis cannot be achieved safely, the clinician should at least try to categorize the condition into one of the major recognized syndromes (listed above). Consideration should then be given to the selection of the most appropriate further tests and procedures. It is unwise and unfair to expect a clinical pathologist, bacteriologist or dermatohistopathologist to support a diagnosis without access to all relevant clinical and historical information. A photocopy of the case record sent with any specimens is very helpful and saves time and effort.

If a diagnosis still cannot be reached, a thorough review of both the clinical and historical features should be performed. (This is made very much simpler if a full standard record has been taken at each examination.) It is often helpful to discuss the case with a colleague or a pathologist who might have different experience and a different perspective on it.

Various dermatological diagnostic tests are available, some are simple and some more complicated. Regular contact with pathologists often provides very valuable information and a good rapport is to be encouraged. Unless the diagnostic tests are standard and performed frequently, it is often very useful to consult a specialist pathologist (or technician) before embarking on them. For example, skin biopsy in particular appears to be simple but there are specific types of biopsy technique or fixatives which may be useful in particular cases (see Chapter 3). A pathologist's decision on the orientation, site and type of biopsy can often be significantly different from the standard clinical approach.

Once a decision has been taken with respect to the selection of further tests, the clinician must obtain all the relevant equipment to perform the procedures. A wide range of tests is available and most of the regular ones are described in detail in Chapter 3.

Regular access to good textbooks and well-illustrated clinical papers in journals is very helpful but cannot be relied upon to provide a diagnosis.

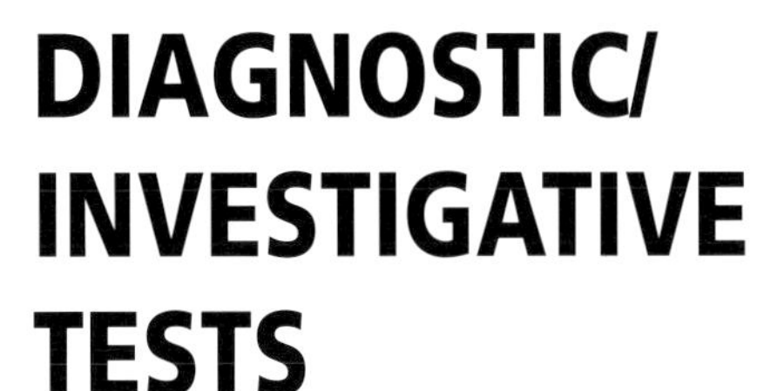

chapter 3

DIAGNOSTIC/ INVESTIGATIVE TESTS

A careful review of the differential diagnosis list will direct the clinician to the most appropriate further diagnostic aids or tests which can be used either to confirm suspicions of a diagnosis or to eliminate specific disorders.

Basic tests, which can be carried out in a practice laboratory by means of a microscope and simple stains, can often provide useful diagnostic information in uncomplicated diseases. However, unless handling and processing of specimens is performed regularly, it may be wiser to send specimens to a recognized veterinary laboratory for assistance with diagnosis. A positive diagnosis from your own practice laboratory can be very rewarding, but a false (negative or positive) may be embarrassing. Most commercial and university laboratories are well equipped and staffed with trained pathologists and technicians. If all relevant clinical information is supplied to them, they can be a powerful ally in establishing a diagnosis in many cases and particularly so in complex or unusual ones. However, as there are few specialist equine pathologists and even fewer equine dermatohistopathologists, some difficulties may be experienced in obtaining a correct interpretation of the specimens. Discussion with an experienced pathologist in such cases is helpful and he or she may have access to colleagues who might also be willing to assist. The use of human dermatopathologists should be considered only in the last resort. They are usually very keen to help but are seldom familiar with horse conditions and, unless they are in active contact with colleagues who can assist them with diagnoses, results can sometimes be very misleading.

A simple practice laboratory should have the equipment listed in **Table 3.1**. This list is basic because sophisticated or expensive equipment is not usually necessary in practice. Procedures which require the more advanced expertise of a pathologist should be sent directly to that specialist. Without the experience or skill required to perform sophisticated tests, possession of sophisticated apparatus is often wasteful and frustrating. There is little merit in sending prepared samples to a pathologist (such as mounted and stained sections) unless a second opinion is being sought – indeed the pathologist may not then be able to establish the true orientation of the specimen and might be unable to explore other stains and other orientations of the sample.

Although it is tempting to take every conceivable sample from every case, this approach cannot be justified. A sensible selection should be made which is economical, relevant and most likely to lead to a diagnosis. Notwithstanding this requirement, groomings, hair samples and skin scrapings should probably be taken from all horses with pruritic skin disease.

Table 3.1 Basic equipment for a simple practice laboratory

- Hand magnifying lens (possibly with a built-in light source)
- Dark ceramic tile
- Simple (preferably binocular) optical microscope with integral light source and ×4, ×10, ×20, ×40 and ×100 objectives
- Stereo dissecting microscope and appropriate light source
- Sterile specimen bottles
- Bottles containing 10% formal saline (and/or other fixatives)
- Histological specimen baskets with appropriate fixatives
- Slides and cover slips
- Pipettes (preferably disposable plastic)
- Potassium hydroxide (KOH) solution (10%)
- Stains suitable for the range of tests routinely performed in the laboratory (including Gram's, Ziel Nielsen, Methylene blue, Wright–Giemsa, Giemsa, Leishman's, Lactophenol–cotton blue, etc.
- Spatula, forceps and platinum loop (for bacteriology)
- Gas or spirit burner
- Bacteriological plates, incubator (and suitable stains) if cultures are to be performed 'in-house'.

Note: Some culture media are simple and commercially prepared kits are helpful. They require little technical skill or knowledge (e.g. Dermatophyte Test Medium (DTM) or *Fungassay* fungal culture medium), but rely on careful reading of the instructions.

SAMPLES FOR DERMATOLOGICAL INVESTIGATIONS

Groomings

Indications

All horses suffering from pruritic disorders should be subjected to this simple and effective test. It is primarily designed to detect ectoparasites such as lice and surface feeding mites such as *Chorioptes equi*.

Method

A stiff brush such as a scrubbing brush or a denture-type toothbrush is used to sweep skin dander, debris and hair particles into a suitable container (such as a plastic Petri dish) (**Fig. 3.1**) or onto a piece of stiff cardboard, thick paper or a dustpan held below an area of affected skin. The groomings can be placed directly onto a dark tile for immediate examination or into a clean, closed, but not airtight plastic container for later examination under the microscope.

Interpretation

Lice and other large parasites may be identified macroscopically (particularly on a dark ceramic tile), but a binocular 'dissecting' microscope is very useful for smaller parasites and their eggs. It allows the examination of a large volume of specimen under ideal lighting conditions. Movement of parasites is often the easiest feature to spot.

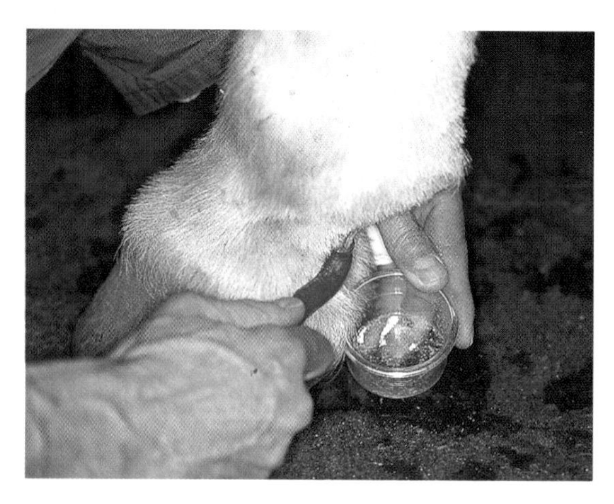

Figure 3.1 Groomings being taken with a stiff (denture) brush from the hind pastern region of a horse affected with chorioptic mange. The groomings are collected in a wide-mouthed, sealable plastic pot held under the area.

Hair sampling

Indications

Hair sampling is indicated when there are altered growth patterns, broken hairs, crusts, scales and actual loss of hair (alopecia). As dermatophytes are associated with hair follicles, there are advantages in plucking the hair with a pair of haemostat forceps (artery clamps) as opposed to using a skin scraping. Horses suspected of dermatophyte (ringworm) or *Dermatophilus* spp. infections are examples in which hair sampling is useful.

Method

1. Pluck hair and associated scabs from the margins of a number of fresh lesions and place in numbered/identified sterile bottles. For fungal culture the bottles should not be airtight as this might encourage overgrowth of saprophytic fungi.
2. Lightly clean the area with 70% alcohol on a swab but do not scrub or abrade the skin.
3. Pluck hair from the cleaned area and place in numbered sterile bottles, leaving the caps slightly loose; if transported, use cellulose tape to secure lids without sealing the container.
4. Examine samples in an appropriate fashion (see below) in the practice laboratory or dispatch to a diagnostic laboratory with a full history.

Interpretation

Positive results are very satisfying, but failure to demonstrate the organisms (false negative results) may be due to the sampling of an old lesion. Further, fresher samples and submission of scabs for culture to the microbiology laboratory can help.

Typical branching mycelia-like organisms and spores attached to or associated with the hair shafts will be seen in positive ringworm samples. Mixed populations of Gram-positive cocci consisting of *Streptococcus* spp. chains and clumps of *Staphylococcal* spp. bacteria may be found in cases of pastern folliculitis. *Dermatophilus congolensis* is a Gram-positive, branching filamentous bacterium. The bacteria divide longitudinally and horizontally, forming parallel rows of coccoid bodies ('railway-line organisms'; see Figure 7.16). Specific details for direct smear examination for *Dermatophilus congolensis* are given below.

Note: Examination of direct smears for dermatophytes can be time consuming and even then may not lead to a positive identification of the species of fungus involved. All specimens should therefore be cultured for positive confirmation (see culture methods later). Examination of hair is facilitated by using mineral oil or, better still, a clearing agent such as 10% potassium hydroxide (KOH) or chlorophenolac or chlorolactophenol. Specific instructions for maximizing the chances of a positive result are given below.

Specific examination techniques for *Dermatophilus congolensis*

- Impression smears taken directly from the underside of freshly removed scabs can be heat fixed and stained with Methylene blue or Gram's stain, Giemsa or Wright–Giemsa (DifQik).
- Place a drop or two of saline on a clean microscope slide. Clip off excess hairs from the crust sample and place the crusts into the saline drops. Gentle teasing out of the sample can hasten the procedure. Allow the specimen to macerate/soften for a few minutes and then remove the larger particles. Crush out the remaining material flat on the slide and allow to air dry. Heat fix the slide by gentle warming to 50–60°C (50°C is just too warm for the back of the hand). Stain with Methylene blue, Gram's, Giemsa or Wright–Giemsa (DifQik) stain.

Direct examination of hair and skin samples for dermatophyte organisms

Materials required

- Clearing agents
  - 10% potassium hydroxide (KOH) solution
  - Chlorophenolac (made by mixing 25 ml liquid phenol, 50 g chloral hydrate and 25 ml liquid lactic acid in a container in a fume cupboard, it should be stored in a dark glass bottle and is ready for use in 2–3 days.)

These agents are seriously caustic – skin/eye contact must be avoided. In the event of skin contact the area should be washed with copious running water. If the eyes are splashed medical opinion must be sought immediately after washing the eye with copious water.

- Fungal stains, e.g. chlorozol, lactophenol–cotton blue

Method

1. Place 'teased-out' specimen hairs on slide and carefully apply a few drops of the selected clearing agent.

2. With chlorophenolac clearing is immediate; apply cover slip and examine immediately.
3. With 10% KOH, warm the slide (do not boil) for 15–20 seconds, apply a cover slip and examine.

Interpretation

Examine under low-power magnification (×4). Locate a normal hair for reference; infected hairs are pale and swollen. Re-examine with higher magnification (×40). Fungal spores are very small and may be present as chains on the hair shaft.

▷ Skin scrapings

Skin scrapings are primarily used to identify burrowing mites (all of which are rare in the horse) and so the technique is not as useful as in many other species. *Sarcoptes scabei* var. *equi* and *Demodex equi* are the only significant burrowing mites and may be identified on scrapings taken from the deeper layers of the skin. The former is very rare but very serious (it was until recently a notifiable disease in the United Kingdom and remains a feared disease in some parts of the world). The latter is probably more common than is appreciated but is probably of no clinical significance except in immunocompromised horses. Nevertheless, it is probably wise to perform a skin scraping in all cases showing pruritus. Skin scrapings may also be useful in the detection of nematode larvae such as *Pelodera* spp. or *Strongyloides* spp. Trombiculid mites ('harvest mite' or scrub-itch mite) are also occasionally seen in a scraping but the mites often fall off after browsing, leaving either a bare (alopecic) patch or a slightly itchy area without the presence of mites.

It is usually necessary to take samples from as many fresh areas as possible owing to the difficulty in obtaining mites in many samples. There is no defined number of samples to take – more is always better than too few. Single samples often provide a false negative result.

Several different types of scraping can be obtained.

Superficial scrapings These collect hair and macerated tissue from the superficial layer of skin. The process does not cause bleeding. *Psoroptes* spp., *Chorioptes* spp. and *Dermanyssus gallinae* (poultry or fowl mite), and lice may be found in these samples under a low-power microscope or stereo (dissecting) microscope. With the aid of higher magnification, dermatophyte organisms (ringworm) may also be seen, but these specimens often require clearing in warm 10% potassium hydroxide first. The clinical significance of a fungal organism seen in these specimens cannot be assessed without culture.

Deep scrapings These collect material from the intrafollicular space and superficial dermis. Sampling is deep enough for bleeding to occur and so blood cells are invariably present in the specimen. *Demodex* spp., *Sarcoptes* spp. and to a lesser extent *Chorioptes* spp. may be found in these samples under low-power microscopy. Fungal organisms may also be identified under higher magnification, but the pathological significance of a fungal organism again depends on culture.

Hair and scab scrapings These are taken to recover the superficial and deeper hair particles and scabs. They are technically very similar to hair pluckings but are obtained by scraping the area. It is a useful technique for fungal and bacterial culture as they may be less contaminated with commensal organisms from the surface layers of the skin.

Method

1. Lightly moisten the area with light mineral oil (liquid paraffin).
2. **Superficial scraping** A new, sterile #23 scalpel blade is held at right angles to the skin. The selected area is scraped and hair and superficial skin are obtained and placed directly on to a microscope slide. Samples can be placed into sterile labelled universal bottles for transport to the laboratory.
   Deep scraping The skin is pinched firmly between finger and thumb and the skin is scraped with a #23 blade held at right angles to the surface until bleeding occurs. The sample is placed on a slide for immediate examination or into a sterile numbered universal container.
3. An extra drop of oil is applied to the slide and a cover slip is placed carefully so as to avoid artefactual air bubbles, etc. The slide is scanned under low power (×4–×10). Most mites will still be alive and movement is then easily seen. If dermatophyte infections are suspected, the sample can be cleared with 10% potassium hydroxide (warmed for 10 minutes) or chlorophenolac.
4. Examine under higher power (×40) to identify mites, mite eggs and any fungal elements.

Interpretation

In most instances positive findings provide a positive diagnosis of disease. However, care should be exercised when *Demodex equi* or *Demodex caballi* are found as they can be an incidental finding in clinically normal horses. Extensive, multiple scrapings can be unrewarding and may suggest a negative result even in positive cases. Multiple samples will minimize but not eliminate the risk of these false negative results. There is no universally effective way of concentrating parasites to make diagnosis more accurate. Although combinations of clearing agents and centrifugation can be helpful in some cases, they can also cause serious damage to the parasites and so make detection difficult.

Swabs for culture

Bacterial culture

The horse's skin carries a very diverse commensal bacterial population. Swabs taken from the surface of lesions are likely to be unrewarding or difficult to interpret and therefore often have a low diagnostic value. Needle aspirates of pus and debris from the deeper layer of the diseased area may be more representative of the pathology. These consistently provide a more restrictive and relevant culture population from which pathogens may be identified and subcultured more easily.

Bacteriological culture and bacterial sensitivity tests are universal laboratory procedures, but both are of limited value in the horse. It is as well to remember that drugs applied topically would usually have to be absorbed into the tissue to reach the organisms and topical antibiotics commonly do not reach the minimum inhibitory concentration, so that sensitivity results need to be interpreted with care. Furthermore, sensitivity profiles issued from laboratories may not take account of the species of animal involved and so there may be significant safety and efficacy implications in the displayed profile information.

Note: Viral culture or detection using electron microscopy or fluorescent antibody methods, etc. often require specialized sample collection methods. If any sample is to be subjected to viral detection methods, the laboratory should be consulted first. Specialized transport media and handling may be required. Dry swabs are virtually useless but scabs and infected tissue packed on ice are often useful for some diseases such as the pox and papilloma viruses.

Method

1. Locate an intact pustule or the most recently infected area which displays the most characteristic clinical signs. For fungal culture, samples must be obtained from the rim of active lesions and placed in a sterile container. Do not wipe or use antiseptic over the area.
2. Obtain a swab by either:
   - using a sterile disposable needle to open the pustule prior to taking the swab for culture, or
   - using a sterile needle to obtain an aspirate for culture from deep within the tissue where deeper infection may be present.
   - Alternatively, use a biopsy sample (see biopsy sampling techniques p. 27) and obtain a swab for culture from the deep portion of biopsy (see Fig. 3.8). This technique should definitely be used if a deep mycosis is suspected.
3. Bacteriological samples are always placed directly into transport medium. Dry swabs are virtually useless as they are liable to desiccation and significant alterations of bacterial culture are possible within hours.
4. In the laboratory:
   - Use the swab to plate out directly onto an appropriate medium or broth or place the swab into transport medium to forward to laboratory. Sensitivity cultures may be useful, but delays are inevitable as they regularly take 24–48 hours longer than the identification of cultures (and sometimes longer if subculturing is required).
   - If anaerobic bacteria, such as *Clostridia* spp. are suspected, samples should be collected into anaerobic transport media for immediate dispatch. Most such media are specialized and need to be freshly prepared. The laboratory should be consulted for suitable anaerobic media and advice on handling the sample before the procedure is performed.
   - A specific method for culture of *Dermatophilus congolensis* is given below.

Interpretation

Apart from *Dermatophilus* spp., *Staphylococcus* spp. and occasional *Streptococcus* spp., the horse's skin abounds with commensal and contaminating bacteria, which reduces the value of skin cultures. However, if a biopsy sample is taken, a small portion can be aseptically removed and placed in transport medium for culture. This is often more useful. Parenteral use of suitable antibiotics as identified by sensitivity testing may be inappropriate or unsafe in the horse, so great care must be used in the selection of suitable drugs for skin conditions. Some laboratories are amenable to setting up specific equine sensitivity profiles employing only those drugs which are suitable for the species but may need to be encouraged to do so.

Examination techniques for *Dermatophilus congolensis*

Isolations from older or healing lesions present more difficulties and the useful, if time-consuming and complex, technique outlined below can be used to confirm the presence of *D. congolensis*:

- Small pieces of the scabs are placed in bijou (5 ml) screwtop bottles, moistened with 1 ml distilled water and allowed to stand open for 3–4 hours on the bench at room temperature.
- The open bijou bottles are then transferred to a wide-mouthed jar and sealed in an atmosphere of about 20% carbon dioxide produced either chemically or by burning a candle within the jar.
- After 15 minutes the bottles are carefully removed and samples are taken from the water surface with a bacteriological loop and seeded onto 5% ox-blood agar.
- Incubation is at 37°C in about 20% carbon dioxide for 24–48 hours.
- Abundant, small, embedding, haemolytic, rough, fimbriated colonies, typical of *D. congolensis* are obtained, usually in relatively pure culture.
- Identity may be confirmed by examining stained smears from the colonies.

FUNGAL CULTURE

Specimens for fungal culture seldom require any transport medium. Specimens for dermatophyte culture should be placed in a paper envelope or a sterile plastic universal. However, where deep mycosis is suspected, swabs may be taken from biopsy specimens and in these circumstances transport medium may be helpful in preventing dessication (see Fig. 3.8). A positive fungal culture is diagnostic for infection and appropriate treatment can then be started.

1. Remove samples from sterile bottles with sterile forceps. Culture directly on dermatophyte test medium (DTM), which is based on Sabouraud's dextrose agar with pH indicator (methyl or phenol red is usually used) and antibacterial agents to prevent overgrowth of bacterial contaminants. Press the sample firmly into the surface of the medium but do not bury it.
2. (a) Incubate at room temperature for 14 days with a loose cap.
   (b) Incubate duplicate set of plates at 37°C for *Trichophyton verrucosum*.
3. Check cultures daily for colour change and growth of fungal colonies.
4. If necessary submit sample to a specialist laboratory for confirmation and evaluation of doubtful samples.

Interpretation

Pathogenic dermatophytes metabolize protein early and the resulting alkaline medium changes the amber medium to a distinctive red colour, usually within 3–5 days (before any colony is actually visible). Saprophytic fungi metabolize carbohydrate and only induce this change after 14 days or more.[2] The dermatophyte colonies are white/beige and are seldom if ever dark in colour. A positive identification can therefore be made in most instances, if at the same time as the colour change occurs (or within 24 hours of it) a white to beige, powdery or fluffy colony begins to appear.[3] Light brown or dark, black/green colonies are negative even if the medium colour changes to red. False results are uncommon, however; the characteristics of the culture are pathognomonic and examination of the macroconidia/spores will also support the diagnosis. Mistakes are usually the result of contamination or errors of interpretation.

▷ Acetate (clear, adhesive) tape preparation

This is primarily used to detect *Oxyuris equi* eggs around the anus, vulva and perineum. It may also be used in an attempt to find surface-living lice and certain parasitic mites and their eggs. Hair should routinely be clipped with scissors to allow the application of the adhesive tape to the skin and base of the hairs.

Method

1. If appropriate, clip hairs short (but do not shave) and gently remove any excessive crust.
2. Press tape firmly and evenly to skin and hair.
3. Remove tape and carefully place, sticky side down, on a microscope slide over a drop of mineral oil so as to avoid air bubbles.

4. Place a drop of mineral oil over the tape and carefully apply a cover slip over the entire mount.
5. Examine for parasites and/or eggs under low power.

Interpretation

This may be a useful exercise to show to clients but it is time consuming and can be unrewarding. Use of hand lens and careful examination initially of ears, base of mane and tail as well as muzzle and legs, may be more rewarding in the search for parasites. Positive identification of *Oxyuris* eggs (90 μm × 30 μm) with their characteristic operculum at one end, or live or dead mites or their eggs is diagnostic. Artefactual bubbles and pollen grains, etc. can be misleading. A negative finding is of course inconclusive.

Tissue biopsy

Biopsy specimens obtained from skin lesions are used for several purposes and the technical aspects of obtaining a suitable specimen will vary. There is considerable merit in consulting the pathologist at an early stage and it is sometimes helpful to ask the pathologist to be present during the procedure so that the surgeon can get the best advice on sampling. For example, it is sometimes very helpful to obtain a particular orientation of biopsy such as a shave biopsy or to use a special fixative. Furthermore, a full history and clinical report should always be provided with the sample so that the pathologist is aware of the true nature of the case and can adjust the investigations so as to maximize the value of the procedure. It is not helpful to 'test the skill' of the pathologist by providing no or scanty information.

The response of skin to a variety of insults can be histopathologically similar. Consequently, results of biopsies are often nonspecific and therefore disappointing to both clinician and pathologist. It is probably unrealistic to expect a single biopsy to provide all the possible results. If a primary diagnosis is required, it is usual to biopsy a representative mature lesion; the exception to this is any vesicular disease, which should be biopsied entire as early as possible in the course of this disease. Self-inflicted trauma is a common event in equine skin disease and is particularly so in pruritic cases. Vigorous or even milder rubbing can cause significant alterations, with primary lesions rapidly being converted into secondary lesions which are, naturally, nonspecific. The salient features of the primary condition may be obliterated completely.

Skin biopsy has certain limitations. It can be very useful for papules or pustules but is much less so for ulcers and crusts. Biopsy of chronic lesions, superficial inflammatory changes and lichenified, crusted dermatoses often reveal little extra information because they are invariably secondarily affected by chronic changes. However, there are no hard and fast rules and regular biopsy usage may provide valuable clinical experience from which long-term benefits can accrue.

Remember that while a definitive diagnosis is ideal, the elimination of other suspect diagnoses can be of equal importance in difficult cases.

Indications

Skin biopsies are taken:

- to establish a specific diagnosis;
- to eliminate other clinical diagnoses;
- to follow the course of the disease;
- to confirm the completeness of excision of a tumour.[4]

Biopsy specimens are used for several pathological purposes including:

- histological diagnosis
- needle aspirate cytology
- special tests
  - immunohistochemistry/immunofluorescence.
  - bacterial/fungal swabs (see above).
  - virus identification (using direct electron microscopy or culture or ELISA tests)

Types of biopsy

Shave biopsy Shave biopsies are particularly useful for the vesicobullous conditions such as pemphigus vulgaris and pemphigus foliaceus.

Punch biopsy A column of tissue is removed with a commercially available disposable biopsy punch. These are available in several different sizes but specimens of less than 6–7 mm diameter are probably less useful than larger ones. Pathologists are often significantly hindered by having very small specimens which may not be fully representative of the diseased tissue.

Wedge biopsy An outward-facing wedge with only a small amount of normal skin may be more sensible in some circumstances. The important portion is the abnormal tissue and the small segment of normal skin serves to provide the pathologist with an orientation of the lesion and an example of the normal skin for comparison. A separate biopsy of adjacent normal skin may be sent if requested by the pathologist.

Excision biopsy This is used when normal and abnormal tissue are required in the sample or when the lesion is so small that biopsy of a portion is difficult. It is also used when the lesion present (e.g. a vesicle or pustule) is likely to be adversely affected by partial biopsy. It is also indicated when malignancy and dissemination of tumour may follow partial biopsy.

Fine needle aspirate This is used to sample cells or fluids from a lesion. Interpretation of cells obtained in this way is a very specialized technique often requiring an experienced cytological pathologist. The method of obtaining the cells is important as they are easily damaged beyond recognition. The pathologist should be consulted on the correct sampling and preservation methods.

Impression smears These have limited value. Many skin lesions have surface bacterial contamination (which may or may not be of clinical significance). Exfoliative and inflammatory cells are regularly encountered and again they may or may not be of significance. Interpretation is particularly difficult and is again a very specialized procedure.

Fixatives

Fixatives require a finite time to exert their effects. This may be dependent on the type and size of the specimen (and the extent of penetration required) but is seldom less than 24–36 hours. Pathologists are justifiably reluctant to process specimens at an earlier stage and more rapid results may require frozen sections.

- Buffered, neutral formol–saline is used routinely. At least 10× volume of fixative to specimen must be present.
- Michel's medium was formerly used to preserve specimens for immunohistochemical investigations. This is now no longer required in many cases and consultation with the pathologist will establish its value in any particular case.
- Frozen sections are sometimes used to obtain a very rapid result. They require particular circumstances and handling of the specimen. Where this is required a pathologist or technician must be present to handle the tissue.

Method

Tranquillization may be needed to allow handling of the horse and safety of the surgeon. Combination of an α_2-adrenoreceptor agonist (such as romifidine or detomidine) and an opiate analgesic (such as butorphanol) often allows minor surgery without the need for extensive local anaesthetic infiltration which itself may adversely affect the results of biopsy.

Do not shave or vigorously clean the lesion prior to biopsy. Sterilize around lesion rather than over it. Owners may be somewhat surprised by the lack of sterilization, but careful instruction should avoid any subsequent complication.

Regional perineural anaesthesia will avoid any possible complications from local injection of an irritant drug such as lignocaine hydrochloride. Alternatively, infiltrate a minimal volume of 2% lignocaine hydrochloride using a 25G needle under small lesions. A ring block of 2% lignocaine hydrochloride can be used for larger lesions or those requiring more extensive biopsy.

Shave biopsy The epidermis is shaved parallel to the surface in layers (**Fig. 3.2**). Use a sterile (new) scalpel blade and *do not* use scissors to cut the sample off. The specimens are very thin and easily traumatized so they should not be gripped with sharp or crushing instruments. Suturing is not required. An accurate diagrammatic orientation of the biopsy should be made immediately to assist the pathologist.

Wedge or excision biopsy A wedge of tissue is obtained by full-thickness incisions with a suitable scalpel blade through the abnormal tissue to include a small rim of normal skin on the wider (outer) edge

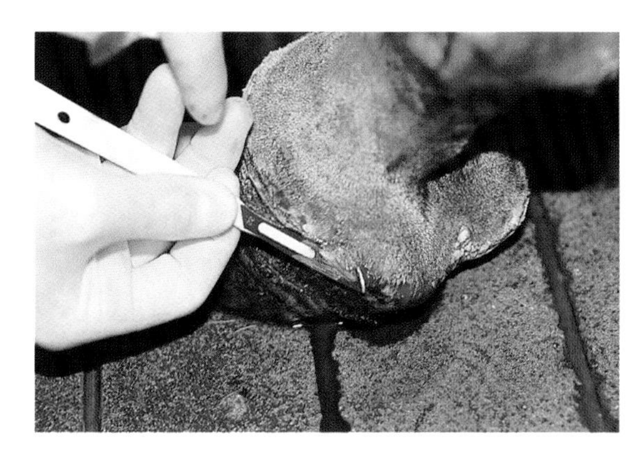

Figure 3.2 A shave biopsy being taken from the bulb of the heel of a horse with a suspected pemphigus foliaceus. The area has been anaesthetized with a palmar digital nerve block.

(**Fig. 3.3**). An excisional biopsy is similar in execution but involves the removal of the whole lesion, which may involve rather more surgery if it is large. An elliptical incision with an appropriate margin for the type of tissue is made with a suitable scalpel to include all tissue down to the cutaneous muscle.

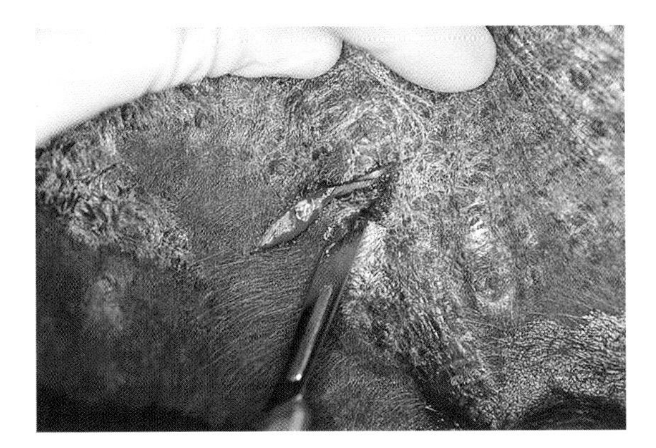

Figure 3.3 A wedge skin biopsy being taken from a suspected sarcoid lesion in the groin of an anaesthetized horse. The site was closed with skin staples.

Always use sterile equipment and *do not* use scissors to cut the sample off. Neither should the specimen be gripped with sharp or crushing instruments. For wedge and excisional samples, sutures, staples or n-butyl cyanoacrylate adhesives may be used to close the wound depending on the size and nature of the defect. An accurate diagrammatic orientation of the biopsy should be made immediately to assist the pathologist.

Punch biopsy A disposable skin punch of varying diameter is used to remove a core of abnormal tissue consisting of epidermis, dermis, subcutaneous fat and panniculus muscle. For equine skin 6–9 mm diameter punches are usually selected (**Fig. 3.4**). The punch is used to incise the skin without significant distortion. The specimen can be easily and significantly traumatized by rat-tooth forceps or by excessive pressure/squeezing by forceps and these should therefore not be used. A 25G needle is used to carefully lift the specimen so that the underlying attachments can be cut with the scalpel blade (not scissors). Remove the specimen from the site without damaging it and place it in fixative. Suturing is not usually required. A specimen of adjacent normal skin may be obtained in a similar fashion for comparative purposes.

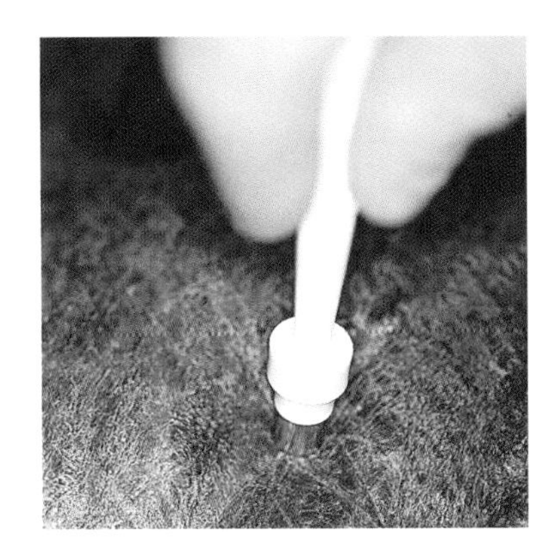

Figure 3.4 An 8 mm disposable biopsy punch being used to obtain a specimen of skin. Systemic sedation and analgesia were all that was required. The site was not sutured.

(Fine) Needle aspirate This is often difficult for a solid lesion. Lay out a series of very clean (new), degreased slides on the bench. A large syringe is attached to a suitable hypodermic needle (usually 19G or 20G). The needle is advanced into the centre of the mass and maximal suction is applied to the syringe repeatedly for a few seconds each time. The needle is withdrawn and air is drawn into the syringe. Repeated jets of air are directed through the needle at the slides. Cells will be obviously delivered to the slides. If advised by the pathologists, smearing of these can be performed but this often results in cellular distortions.

Samples for cytological examination should be placed directly on a slide and smeared in an appropriate fashion. It is sometimes better to fix the sample immediately (consult with pathologist). Among the solid tumours only the melanoma provides an instant diagnosis – the black material is easily recognized even in unstained aspirates. Cells from fluid-filled cavities (including bullae and abscesses) can be obtained using fine needles (**Fig. 3.5**). It is often helpful to identify fluid cavities by ultrasonography at the same time. This avoids indiscriminate and random exploration. The sample obtained should be treated according to its purpose. Thus, samples for virus identification must be treated accordingly (consult with pathologist or virologist) while those for bacterial culture can be introduced directly into either biphasic (blood culture) bottles or other transport media.

Impression smears These are obtained by pressing a clean (new) glass slide onto the surface of a

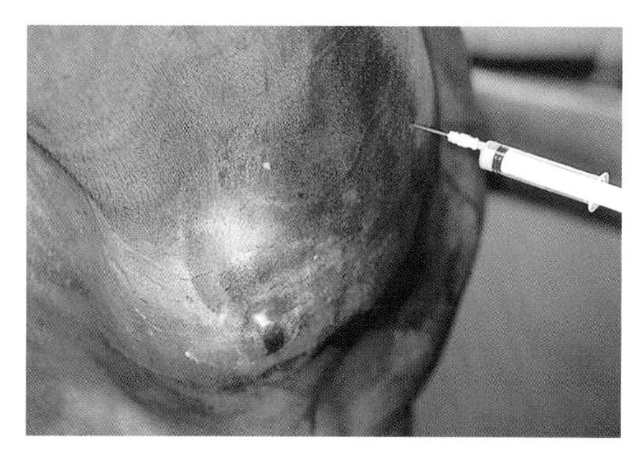

Figure 3.5 A needle aspirate being taken from a fluctuant cutaneous swelling. Culture and direct examination of a Gram-stained smear of the material confirmed that the swelling was an abscess.

suitably representative lesion (often after a scab or surface exudate has been gently removed). The slides are heat or alcohol fixed immediately and stained appropriately before being examined. Impression smears may be helpful for fresh *Dermatophilus congolensis* lesions. Some tumours and subcutaneous nodules may require to be incised before the smear is taken (**Fig. 3.6**).

Note: As many biopsies are quite correctly taken without surgical preparation (which may distort or alter the results), a suitable systemic antibiotic can be administered immediately after the sample has been taken. Topical antiseptic medication is also probably a wise precaution.

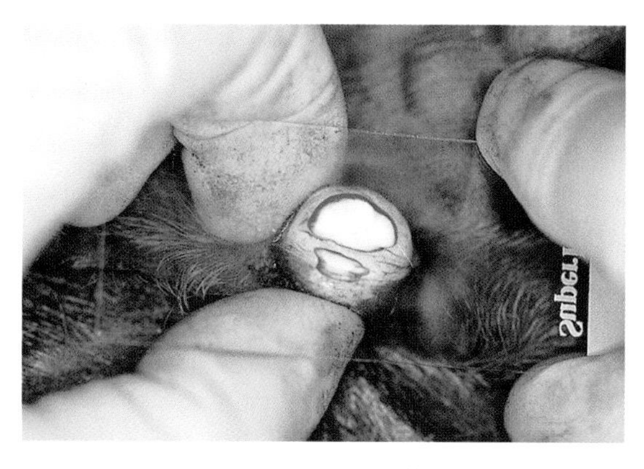

Figure 3.6 An impression smear being taken from an incised skin nodule. The smear was unrewarding. Only very few cells were identified among the blood cells.

Specimen handling

Biopsy samples of skin which might become distorted during fixing should either be placed dermis down on a small square of cardboard for about 1 minute to adhere to the cardboard before being placed in fixative or should be pinned gently to a piece of card in its natural shape. Alternatively, a specimen basket can be used to avoid distortion of tissues as fixation occurs (**Fig. 3.7a,b**). These are simple and efficient means of preventing distortion without the need to pin the sample and are highly recommended.

1. Sample specimen with sterile swab for bacteriology and fungal culture if indicated (**Fig. 3.8**).
2. Place sample in appropriate fixative solution.
3. A further sample should be taken if a possible diagnosis of onchocercal microfilariasis (*Onchocerca cervicalis*) is suspected. The sample should be preserved fresh in a cooled container.

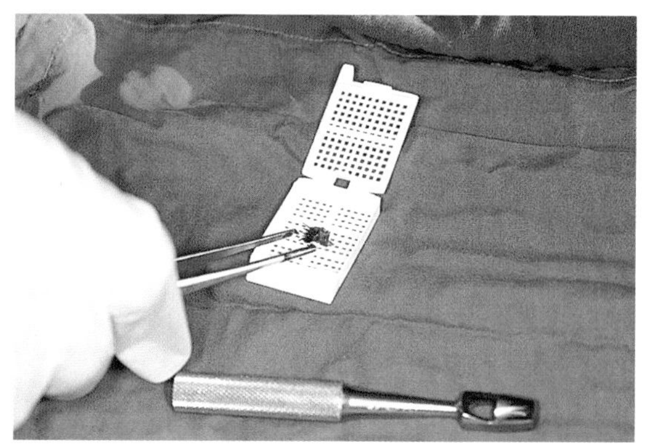

a

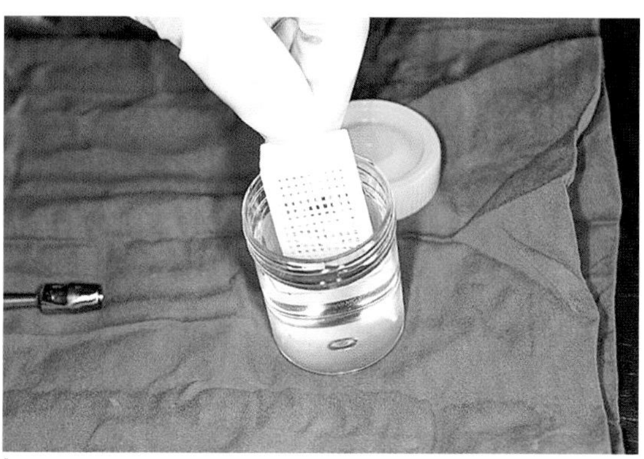

b

Figure 3.7 (a) A biopsy specimen being loaded into a specimen mesh to prevent distortion. (b) The specimen enclosed in the mesh being inserted into the fixative solution for dispatch to the pathologist.

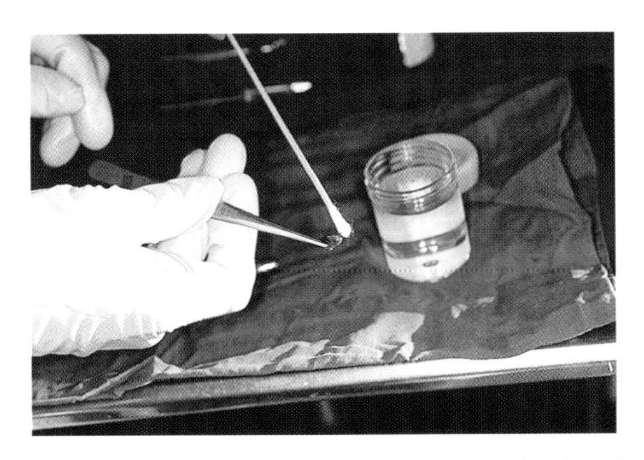

Figure 3.8 A swab being taken from the depths of a biopsy specimen prior to the specimen being placed in 10% buffered formalin solution. The swab is then placed in suitable transport medium.

Specific examination for *Onchocerca*

Sample affected or suspect areas by punch or excision biopsy technique as outlined above. As many horses in endemic areas have accumulations of *Onchocerca* located in the ventral midline region without apparent pathological effect, lesions away from this should be sampled, e.g. head and face between the eyes and ears, neck, thorax and proximal regions of the front legs. In nonendemic areas there may be justification in sampling any lesion regardless of the area.

Method

1. Use 6 mm biopsy punch as described above to obtain several samples from lesions.
2. Place half of (each) biopsy in 10% buffered formalin for normal histology.
3. Place the second half (or halves) in a cooled plain container on ice. At the laboratory the sample is finely cut up (minced) and suspended in Tyrode's solution or phosphate buffered saline at 37°C for 3 hours. Filter through a 250 μm sieve and centrifuge at 3000 rpm for 3–5 minutes. Discard supernatant. Examine the resuspended deposit with a 'hanging drop' or on a glass slide with ×60 to ×100 objectives.

Interpretation

Live larvae are very easy to identify from the movement they cause in the drop or on the slide. A positive larval finding from the biopsy site must be evaluated with the clinical signs shown by the horse. A diagnosis can be confirmed where the clinical condition of skin lesions with pruritus is substantiated by the presence of larvae in the biopsy sample. Histopathological detection of the larvae is rather more difficult and they can easily be missed. However, if one or both is positive the diagnosis can be considered to be safe.

PRECAUTIONS

Measures to improve the quality of the results from tissue biopsy include the following.

- Do not stretch the skin during biopsy. This causes distortion both on a macroscopic and microscopic scale.
- Use a scalpel, not scissors. This eliminates crushing artefacts along the line of incision.
- Try to avoid over-handling of the specimen and use fine plain forceps very gently or, preferably, a fine hypodermic needle to remove/handle the specimen.
- Try to reduce specimen size to less than 1 cm to allow rapid and proper fixation.
- Large samples should be serially cut into pieces <1 cm and preserved in numbered separate containers with a diagram to help the pathologist orientate the specimen correctly.
- Avoid *too small* specimens. Samples less than 4–6 mm in diameter are probably barely adequate and are particularly liable to artefactual distortions from stretching, compression or crushing during sampling and may be difficult to handle when fixed.
- Multiple sections are useful from large lesions and in some circumstances the complete specimen should be sent in a suitable container with at least 10 times the specimen volume of fixative. Solid intact specimens require to be cut open and advice should be obtained from the pathologist as to the best way of handling such a specimen.
- Remember that specimens will need to be removed from the container. A narrow-mouthed container (such as a glass bottle) means either that the specimen has to be handled roughly or that the container needs to be broken to get the fixed specimen out. Therefore, a suitable wide-mouthed, inert, clean container must always be used.
- Samples which have to be sent by post and for which there is no urgency can be fixed for a suitable time before being drained of fixative prior to posting. A day or two without the fixative will not usually harm the specimen – remember

though to ensure that it is packed suitably to prevent dessication. The pathologist will need to know that the sample has no fixative.

SPECIALIZED TECHNIQUES

Restriction/provocation tests

In cases where a feed allergy or reaction is suspected it may be useful to attempt to identify the cause by use of an exclusion/provocation test. Alfalfa or ryegrass hay are generally regarded as the starting point (although whether they could be regarded as hypoallergenic is debatable). The horse should be fed exclusively on a single dietary substance for 2–4 weeks (but it may be longer). Once the basic diet substance is tolerated and standardized, individual other components including the suspected material can be added at 2-week intervals. It is important to realize, however, that there are few recorded cases of confirmed diet-related skin disease. Environmental and other factors may need to be considered and the overall complexity of the problem can be very difficult to sort out.

Immunofluorescence

Tests using these techniques are available in specialized pathology laboratories. Some pathologists question the value of direct and indirect immunofluorescence methods in horses and prefer to rely on characteristic conventional histopathological changes. Biopsy samples should be placed in appropriate fixatives after discussion with the pathologists. In the absence of any guidance each biopsy should be divided into two and placed both in 10% formal saline and in Michel's solution.[5]

Antinuclear antibody (ANA) testing

The antinuclear antibody (ANA) titre and lupus erythematosis (LE) cell preparation may assist in the diagnosis of systemic lupus erythematosus-like syndrome of horses (SLE). This test was originally developed to diagnose LE, but it may give positive reactions in a number of other conditions. It is a test performed on serum and detects antibodies directed against nucleolar DNA. High ANA titres (exceeding 1:160) are indicative of immune-mediated disorders. A high titre in combination with multisystem clinical signs is highly suggestive of a positive diagnosis for SLE.[6] While neither test is specific for SLE, a positive result serves to indicate a possible autoimmune dysfunction.

Although the ANA test is the best test available for SLE[7] there is some doubt as to its relevance because some cases which present all the clinical features of the disease fail to show any detectable ANA antibody and others may develop the antibody, particularly subsequent to drug administration, without showing any cutaneous or systemic signs.

Serum (10 ml) or freshly clotted whole blood (20 ml) is required. It is probably wise to consult with the laboratory regarding the collection of the sample as some do not perform the test.

Allergy testing

Intradermal (in-vivo) skin testing

Intradermal skin testing in horses has been used in a very limited way. It requires the availability of specific allergens and experienced personnel to conduct and read the test. It should be read and interpreted in the light of the history and general examination of the horse. False negative and false positive tests do occur and some horses even show detectable reaction to the blank test sites. Clinically normal horses can also show marked positive skin reactions, giving a misleading impression of the relevance of the test. However, most dermatologists regard skin testing as the ultimate test of atopic disease[8] but this condition is probably singularly rare in the horse anyway.

Prior to skin testing the patient should not have been treated with drugs such as corticosteroids, antihistamines, tranquillizers or anaesthetics and nonsteroidal anti-inflammatory drugs – a drug-free period of at least 6–10 days is advisable. Fractious animals can be safely and effectively sedated with an α_2-adrenoreceptor agonist (such as xylazine, detomidine or romifidine) immediately prior to the procedure. Phenothiazine ataractics (such as acepromazine) may have a significant suppressive effect on the test.

Many substances such as grass, tree and weed pollens, moulds, stable dust, dust mites, feathers and dander have the potential to cause inhalant allergies resulting in atopic pruritus and may be detected by intradermal testing.

Method

1. Two days before the test is to be performed, the hair over the lateral neck should be clipped (avoiding any areas with obvious

lesions) and gently washed with a bland soap. The area prepared depends on the number of agents to be tested. Each will need an area of about 3–4 cm radius to avoid possible overlapping reactions.

2. One day before the test, 0.05 ml of 1:100 000 histamine phosphate solution is injected intradermally into a site just outside the test area. Normally a weal approximately 1–2 cm in diameter should develop within 30 minutes. No response suggests that the horse is 'non-responsive' and the test should be postponed until a reaction can be elicited by this test. If an inordinate reaction develops the procedure is probably unwise.
3. Prepare all reagents required, including emergency adrenaline. Fortunately, untoward reactions in the horse (anaphylaxis or urticaria) are very rare.
4. The full required range of allergens is reconstituted. Lyophilized allergen panels are available commercially. Once reconstituted they must be refrigerated and used within 3 months. It is not wise to use compounded (multiple) allergens containing several different substances as this fails to provide the narrow diagnosis which is required for subsequent desensitization.
5. The sites for the injections are identified by a nonirritant, indelible felt-tip marking pen and numbered (either on the animal or on a prepared 'map' of the site. If palpable variations in skin thickness are present, the thickness of the skin at each site (as measured by dermal calipers) should be recorded. Tuberculin testing calipers are crude but effective. More accurate mechanical or electronic skin testing calipers are available.
6. Small amounts (usually 0.05 ml) of the various suspect allergens are then injected intradermally using a 25/26G 10 mm (intradermal) needle and a 1 ml tuberculin or insulin type syringe. Histamine (positive) and N. saline (negative) controls are also used.
7. The extent of reaction at each numbered and identified site is measured (using skin testing calipers) and recorded after 15 and 30 minutes and at 4 hours post injection (**Fig. 3.9**). Reaction to allergens can then be compared with the two control sites.

Interpretation

A positive result is indicated by swelling at the site of the injection. By convention a significant

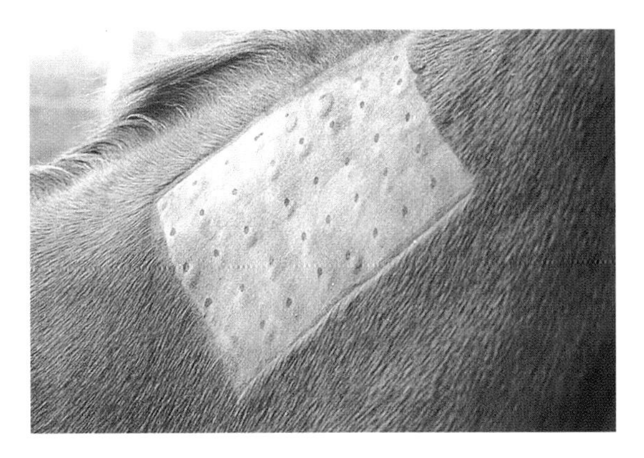

Figure 3.9 The appearance of a multiple allergen skin test performed in a horse some 3 hours previously. Note the positive oedematous nodular reactions shown as swellings at the site of the intradermal injection. The control and the negative sites show little or no reaction.

response is taken to be a swelling greater than, or equal to, twice the average increase between the negative and positive controls. A positive response does not necessarily correspond with pathological allergy but when considered with the clinical syndrome and the history it can be a useful additional help. Furthermore, the extent of the positive reaction is not necessarily proportional to the severity of the allergy.

Note: Allergy neutralization testing and therapy involves the use of serial dilutions of the allergen to establish a dilution at which the allergen fails to induce a reaction in the skin. This is, somewhat surprisingly, often some way between the highest and lowest concentrations which show significant reactions. This dilution is then used by subcutaneous injection to 'neutralize' the allergic response. Good results have been claimed in the human and with equine respiratory allergies, but the value for dermatological responses to inhaled or ingested allergens in the horse has yet to be established.

In vitro allergy testing

Commercially available tests on serum use either the radioallergosorbent test (RAST) which employs radioimmunoassay with isotope-labelled antisera, or an enzyme-linked immunosorbent assay (ELISA) which uses antibody coupled to enzymes. The 'extent of allergy' to an inhaled or ingested allergen is supposedly correlated with the amount of allergen-specific antibody (IgE) present in the serum sample. The responses may be very different in contact allergies. Very careful evaluation of results is necessary. There is little standardization between individual laboratories and so results can vary widely. Both RAST and ELISA methods, while offering some extra information, must be interpreted very cautiously in the horse.[9] There have been insufficient published reports and results to allow true evaluation of its value in equine dermatology at the present time.

Serum (10 ml) or freshly clotted whole blood (20 ml) is required for either testing procedure.

chapter 4

PRINCIPLES OF DERMATOLOGICAL THERAPEUTICS

The treatment of skin disease provides many challenges for the clinician. These include the type of disease and the practicality of many of the normal therapeutic options in such a large animal. In selecting a treatment method the clinician should consider its likely benefits and any possible undesirable consequences. Thus, a surgical option might present itself, but the wound resulting might be impossible to close, or the resultant scar might cause more serious consequences than the condition itself.

Drugs are commonly used to treat skin disease but many of them have significant undesirable consequences, some of which may be life-threatening. For example, the use of a corticosteroid to treat a minor skin disorder in a pony with a tendency to laminitis may precipitate a catastrophic acute laminitic episode. Amitraz is commonly used in dogs and cattle for treatment of ectoparasites, but its use on a horse is likely to be catastrophic – it is extremely poisonous to horses. The number of therapeutic options available in any particular part of the world will necessarily vary and clinicians will need to make themselves aware of the proprietary names of the therapeutic agents and compounds mentioned below. Regulations concerning the residues in tissue may be very important in some regions and irrelevant in others. However, every effort should be made to use the most effective treatment method for the specific condition. There is little more wasteful use of resource than using a treatment which does not work, whether this is an expensive or cheaper option. Time is wasted and the condition might get worse in the interim or the drug might have unwanted side effects which make the case even more difficult to treat.

Pharmaceuticals described in this chapter refer specifically to their use in dermatological treatment in the horse. However, many of the compounds have not been researched or tested effectively in horses. Data extrapolated from other species may be useful in some cases, in others it may be less so. Furthermore, some drugs either are not available or have licensing problems in many individual countries. Where specific licensing problems exist the reader is advised to check carefully with the regulations in force in his or her locality to avoid any problems with the use of unlicensed products. New drugs are being developed and others are being withdrawn from the market for safety or financial reasons (or both) and the list given here cannot therefore be complete. Generic drug names are used throughout in this text.

ANTI-INFECTIVE PHARMACEUTICALS USED IN DERMATOLOGY

Antiseptics/disinfectants

Many of the modern antiseptic compounds have good virucidal, bactericidal and fungicidal effects and some have strong sporocidal effects for spore-forming bacteria and fungi. The commonest compounds used in equine dermatology and wound management include chlorhexidine, povidone-iodine, iodophor, quaternary ammonium compounds, halogenated tertiary amines, inorganic peroxygen compounds and acidic iodines. Some antiseptics and disinfectants can be used on the skin but others are harmful. Manufacturers' instructions should always be followed implicitly. The antiseptics are variously used for their antibacterial properties prior to surgical interference in aseptic surgery and also as wound antiseptics. Most compounds will have some harmful effect on the skin when used in abnormally high concentrations and the specific dilution instructions are vitally important. In any case, many of the iodine-based compounds work more effectively at lower concentrations than at the higher ones and it is very important to ensure correct dilution.

Most agents will have less or more activity against various microbes and the correct selection will enable a more rapid resolution or effect to be gained. Thus, chlorhexidine probably has less antifungal activity than povidone iodine and some of the newer quaternary ammonium compounds and halogenated tertiary amines have a very wide range of activity against viruses, bacteria and fungal organisms but some are irritant if applied to the skin. Care must be taken to read the labels to check for the range of activity and the value and dangers of application to the skin. Some agents are used solely as environmental disinfectants in order to reduce the microbial challenge to animals.

Chlorhexidine diacetate/gluconate is a phenol-related biguanide antiseptic-disinfectant with few problems and no apparent systemic absorption or local effects. It has a wide range of antibacterial activity and probably superior control over *Staphylococcus aureus* than povidone iodine. It has little or no fungicidal effect except at high concentrations and is used primarily as a surgical scrub and antiseptic solution (in spirit). The presence of pus or organic material does not diminish its activity and it has good tissue properties with some residual effects in tissues providing prolonged activity. Routine use of 0.5% is recommended, but as a wound irrigation solution concentrations of 0.05% should be used. It is important to dilute the concentrate with water rather than saline or other electrolyte solutions which may cause significant precipitation of the compound in solution and consequent loss of effect.

Povidone-iodine is a non-irritating, non-staining, iodophor which comprises iodine solubilized by surface-active agents. It has a broad spectrum of activity with virucidal, bactericidal (and sporocidal) and fungicidal effects which are not affected by blood, serum, necrotic tissue or pus. The rapid bactericidal effects are better at lower dilution – higher concentrations result in reduced bactericidal effects and greater tissue toxicity. The mild tissue toxicity effects are minimized by dilution to less than 0.05%. Solutions of 5% or more actively inhibit leukocyte migration into wounds, while very weak solutions appear to encourage neutrophil and monocyte migration. One per cent solutions cause death of fibroblasts but 0.01% has no detectable harmful effect on these cells.

Acetic (and malic) acid are natural highly acidic chemical solutions which are widely marketed as wound irrigants. They are effective in the control of *Pseudomonas* spp. infections on skin and their use should be restricted to old wounds infected with this organism and use as a debriding agent. The solutions should not be applied to a fresh wound or wounds without *Pseudomonas* spp. complications as it causes severe deleterious effects on all cells associated with wound healing.

Hydrogen peroxide, available in various dilutions, has been used widely for its disinfectant properties. It has only weak germicidal effects but an impressive foaming and deodorizing property as a result of liberation of nascent oxygen. The oxygen release can be employed usefully in the control of deep anaerobic infections. Concentrations higher than 5 vol (v/v) are damaging to tissues, with worse cytological effects against tissue cells (including fibroblasts) than against bacteria. As the chemical can cause microvascular thrombosis, it can retard healing. It can, however, be effective at higher concentrations in the treatment of thrush in the cleft of the frog.

Hexachlorophene is used primarily in medicated shampoo but it is possibly less effective than many of the other agents and is becoming less available owing to its potential long-term toxicity.

The specific properties of the common agents are described in **Table 4.1**.

Table 4.1 Relative activity of some of the common disinfectant compounds used in veterinary practice (the more stars the greater the effect)

Agent	Antifungal activity	Antibacterial activity	Antiviral activity	Value as dermatological therapeutic
Chlorhexidine	*	***	–	***
Povidone-iodine	**	***	–	***
Halogenated tertiary amine	****	****	****	Uncertain
Inorganic peroxygen compound	***	****	****	Uncertain
Acidic iodine	**	****	****	Not for topical application

Fumigation of tack and equipment using formaldehyde gas

This is a very useful technique for sterilizing equipment and tack without damaging it and without the need to handle every single piece of it. The method and precautions outlined below make the procedure both safe and effective.

Equipment required

- Protective clothing and mask are advisable.
- Suitable amount of potassium permanganate (Condy's crystals) (usually about 100 g).
- Suitable volume of 40% (strong/neat) formalin solution (for the 100 g of permanganate about 250 ml is required).
- Air-tight plastic bags of suitable size.
- Sealing clips for bags.

Precautions

Note: Although the precautions outlined below may initially be daunting, they are sensible. However, the method is really very simple, very practical and highly effective. With reasonable care it is entirely feasible in almost every stable situation.

- All procedures should be carried out in the open air under cover (ventilation is extremely important as the gas is very toxic).
- Ensure that bags are air tight.
- Avoid contact with either permanganate or formalin solution. It is advisable to wear a mask, gloves (preferably up to the elbow), rubber boots and protective waterproof clothing.

Method

1. Place the articles to be sterilized in a large plastic bag.
2. Place a plastic bowl with potassium permanganate crystals (Condy's crystals) into the bag.
3. Pour 40% formalin onto the crystals.
4. Quickly seal the bag.
5. Leave undisturbed for at least 12 hours.
6. Open the bag in fresh air without breathing fumes.
7. Leave the bag open for 12 hours before handling any equipment inside it.

Note: Although this is an excellent method for disinfecting equipment it can be a dangerous procedure. Formaldehyde gas can be seriously toxic to humans if inhaled in quantity or on repeated occasions. The strong formalin solution is also toxic and should not be touched.

Antiviral agents

There are few if any specific antiviral agents currently in use in horses. In theory at least some of the new antiviral drugs (such as acyclovir and vidaribine) would be expected to have significant benefits on virally induced skin disease and in particular the herpesvirus conditions. Only acyclovir has any equine reputation and this is limited to treatment of putative herpetiform keratitis. Its action is specifically against herpesviruses. Topical applications of a 5% cream can be used on painful coital exanthema (EHV-3) lesions. Oral dosing of acyclovir can also be used but no information is available as to its safety or efficacy.

The modern acidic iodine, tertiary amine and inorganic peroxygen disinfectants have strong antiviral properties but many are highly irritant to the skin.

However, some tertiary amine compounds have been formulated into surgical scrub solutions and can therefore be justifiably used on the skin.

PRINCIPLES OF ANTIBIOTIC THERAPY IN SKIN DISEASE – THE USE OF ANTIMICROBIALS IN WOUND MANAGEMENT AND SKIN DISEASE

A full understanding of the action and function of antibiotics can be obtained from pharmacological texts. Antibiotics are commonly used by veterinarians in their daily practice – often to treat defined or suspected infections or as prophylaxis for various medical and surgical procedures. Antibiotics do not eliminate infection, rather they reduce the rate of bacterial replication to a degree which allows the host defences to eliminate the infectious agent. The use of antibiotics carries risks of potentially harmful side effects and therefore they should be used with care. Potential side effects include:

- Bacterial resistance
- Anaphylactic/hypersensitivity reactions
- Delayed drug related skin eruptions
- Immunologically mediated systemic effects
- Overgrowth of other bacteria or fungal species
- Gastrointestinal disturbances deriving from alteration of large bowel flora and fauna

Since potential risks are involved in the use of antibacterial and antifungal drugs, it is important to continue asking the following questions to ensure correct and appropriate usage:

1. Is an antibacterial agent really indicated either prophylactically or therapeutically?
2. Should a culture and sensitivity test be performed before embarking on the medication and is there sufficient justification for the inevitable consequent delay in institution of the therapy?
3. Is the chosen agent appropriate for the case and the suspected (or confirmed) condition?
4. What are the correct dose, dosing interval and route of administration?
5. Is its use likely to result in early resistance and are there measures which can be taken to minimize this risk?
6. Is the duration of therapy appropriate and should any monitoring procedures be performed (to assess either resistance of pathogen or harmful side effects on the patient)?

Prophylactic antibiotic therapy

The use of prophylactic antibiotics is necessary for surgical procedures that carry a significant risk of postoperative infection such as with wounds on the lower limb, in the perineum or around the mouth. Clean procedures are associated with a low risk of postoperative infection and therefore require less than 24 hours of antibiotic coverage. Since in all but surgical skin wounds some infection is likely, elective procedures involving skin wounds should be preceded by at least one full therapeutic dose of a suitable antibiotic. If full aseptic technique can be sustained throughout the procedure (such as in a surgical wound resulting from excision of a small tumour), additional therapy should not usually be necessary. If any break in aseptic technique occurs or the procedure involves complicating factors such as a synovial structure, continued antibiotic administration for up to 5 or more days may be prudent. The aim of prophylactic therapy is to achieve high levels of antibiotics in the skin at the time of surgery. Ideally the concentration of the agent should be 4–8 times the minimum inhibitory concentration (MIC) for the potentially infective bacteria. This requires administration of antibiotics about 30 minutes preoperatively for intravenous dosing and 1–2 hours preoperatively for intramuscular dosing. Care should be taken to ensure that antibiotic administration does not interfere with the anaesthetic protocol (for example, potentiated sulphonamides should not be used concurrently with injectable α_2-adrenoreceptor agonist sedatives because the combination might induce cardiac dysrhythmias). In addition, the potential systemic toxic effects and the cost of the antibiotic should be considered.

Therapeutic antibiotic therapy

Antibiotics are required when suspected or confirmed infection is present. Confirmation is obtained by culture of swabs taken from the site (see above) and subsequent culture, Gram stain and antimicrobial sensitivity test. In the absence of confirmation of an infection, clinical signs of inflammation (heat, pain, swelling, redness) or lack of response to supportive therapy are sufficient to warrant the use of antibiotics. As cultures often take several days to perform, it is often wise to preempt the findings by administration of a suitable and logical antibiotic and adjust the drug if necessary when results become available. A clinical judgement of the likely infectious organisms based on experience can usually be made.

In most equine skin conditions *Streptococcus*

spp. are usually the most common organisms involved and most of these are fully or partially sensitive to penicillin. Therefore it has become common practice to use full therapeutic doses of penicillin as a primary approach to skin antimicrobial therapy. This is entirely justifiable.

Both prophylactic and therapeutic antibiotics in skin disease rely on the delivery of the drug to the skin in therapeutic concentrations. Few antibiotics have been shown to be delivered in effective dosages to the skin of the horse and so careful appraisal of the effects of therapeutic measures must be taken. The distribution of antimicrobial drugs in the skin depends on its formulation, lipid solubility, state of ionization, protein binding capacity, route of administration and the delivery efficiency to the site. For instance, a drug that is more soluble in lipid may have better intracellular penetration and therefore prove more effective for use against intracellular bacteria.

Failure of a detectable therapeutic response to antibiotic therapy may result from:

- inappropriate drug selection for species of bacteria involved;
- resistant (strains of) bacteria;
- inappropriate drug delivery dynamics;
- inability of the drug to reach the site due to a compromise in the blood supply or the presence of fibrous tissue;
- inactivation of the antibiotic due to enzymatic inactivation or the pH of the tissue. Local factors such as the presence of destructive enzymes, acidic pH, low oxygen tension and intracellular organisms can have a marked effect upon the *in vivo* efficacy of the drug.

Culture and sensitivity results allow the use of antimicrobials to which a particular bacterium is most sensitive *in vitro*. Enzymatic and pH-related inactivation can usually be avoided if abscess cavities are drained or if septic synovial structures are flushed to remove the acidic debris.

Rapid identification of the infecting organism can sometimes be made from a Gram-stained impression smear from the surface of infected skin, but in dermatological disease the heavy normal commensal bacterial flora of equine skin makes the interpretation difficult. Gram staining may only indicate the type of bacteria, whereas a culture will usually provide a positive identification. Specific organisms involved in skin disease such as *Dermatophilus congolensis* benefit from specific culture methods (see page 26) and the correct method of sampling (see above) should always be observed so as to avoid errors of omission or commission. Many factors influence the function and efficacy of the drugs and the clinician needs to consider carefully the whole case and make a reasoned selection.

Sensitivity testing by disc diffusion or microdilution methods can be used to establish whether the bacteria are susceptible, moderately susceptible, or resistant. The minimum inhibitory concentration is the lowest concentration that inhibits bacterial growth and is calculated from serial dilution of the bacteria grown. The antibiotic dose necessary to achieve 4 times the minimum inhibitory concentration in the blood can be calculated and administered, but delivery to the site may still be a problem.

Ideally, choice of antimicrobial agent will be based on culture and sensitivity results. However, the decision regarding immediate antibiotic administration must invariably be based on clinical judgement. This requires an assessment of the location and nature of the condition, and more importantly a knowledge of the organism(s) most likely to be present. For instance, a kick wound may have a significant infection with *Escherichia coli* resulting from direct contamination but could also have pathological skin contaminant bacteria such as *Staphylococcus aureus*, *S. intermedius* or *S. epidermidis*. Once the potentially useful antibiotics are selected, the final choice may be based on the route or frequency of administration, the location of the infection, the pharmacokinetics of the drug, the cost of the drug, and the clinician's preference.

The pharmocodynamics and kinetics should be considered before any antibiotic is administered to a horse. A drug administered to treat a dermatological problem needs to be delivered to the skin in an effective concentration without any untoward effect on other organ systems. The extent of local irritation, the rate of uptake from the site and the excretion pathways carry significant risks if an inappropriate drug is administered. Thus lincomycin and possibly oxytetracycline may have profound harmful effects on the bacterial flora and fauna of the large colon and intractable diarrhoea may ensue. Similarly, amitraz is an effective ectoparasiticide for dogs and cattle but is extremely toxic to horses, causing severe colic as a result of complete and irreversible gut stasis.

The extent of protein binding can also influence the efficacy of a compound. A highly protein-bound drug is unlikely to reach effective concentrations in the skin without very high systemic doses. A horse suffering from low blood proteins might sustain higher plasma concentrations for longer than a normal healthy horse, but effective uptake from the site of injection may be significantly delayed. The overall clinical status of the horse is therefore important when considering the drug and route of administration.

When should antibiotics be used in skin disease?
The number and type of bacteria in a wound or skin lesion are the major considerations governing wound contamination and infection.[10] These can be further complicated by tissue trauma and necrosis. Impairment of the local blood supply and hence lowered delivery of immunoglobulins and leukocytes as well as the general condition of the horse are also important considerations. Old, debilitated horses often have poor responses to skin injury or insult. The use of systemic glucocorticoids also increases the risk of more severe bacterial invasion of the tissues.

For how long should antibiotics be used?
This is often related primarily to the tissue involved. Involvement of bone, joints and tendon sheaths may require prolonged therapy (often up to 2–3 months), whereas, in superficial skin wounds, parenteral medication can usually be terminated once granulation has commenced. Where poor blood supply to a wound can be identified, therapy should nevertheless be prolonged rather than shortened.

What are the best routes for administration of antibiotics?
Prolonged intramuscular or intravenous medication can be distressing for some horses. Resentment can develop at or after even the first injection, with increasing subsequent difficulty, particularly if the injection is painful. Pain can result from the material itself or from the volume of drug deposited at a single site or from incorrect injection technique (including errors of route). The benefits from multiple-site injections with a reduced individual volume have to be considered against the possible resentment arising from multiple injections.

There are few effective oral antibiotics for use in horses and there have been few attempts to establish pharmacodynamics of the common oral antibiotics. Some drugs carry serious risks while in others there seems to be much less risk. However, anecdotal reports of serious complications arising from oral-administration (and some parenteral) antibiotics makes the selection difficult. In practical terms the only available economical, safe, proven antibacterial agents in horses are the potentiated sulphonamides. These are used widely, being convenient, safe, easily administered and largely effective, although the distribution to the skin may be less efficient and achievement of effective antibacterial concentrations may be difficult.

How can the best (most effective) and most convenient antibiotic be selected?
Various factors to be considered when selecting an antimicrobial drug.

- The sensitivity of the bacteria involved (or suspected). The *in vitro* sensitivity to a given antibiotic does not guarantee *in vivo* efficacy. Lack of response may be related to tissue concentrations of the active agent as well as the extent to which the organism is in contact with the drug. Thus, some organisms are largely intracellular and may have a lipid capsule which prevents antibiotic effects. Positive identification of the organism and its antibiotic sensitivity provide the best selection. However, some laboratories do not limit sensitivity tests to those antibiotics which are safe and available for horses and results should therefore be interpreted with some care.
- Antibiotic blood levels affect the tissue levels because passive diffusion appears to be the most likely method of delivery of most antimicrobials. Efficacy is then subject to the activity in the presence of pus, tissue enzymes, acidity/alkalinity (pH) and fibrinous exudate, each of which can influence the clinical response.
- The relative benefits of bactericidal or bacteriostatic effects are important. Bactericidal antibiotics are usually preferred for skin diseases and wounds. There is then less reliance upon the body's own defence mechanisms. However, many bactericidal antibiotics are not effective, or are contraindicated in horses, or fail to reach the desired concentration in the desired site. This promotes the development of antibiotic resistance within the wound.
- Safety and freedom from side effects and idiosyncratic reactions are obviously important. Unpredictable (idiosyncratic) side effects such as urticaria, anaphylaxis, etc. are entirely possible with any antibiotic but for the most part are commonest with the penicillin groups. Other drugs (such as lincomycin) have more predictable harmful side effects (such as diarrhoea). Drug eruptions involving dermatological and systemic effects (such as immune-mediated vasculitis, systemic lupus erythematosus-like syndrome and thrombocytopenia) are less

predictable and may follow the administration of any drug (although antibiotics probably have the greatest tendency to induce this) over a period of weeks or months.
- The cost of the drug will also influence the choice. Many of the most effective, dermatologically active antibiotics are very expensive and involve regimens of treatment which make their use impractical. The cheapest drugs are usually basic penicillin, oxytetracycline and the potentiated sulphonamides. Fortunately, these are commonly sufficiently effective as to make them valuable in the treatment of skin diseases.

In general the first-choice antibiotics are the simple penicillins as many dermatological infections in the horse are of *Streptococcus* spp. and most of these retain good or moderate sensitivity to penicillin. The synthetic penicillins such as ampicillin, amoxycillin and cloxacillin are less commonly used, often because of local reactions or impractical administration requirements. Aminoglycosides (such as neomycin and gentamicin) or cephalosporins (such as ceftiofur) are more useful if Gram-negative organisms are involved. The advanced, later-generation aminoglycosides such as amikacin are extremely expensive and usually impractical for dermatological cases. Long-term therapy is effectively limited to potentiated sulphonamides by mouth. These have the added advantage that courses of treatment can be started parenterally and continued for long periods.

Spectrum of activity

Some drugs have particular affinity for certain tissues, but unfortunately most seem to have a low affinity for skin. This may relate to the relatively low blood supply or other factors as yet undefined. Delivery of adequate therapeutic concentrations of antibiotics in the skin is often difficult and often requires very high doses at frequent intervals.

Most equine skin diseases and wounds carry mixed infections but almost all will have a significant *Streptococcus* spp. component. Most if not all equine streptococci are penicillin sensitive or partially sensitive and so penicillin is widely used as first line of treatment in skin injuries and disease. However, kick injuries and wounds contaminated by faecal material will most likely have significant Gram-negative infections. Specific infections involving defined organisms may have characteristic sensitivity to antibiotics, but the widespread use of broad-spectrum antibiotics (often in unjustified circumstances) makes resistance a serious potential problem. In general, penicillin is ineffective against Gram-negative organisms but synthetic penicillins have improved activity. β-Lactamase-producing bacteria are resistant to penicillin and so infections with these organisms do not respond to it. Gram-negative organisms usually require aminoglycosides (preferably gentamicin); however, care must be taken to ensure delivery to the skin, which may be less than ideal.

The spectrum of activity also includes the activity of the drug against anaerobic or aerobic organisms. Metronidazole is a very useful drug for treatment of suspected or confirmed anaerobic skin infections (and is particularly useful topically in the foot region).

Route of administration

The route of administration of an antibiotic may be dictated by the wound location, practitioner preference, environment of the animal, patient or owner compliance and economics. The duration of therapy needed may also influence the decision, since long-term intravenous administration requires a long-stay catheter, hospital environment and normal patent jugular vein(s).

The standard options available for administration of antibiotics to horses include: parenteral route (intravenous; intramuscular), topical application, and oral administration.

Intravenous administration provides a rapid, high plasma concentration. This route often requires frequent dosing and special training to administer, and is usually therefore expensive. The need for special training can be avoided by the placement of an intravenous catheter; however, this may not be feasible outside the hospital and in any case catheter management can be difficult. Recently, it has been found that gentamicin can be administered effectively using 6.6 mg/kg once daily[11] rather than 2.2 mg/kg three times daily and this will clearly make its administration more economical.[12]

All drugs administered to horses by the intravenous route should be suitably formulated and given slowly to avoid damage to the vein and possible delivery of a bolus of potentially irritant drug to any internal organ. The intravenous route may be chosen to avoid complications associated with tissue damage and local irritant/pain effects.

Possible side effects of intravenous drug administration include:

- jugular thrombosis/thrombophlebitis;
- accidental intra-arterial injection;
- accidental extravascular injection with local tissue effects on skin, connective tissue and other structures in the vicinity of the vein, for example the vagosympathetic trunk;
- bolus effects from over-rapid injection of a drug which might have effects on the heart or brain;
- anaphylactic reaction.

Intramuscular administration may achieve good plasma concentrations but these may not be attained until 1–2 hours following administration. Slower absorption, distribution and elimination require less frequent dosing than the intravenous route but levels may fluctuate. Although some special training is necessary for safe administration, clients can usually be trained to give intramuscular injections. The expense is usually less than for intravenous medication. Large volumes of drug are, however, needed and these can be painful or warrant division of the dose into several sites. Patient resistance can make it difficult to complete longer courses.

Unwanted side effects are rare but include:

- local swelling;
- abscessation (either sterile or infected);
- anaphylaxis. (This is fortunately very rare but the risk is always present whenever a drug is administered parenterally.)

Oral administration is perhaps the easiest for the client and the least traumatic for the animal. However, plasma levels of the drug are achieved slowly and it may be prudent to administer a loading dose of the drug by injection (if such a formulation exists). Furthermore, there are few antibiotics which can be given to horses by mouth. The logistics of administration of the doses which would be required are also problematical for many of the drugs used by this route in other species.

Where the oral route can be used the expense will vary with the medication used, but economies can be made simply by home administration. The cost of hospitalization and intravenous catheter placement can be avoided. Patient compliance is usually good and side effects are usually minimal. Some drug interactions are important, such as the cardiac effects which are reported to occur when α_2-adrenoreceptor agonist sedatives (such as romifidine and detomidine) are administered with potentiated sulphonamides.

Topical antimicrobials are usually in the form of antiseptic solutions, antibiotic creams (often combined with various other pharmaceuticals such as corticosteroids or local anaesthetic agents) and so-called triple antibiotic ointment (a combination of bacitracin–neomycin–polymixin in ointment base). Topical antibiotics may be useful as a method of antibiotic prophylaxis in surgery. However, it is preferable to apply them to the tissues at the time of incision. This will provide for maximum effect.

Duration of therapy

The duration of antibacterial therapy depends on the situation. In elective procedures, prophylactic antibiotics are useful when administered prior to surgery so that the skin concentrations are high at the time of the surgery. A refined clean procedure may require as little as one preoperative dose. By contrast, severely contaminated wounds involving synovial structures can require in excess of 21–28 days of intensive treatment. Although intravenous or intramuscular administration may be used initially, there are clear advantages in changing to the oral route. However, there are severe limitations in choice and resistance or non-response to the oral formulations available for horses make long courses difficult. The change to the oral route should probably be delayed until patent sepsis has cleared. For traumatic wounds that do not involve bone or synovial structures, 3–5 days of treatment is usually sufficient. If a drain has been placed, therapy should continue for at least one day beyond the time of drain removal. If signs of infection are present, antibiotic therapy should continue for 2–3 days following resolution of the signs. Usually once drainage is established at the site of an incisional abscess, signs of infection will resolve rapidly.

Table 4.2 shows the commonly used antimicrobial agents and gives a summary of the regimens for their use. It is important to remember that none of these can be definitive and the clinician must make a careful assessment of the case as above before embarking on any therapeutic course. Furthermore, the clinician should be satisfied as to the safety and relevance of the regimen to be used.

ANTIFUNGAL AGENTS

A variety of antifungal agents is used in equine dermatological disease. These are either administered topically (several of the konazoles, nystatin, natamycin and benzuldasic acid) or by mouth

Table 4.2 Commonly used systemic antibacterial agents used in equine dermatological disease[a]

Drug group	Agent	Route[b]	Dose (mg/kg)	Dosing interval (q–*h)	Notes
Penicillins	Sodium/potassium penicillin	i.v. / i.m.	20–30[c]	6–8	Few problems
	Procaine penicillin	i.m.	20–30[c]	12–24	Few problems
	Benzathine penicillin	i.m.	20–30[c]	24–36	Few problems
	Ticarcillin	i.v.	50–75	6–8	Very expensive
	Ticarcillin + clavulinate	i.v.	50–75	6–8	Very expensive
	Ampicillin	i.v. (i.m.)	30–100	8	Risk of site reaction
	Amoxycillin	i.m.	30	6	Risk of site reaction
Aminoglycosides	Neomycin	i.m.	4–5	8–12	Possibly nephrotoxic
	Amikacin	i.v.	5–7	8–12	Possibly nephrotoxic; *very* expensive
	Kanamycin	I.v.	5	8	*Very* expensive
	Gentamicin	i.v. (i.m.)	3.3 (6)	8–12 (24)	Nephrotoxic; expensive
Cephalosporins	Ceftiofur	i.v. (i.m.)	2	6–8	Site reaction i.m.
	Cephalexin	p.o	25–30	6–8	
Tetracyclines	Oxytetracycline	i.v.	5–10	8–12	Risk of shock if i.v. and diarrhoea
Amphoterics	Chloramphenicol	i.v.	30–50	6–8	Risk of bone marrow suppression/resistance
Sulphonamides	Potentiated sulphonamides	i.v./i.m./p.o.	30 (total)	24	Site reaction Do not use with the α_2-agonist group sedatives Very safe even with prolonged courses
Nitroimidazoles	Metronidazole	p.o./i.v.	15–25	6–8	Risk of diarrhoea
Macrolides	Erythromycin	p.o.	25	8	Risk of diarrhoea

[a] Uncomplicated superficial infections are probably best treated initially with penicillin or potentiated sulphonamides unless there is reason to suspect a Gram-negative or anaerobic infection. Use of other agents should be based on culture and sensitivity results but inevitably there will be occasions when other agents will be preferred. Antibiotic dosage regimens for horses are suggested but not definitive and may need to be adjusted in various clinical circumstances.
[b] Route: i.m., intramuscular; i.v., intravenous; p.o., by mouth.
[c] Dosages for penicillin are given in 10^3 i.u./kg.
Dosing interval (q–*h), to be repeated hourly.

(griseofulvin and potassium or sodium iodide) or by injection (amphoteracin B and sodium iodide). Generally antifungal agents work best when applied directly to the lesion, but extensive disease or deep mycosis are likely to resist topical application alone.

Sodium iodide and **potassium iodide** are underutilized, effective and safe antifungal agents when administered by intravenous and oral routes, respectively (the potassium salt must not be administered by intravenous injection). A dose of 10 g per 450 kg bodyweight twice daily given in the feed has a detectable antifungal effect against *Aspergillus* spp. It is convenient and accurate to use a twice daily dose of 25 ml of an aqueous solution of 160 g of potassium iodide dissolved in 400 ml of water. The solution can be mixed easily with the food and is generally totally unnoticed by the horse. Lesser doses can be effective also. The drug can be continued until obvious signs of iodism develop (lacrimation is the first sign in most cases, and later a scurfy, flaky skin). The compound is then withdrawn for 7 days and re-administered if needed. The effects are slow to develop and dramatic responses are unlikely in any deep-seated fungal infection.

Amphotericin B is a very expensive drug which can be administered topically or intravenously. It has a wide antifungal range (*in vitro* activity against *Blastomyces*, *Aspergillus*, *Histoplasma*, *Cryptococcus*, *Sporothrix* and *Zygomycetes*). It is fungistatic at low doses and fungicidal at high doses. It acts by binding to sterols in cell membranes and allows intracellular electrolytes (potassium in particular) to leak out. As bacteria and rickettsia have no sterols it is not active against these organisms. It is highly bound to plasma proteins and has good distribution to all organs including skin. It is used most often for treatment of phycomycosis and other deep fungal infections. As there is a significant risk of systemic toxicity, all cases receiving parenteral doses must be carefully assessed to confirm its value and to check for ongoing systemic toxicity. Topical creams are also useful for application to localized fungal lesions.

Griseofulvin is a microsized-particle antifungal agent used in the treatment of superficial mycosis (such as dermatophytosis/ringworm). The drug has been used for many years and has gained a good reputation but recent results are not as satisfying. Reports of the efficacy of griseofulvin are anecdotal – no extensive trails have been reported in support of this. This may be due to resistance or another factor not yet established. It is a tasteless powder which is well tolerated for prolonged courses: courses of up to 30–40 days may be required in some cases. There is no detectable effect against *Aspergillus* spp. or other deep mycoses. It is potentially teratogenic and so should not be used during pregnancy.

The **conazoles** (including **miconazole**, **ketoconazole** and **enilconazole**) are used widely in the treatment of fungal infections and particularly in superficial mycoses such as trichophytosis and microsporosis (ringworm). The drugs do have a useful effect on *Aspergillus* spp. but delivery to the site may be more difficult. Topical application and systemic dosing can be used with relevant formulations.

Ketoconazole has some potential in the treatment of *Sporothrix schenckii* but its action is poorly documented. The drug is administered by mouth at 30 mg/kg twice daily. It is extremely expensive and has already largely been replaced in human medicine (for treatment of sporotricosis) by itraconazole, which can be given to horses at 3 mg/kg twice daily by mouth. Again its expense is likely to limit its use to those fungal infections which fail to respond to other agents (including iodine salts). A commercial mixture of 2% miconazole with 2% chlorhexidine has been shown to be useful as a whole-body antifungal shampoo and an environmental anti-fungal agent.[13]

Enilconazole is very effective when applied topically to ringworm-infected horses.[13] It is applied directly to the lesions and the surrounding skin every 3 days for 3 or 4 applications. Alternatively, the horse can be sprayed with the diluted solution. The drug is not absorbed from the skin and has no significant toxicity apart from the irritant effect of very strong solutions incorrectly applied.

Nystatin is a naturally derived antifungal antibiotic which is available for topical use as a powder or a cream. Oral use is not effective as the drug is not absorbed from the gut. Although it is anecdotally reported to be particularly effective against *Aspergillus* spp. and *Candida* spp. there are no reports of efficacy trails in horses.

Natamycin is an insoluble powder which, in suspension, is used to treat superficial mycosis and in particular *Trichophyton* spp. and *Microsporum* spp. infections (ringworm). The suspension is very safe and non-irritating and is therefore widely used. In high concentrations it can, however, cause skin inflammation and so strict adherence to manufacturers' instructions is required. Its strong sporicidal activity makes it very useful both for the direct treatment of affected horses and for sterilizing the stable and harness, etc. Again there are no reports of efficacy trials. Unless previous personal usage has given uniformly good results, natamycin and nystatin should be used with care until appropriate data is established.

Potassium monopersulphate can be used to control environmental fungal infections[13] and many of the available disinfectants (see above) have strong antifungal and sporocidal effects.

The common antifungal drugs and agents are shown in **Table 4.3**.

(ECTO)PARASITICIDES

This is an important group of therapeutic agents in dermatology but unfortunately the therapeutic options have been decimated with the removal of many organophosphate and chlorinated hydrocarbons from the drug lists. There are few, if any, licensed ectoparasiticidal products for topical application to horses in Europe, Australasia, the United States and Canada. In other parts of the world some of the more effective (but environmentally harmful) compounds remain in use. There is no doubt that many of the problematical compounds have been abused (environmental considerations are very important) but their value in veterinary treatment and the relief of animal suffering has been considerable. Furthermore, there are some compounds including amitraz and arsenical cattle dips which are very harmful to horses and should never be used in any case.

The treatment of ectoparasites can be performed by systemic or topical means. The correct selection of the approach depends upon the nature of the drug and the desired effect. For example, there is little merit in treating a single small local lesion with systemic treatment involving high systemic doses of a drug, and conversely topical application to large areas may be difficult and impractical and a systemic option might be more appropriate.

Chlorinated hydrocarbons

In most countries production and use of these compounds is prohibited due to toxicity and residue problems. Gamma benzene hexachloride and bromocyclen are probably the last of these compounds which are available in some countries. There is little doubt that the compounds were effective and that their loss has a significant implication in the treatment of parasitic infections. Some human antiparasitic washes and shampoos, however, still have the chemicals and some of these may be safely used on horses where such an approach is legally and ethically acceptable.

Organophosphates

These compounds are now banned in many parts of the world due to the toxic effects of prolonged or repeated exposure. Many of them are, however, still used in the control of insect pests on domestic pets and on agricultural crops and garden plants.

Commonly used insecticidal compounds which have been used for horses include dichlorvos; diazinon; malathion; phosmet; and chlorpyrifos. These compounds are potentially very toxic if used improperly. All have been used topically in horses (usually as washes or dips but occasionally as pour-on compounds) and have good anti-ectoparasitic effects. Most of the compounds have a potent anticholinesterase activity but vary in their toxicity. Application must be strictly according to the manufacturer's instructions. Clinical signs of toxicity can develop rapidly following their use, particularly in overtired/exhausted horses or in hot humid weather or as a result of overfrequent dipping or from overstrength applications. Signs of toxicity include salivation, trembling or convulsions, constricted pupils, diarrhoea and collapse. Simultaneous use of other organophosphates (such as dichlorvos-based anthelmintics) makes toxicity even more likely. Treatment of the toxic signs include administration of atropine sulphate by injection and control of convulsions.

Natural insecticidal compounds

A number of natural compounds with variable insecticidal properties have been used over many years in treatment of ectoparasitism in horses. These include rotenone/derris; lime sulphur; and natural pyrethrins. These compounds are usually derived from plants or naturally occurring chemicals. They are almost all very safe and nontoxic but their effects are often marginal. All these substances have a limited duration of effect which limits their therapeutic value. Lime sulphur has a particularly unpleasant smell and can cause burning and irritation of the skin when used in strengths over 5% but it has a significant effect on surface-feeding mites and on some dermatophytes.

Table 4.3 Commonly used antifungal drugs for use in treating fungal skin infections in horses.

Drug group	Agent	Route	Dose (mg/kg)	Dosing interval (q–*h)	Notes
Iodines	Potassium iodide	Oral	10 g total dose	12	Safe and cheap but somewhat unreliable Cease if signs of iodism occur (lacrimation/scurfy coat) Activity against *Cryptococcus* spp., *Histoplasma* spp., *Blastomyces* spp., *Aspergillus* spp.
	Sodium iodide	Oral i.v.	10 g total dose	24 (4 days only for i.v)	Safe and cheap but somewhat unreliable. Cease when signs of iodism occur (lacrimation/scurfy coat) Activity against *Cryptococcus* spp., *Histoplasma* spp., *Blastomyces* spp., *Aspergillus* spp.
	Povidone iodine	Topical	Dilute	n/a	More dilute solutions are better Activity against *Cryptococcus* spp., *Histoplasma* spp., *Blastomyces* spp., *Aspergillus* spp., *Trichophyton* spp., *Microsporum* spp.
Polyene agents	Griseofulvin	Oral	10 mg	24 (×10–30)	Activity against *Trichophyton* spp., *Microsporum* spp. *only*
	Nystatin	Topical			Very toxic parenterally Activity against *Candida* spp., *Cryptococcus* spp., *Histoplasma* spp., *Blastomyces* spp. *Trichophyton* spp. *Aspergillus* spp.

	Natamycin	Topical			Activity against *Trichophyton* spp., *Microsporum* spp. Useful sporocidal activity
	Amphotericin B[1a]	Topical i.v. as solution in 5% dextrose (*not saline*)	0.3 mg 0.5 mg 0.6 mg 0.6 mg	Day 1 Day 2 Day 3 q48h for 3 days per week	Renal and hepatic toxicity. Used for phycomycosis and other deep/systemic mycoses *Cryptococcus* spp., *Histoplasma* spp., *Blastomyces* spp., *Aspergillus* spp.
Imidazoles	Miconazole	Topical			Active against *Candida* spp., *Cryptococcus* spp., *Histoplasma* spp., *Trichophyton* spp. (with chlorhexidine)
	Ketoconazole	Topical			Active against *Candida* spp., *Cryptococcus* spp., *Histoplasma* spp., Trichophyton spp., *Microsporum* spp.
	Enilconazole	Oral			Active against *Candida* spp., *Cryptococcus* spp., *Histoplasma* spp., *Trichophyton* spp., *Microsporum* spp.

[a] Manufacturer's data sheet *must* be consulted carefully before using this drug. Preparation of the solution and rate of administration intravenously *must* be accurate.
Dosing interval (q–*h), to be repeated hourly.

As the more effective drugs are discontinued the value of these compounds may need to be reviewed.

Synthetic pyrethroids

Commonly used compounds include: deltamethrin; permethrin; cypermethrin; and fenvalerate. These compounds have almost no known toxicity at any dose and so are extremely safe. They are frequently used topically against skin parasites. They have a higher efficacy and longer duration than the natural pyrethrins which they have largely replaced. The synthetic pyrethroids are particularly useful as repellents for *Culicoides* spp. midges and a few species of fly but must be applied at least weekly and immediately after rain wetting in order to achieve continuous protection. Cypermethrin and permethrin have been used as repellents in fly fringes and tags for attachment to head collars and the mane and tail hair.

Other agents

1. **Selenium sulphide (1%)** A shampoo for the treatment of seborrhoea in pet animals has been applied to the treatment of lice in particular, in horses.[15] It is claimed that the shampoo also reduces the secondary seborrhoea which is characteristic of lice infestation.
2. **Avermectin compounds** These are commonly used for the treatment of helminth and bot (*Gastrophilus* spp.) parasites. Ivermectin administered orally has been shown to have an effect in reducing the extent of egg laying by lice (*Damalinia equi* and *Haematopinus asini*) and mites (*Chorioptes* spp., *Sarcoptes* spp. and *Psoroptes* spp.) and is anecdotally reported to have some effect against the adult stages themselves, but the effects are unpredictable and generally it seems that it is unlikely to eliminate the parasites.[16] It is possible that later-generation avermectin compounds will be found to have a greater effect when administered either by mouth or by injection. There are no published trials of these (or any of the other compounds) in horses.

CORTICOSTEROIDS

General considerations for the use of corticosteroids

Corticosteroids are anti-inflammatory, immunosuppressive drugs which are frequently used in immune-mediated and pruritic skin diseases and in diseases where noninfective inflammation plays a major role in the aetiopathogenesis. They are powerful drugs and must be used carefully and correctly. Oral medication is usually preferable to parenteral injection as the former provides a better sparing effect on the pituitary–adrenal axis and thereby minimize their secondary, undesirable effects.

The drugs are commonly employed in the treatment of insect bites, insect hypersensitivity, habronemiasis, allergies and in some immune-mediated diseases including vasculitis, urticaria, pemphigus (in all its forms) and sarcoidosis.

Specific diseases do not always respond to standard treatment regimens and may require either a higher or lower than normal dose rate. Once remission is established, the dose should be gradually reduced over 2–3 weeks to the lowest dose which maintains the desired therapeutic effect. Once this dose is established, an attempt should be made to use alternate-day treatments as this will have a negligible effect on the pituitary adrenal axis and will minimize side effects.

Some of these drugs do not always have the expected effect in every case and alternatives should then be tried. Thus, it is usual to institute treatment with prednisolone as it has the fewest problems and is conveniently administered by the oral route. Dexamethasone should then be used if no effect is detectable within 24–48 hours. Again it is important to reduce the drug dose to a minimum effective dose as soon as possible.

Whenever prolonged corticosteroid treatment courses are unavoidable, alternate-day therapy should begin as soon as the case becomes stable. Prednisolone and methylprednisolone can be used in this way and so are the preferred choice in most cases. Dexamethasone and betamethasone have a longer duration of effect and so have less sparing effects but can still be used in alternate-day regimens. Anti-inflammatory (low) doses of prednisolone may not cause side effects, whereas immunosuppressive (high) doses administered daily carry significant risks including immuno-suppression (with a risk of infections), laminitis, polydipsia, polyphagia and behavioural alterations.

Prolonged (or sometimes even short) high-dose (or low-dose) courses may induce acute, often life-threatening laminitis, although there are few recorded confirmed scientific reports to this effect. The risks of laminitis should not be underestimated but are probably not as great as once feared. The risks appear to be much higher in cases which have active laminitis or which have had, or are susceptible to, laminitis. Under these conditions the use of corticosteroids should be considered particularly carefully. Triamcinolone seemingly has a greater potential for causing laminitis than other members of the group but is commonly only used in very small doses for the intralesional treatment of collagen necrosis nodules (and occasionally for intra-articular injections).

Complete failure of corticosteroid therapy should be followed by a careful reassessment of the case and, if the diagnosis is confirmed, treatment with aurothioglucose can be attempted as an alternative approach with the same objective.

Systemic corticosteroid therapy[17]

Clinical effects

The effects of corticosteroid therapy can be divided into three major categories. Each of the compounds has a slightly different bias in terms of both the desirable and the undesirable effects but these are probably of little overall clinical significance. However, some specific compounds such as triamcinolone may have potentially more dangerous side effects. As a general principle, glucocorticoids are catabolic because they enhance the breakdown of protein tissues and they generally induce an increase in blood glucose levels by stimulating gluconeogenesis and glycogenolysis.

1. **Anti-inflammatory effect**
   - Decreased leukocyte activity (prevent release of lytic enzymes which would destroy cells and attract other inflammatory cells to areas of tissue damage)
   - Decreased leukocyte accumulation (monocytes and lymphocytes are sequestered into tissues)
   - Vascular stabilization (reduced capillary permeability)
   - Suppression (sequestration) of eosinophils
   - Stabilization of mast cells
   - Blockage of prostaglandin release
2. **Immunosuppression effect**
   - Lymphocytopenia
   - Decreased T lymphocyte function
   - Decrease in immunoglobulin and complement levels
3. **Antimitotic effect (retarded cell division)**
   - Specific inhibition of fibroblasts

Drug type

The types of corticosteroids available for use in horses can be divided into those which act for shorter or longer periods.

1. **Short-acting** (biological effects last for less than 12 hours), e.g. hydrocortisone, cortisone
   - Very rapidly metabolized
   - Little pharmacological effect and little clinical application
2. **Medium-acting** (biological effects last for 12–24 hours), e.g. prednisolone or prednisone, triamcinolone, methylprednisolone and isoflupredone
   - Given daily at beginning of treatment
   - Suitable for alternate-day therapy
3. **Long-acting** (biological effects last for over 48 hours), e.g. dexamethasone, betamethasone, flumethasone
   - Long half-life, smaller dosage required
   - Potential additive effect
   - Not usually suitable for alternate-day treatment
4. **Slow-release,** e.g. methylprednisolone acetate
   - Convenient for general use
   - Can be used intralesionally
   - Possibly increased risk of side effects including laminitis

Route of administration

The preferred route of administration for each of the compounds varies.

Parenteral/injection The drug is injected intravenously, intramuscularly or subcutaneously. Over the period during which the drug remains in the bloodstream it exerts a continuous effect on the area of inflammation. There will also be continuous adrenosuppressive and mineralocorticoid effects. These will remain for as long as the drug is at concentrations capable of exerting the effect (even very low doses can have significant effects on the pituitary–adrenal axis). There will be a progressive, slow reduction in circulating drug concentrations and so there is no abrupt withdrawal of the drug.

Intralesional injection Very high local concentrations of the drug can be achieved locally without large overall doses and can therefore provide prolonged local effect. It is applicable to nodular lesions in particular.

Oral This route is generally considered to be safer. The action of the drug stops when therapy ceases. Therefore it is useful for alternate-day therapy and has minimal adrenal–pituitary axis suppression. There are also minimal mineralocorticoid side effects such as polydipsia-polyuria, hyperglycaemia and alterations in appetite.

Topical Topical application of corticosteroids is commonly practised. The local concentration of the drug is high immediately after application but falls rapidly thereafter as the drug diffuses into the bloodstream. Systemic effects are minimal but maintenance of therapeutic effect requires repeated applications at short intervals. It is not often used in the horse except for localized single inflammatory lesions. The antimitotic effects are sometimes used in the control of abnormal cell replication in exuberant granulation tissue or superficial skin neoplasms.

Duration of therapy

Long-term therapy with corticosteroids can be required in some disorders, although it is generally accepted that this is undesirable. Where no alternative drugs class can be used and where long courses are unavoidable, 'the shorter the course the safer the regimen' is probably a justifiable maxim. The treatment course should be carefully monitored to ensure that the drugs are being administered in the most efficient manner while minimizing the risk of untoward effects.

1. Induction and daily dose are high until clinical signs regress.
2. The daily dose is tapered off to obtain a minimal (effective) daily dose (MDD).
3. The maintenance dose is established by using double the MDD every alternate-day and this is then adjusted (downwards usually but sometimes upwards) to establish the effective alternate day dose (EADD).
4. The EADD is maintained to stabilize the condition.
5. Decrease dosage progressively to establish the minimal effective alternate-day dose (MEADD).

Dose factors

The individual drugs have dosages which are usually (although not invariably) effective, but this varies with the purpose for which the drug is being used.

1. **Anti-inflammatory activity**
    - Prednisolone/prednisone
        - Induction dose 0.8–2.2 mg/kg
        - Maintenance dose 0.4–1 mg/kg
    - Dexamethasone
        - Induction dose 1 mg/15 kg
        - Maintenance dose 1 mg/60 kg
2. **Immunosuppressive activity**
    - Prednisolone/prednisone 5–7 mg/kg
    - Dexamethasone 0.1–0.2 mg/kg

Note: Treatment with either drug is continued until remission is obvious. If no change occurs within 10 days, an alternative treatment should be attempted. Once remission is present, the dose should be reduced by 20% every second week until a maintenance dose is achieved (this is usually 20% higher than the minimal effective dose).

Side (or undesirable) effects

Side effects are not common but are invariably important when they are present. They include:

- Suppression of the pituitary–adrenal axis by negative feedback mechanisms.
- Polydipsia and polyuria (mineralocorticoid effects).
- Mood changes.
- Increased susceptibility to infection (immunosupression). This effect is of very doubtful importance in horses.
- Catabolic effects reflected in weight loss and poor hair coat and skin quality (this is usually a marginal effect in horses).
- *Withdrawal syndrome*: Abrupt withdrawal of the drug (even after a relatively short course) may, in theory, result in an adrenal insufficiency syndrome similar to Addison's disease (hypoadrenocorticism). This has, however, not been well documented in the horse which would seem to be less susceptible to the effects than most other species. Nevertheless abrupt withdrawal of the drugs is not advisable.
- *Laminitis*: The true incidence of laminitis following directly from the administration of corticosteroids is hard to establish. There are anecdotal reports of catastrophic laminitis following even small doses, but many horses receive these drugs (even in very high doses) without any untoward effect.

The major factors which appear to predispose to the iatrogenic occurrence of laminitis include:

- combinations of drugs used simultaneously or alternately;
- active laminitis (acute, chronic, refractory) at the time of administration;
- previous history of laminitis;
- predisposing hoof conformation (large horse with small feet).

CYTOTOXIC/ANTIMITOTIC THERAPY

Antimitotic therapy can be divided broadly into topical and systemic applications. Although, in theory, systemic antimitotic drugs such as cyclophosphamide and vincristine can be used to treat neoplastic and autoimmune skin disease, they are probably impractical in the horse under normal clinical conditions. Applications to skin neoplasia is even more restricted. Furthermore, the most aggressive tumours of the lymphosarcoma group are not currently considered treatable. Cutaneous histiocytic lymphosarcoma carries a somewhat better prognosis anyway and systemic therapy probably has little effect on the outlook.

Topical therapy

Topical cytotoxic and antimitotic agents form an important group of pharmaceuticals. Several forms are available but are currently effectively limited to treatment of viral papilloma, equine sarcoid, melanoma and some squamous cell carcinomas. Many and varied compounds of inorganic tissue poisons such as arsenic, mercury and antimony and combinations of these have been used to treat the equine sarcoid in particular. More recently the use of podophyllin, methotrexate, fluorouracil and thiouracil and cisplatin have been described. All require some form of repeat applications, some on a daily basis for as long as 30 days.

Podophyllum Effective against a few localized and very small verrucose sarcoids and viral papilloma situated on the eyelids and periorbital skin. Limited effects make this almost a waste of time.

Cisplatin (Platinol, Bristol Myers, USA; Cis-Platin, Baker Pharmaceutical, UK) An inorganic platinum-containing molecule with strong antineoplastic properties which are independent of the cell-cycle. It is water-soluble: 1 mg will dissolve in 1 ml of saline. It is indicated for the treatment of several neoplastic diseases including some types of sarcoid, squamous cell carcinoma and melanoma. There are few analytical reports of its use but it has been shown to be effective when administered under a strict protocol which includes safety measures for the operators. Aqueous solution–vegetable oil emulsions have been used to enhance the duration of the activity of the drug and so reduce the number of injections which are needed to treat the tumour.[18] Repeated intralesional injection is required. The drug is seriously toxic (nephrotoxic) and should be limited in overall volume/weight at any one time, although the small amounts used to treat localized tumours are probably unlikely to have any material harmful effect. It has a limited availability.

The drug is potentially carcinogenic and so suitable safety precautions must be taken when handling it (gloves and goggles are advisable).

Arsenic paste A soap-based paste containing up to 25% white arsenic trioxide has been used particularly for the treatment of equine sarcoids for over 100 years. Neat arsenic trioxide powder has also been dusted onto ulcerated tumours. The corrosive nature of the material makes it extremely dangerous topically with uncontrollable tissue necrosis. It is also extremely toxic systemically and there are serious safety issues with the handling of the chemical (especially in powder form).

5-Fluorouracil Ointments containing 5–20% 5-fluorouracil (Efudex, Roche, UK) have been found to be effective in the treatment of some very superficial occult and verrucose sarcoids and localized squamous cell carcinomas. Repeated treatments are needed (at least twice-daily applications over several weeks). Remissions are slow, but persistent treatment can be successful in some cases.

AW(3)4-LUDES This material is an experimental combination of cytotoxic and antimitotic drugs, natural oils and steroids in various concentrations which has been shown to have some promise in the treatment of equine sarcoids. It appears to have little or no value in the treatment of other forms of cutaneous neoplasia. Major complications can arise from extensive local cicatrization. Deep muscle damage can also be caused when treating periocular fibroblastic sarcoids (especially where these have been unsuccessfully treated previously by other means). Up to 70% resolution of individual treated lesions has been obtained in trials at Liverpool University. The best results were obtained when AW3-LUDES (the forerunner to AW4-LUDES) was used as an initial treatment method. Repeat treatment and treatment of previously treated and unresolved lesions is much less successful. However, repeated treatments in these refractive cases are still recorded as being more likely to be successful than other compounds and treatments commonly used.[19]

Prednisolone/corticosteroids These compounds have a detectable antimitotic effect and can be used as supplement to other therapy for proliferative dermatological and conjunctival lesions. The usual precautions must be taken before and during use (checking for fungal/viral/bacterial infections and, in the eye region, corneal ulcers). The compounds have a specific inhibitory effect on fibroblasts.[20] Corticosteroid compounds applied topically to exuberant granulation tissue have a marked inhibitory effect on fibroblast replication but probably have no effect on sarcoid fibroblasts.

Systemic therapy

The range of systemic antimitotic drugs for use in horses is very limited. The specific antimitotic drugs used for treatment of generalized or extensive neoplasia in small animals and humans are not feasible in the horse under normal conditions for reasons of cost and toxicity. However, cimetidine (an H_2-receptor blocker used in the treatment and control of gastric ulceration syndrome in adult horses and foals) has been shown to be beneficial in some melanoma tumours. The mode of action is uncertain at present but its antineoplastic properties seem to depend on the antiserotonin effects. It seems likely that activation of suppresser T cells (which are thought to alter the natural antineoplastic mechanisms in the body) is reduced by the drug. This allows the expression of the natural mechanisms which might be expected to control the development or proliferation of melanoma. Oral treatment at up to 3.5 mg/kg three times daily (or somewhat less effectively 9 mg/kg once daily) should continue for 6 weeks; if there is no material change there is little value in continuing. However, if a detectable improvement is evident then the drug should be continued for 3–4 weeks after no further improvement is evident. Repeated courses may have a similar or different effect.

MISCELLANEOUS DERMATOLOGICAL DRUGS

Antihistamines

Antihistamines act by competitively inhibiting histamine at H_1-receptor sites. They do not inactivate or prevent the release of histamine but rather control the effect of the histamine on cells. They may also have significant sedative and anticholinergic effects. Antihistamines appear to have little or no significant pharmacological effects in equine dermatology; their best effects are available before histamine is released (i.e. as a prophylactic measure) and this state is seldom applicable in the horse. Tripelennamine hydrochloride and hydroxyzine hydrochloride are the only specific antihistamines with any clinically significant effects in horses. However, an effective antihistaminic effect is also shown by certain phenothiazine ataractics such as acepromazine and by corticosteroids in general.

Tripelennamine hydrochloride This is an ethylenediamine derivative with strong antihistaminic activity. It acts by blocking the effect of histamine on H_1-receptors on the cell but it does not inactivate the histamine or reduce its release from cells. It has limited effects at a dose rate of 1.1 mg/kg by intramuscular injection (at multiple sites) once or twice daily. The drug should not be administered intravenously (seizures, collapse or disorientation are possible). Intramuscular injection is often painful and causes significant swelling (and risks of abscessation).

Hydroxyzine hydrochloride This is an effective prophylactic antihistamine at a total dose of 600 mg three times daily for a 450 kg horse. The dose should be reduced to a minimum daily level to control reoccurrence of the problem. Once this occurs the dose should be reduced to twice daily and then to once daily. Major side effects can be sedation or hyperactivity. It cannot be given to pregnant mares as it has teratogenic properties.

Aurothioglucose Where horses do not respond to glucocorticoids alone or laminitis is a high risk factor, the use of gold salts (aurothioglucose) therapeutically may be of advantage.[23] These compounds possibly decrease histamine release from mast cells and inhibit prostaglandin formation. It is particularly used to treat severe immune-mediated skin problems such as pemphigus in its various forms. An induction dosage of 20 mg aurothioglucose administered intramuscularly is followed by 50 mg 7 days later. Maintenance dosages of 1 mg/kg aurothioglucose in multiple intramuscular injections at weekly intervals can be continued until the disease is in remission (often after 6–8 weeks). Thereafter the aurothioglucose is decreased in frequency to every 2–4 weeks. Gold therapy should be discontinued if any untoward signs appear.

Immune stimulants

Immune stimulants and immunomodulating compounds are an attractive concept. Immune-mediated diseases or those in which the immune process is in some way impaired (such as sarcoidosis) seem to be the ideal theoretical objective of such therapy. The major problem is that no work has established the certain value of any of these chemicals. The commonest of these compounds in use in the horse is levamisole. This compound is used widely as a livestock anthelmintic and is cheap and available. The efficacy of the drug is very doubtful, with little clinical evidence of improvement in immune process. A number of protein derivatives of mycobacterial cell wall are used as general, systemic stimulants of the immune system. They are injected intramuscularly or subcutaneously and have ill-defined biological effects. Most of the commercially available compounds have shown a singular lack of predictability of effects and side effects and have been withdrawn from the market. There are, however, some good reports of their effect on tumours.

General immune stimulation of a scientifically unreported nature is supposedly derived from administration of several homeopathic medications. There are extensive anecdotal reports of the value of Aloe Vera in particular but these are widely viewed with some scepticism. The wide range of therapeutic claims for this and other natural medicines suggest that there is a basic biological response which could be beneficial under some conditions. The absence of critical scientific analysis of the effects of the materials needs to be addressed.

PRINCIPLES OF SURGICAL TREATMENT OF SKIN DISEASE

Surgical therapy most commonly applies to proliferative or neoplastic skin diseases. Before embarking on a surgical approach, careful consideration must be given to the prognosis. The type and character of a tumour has a profound bearing on the feasibility of surgical options. The character of the problem may render surgical options fraught with difficulty. Surgical excision may appear to be an attractive and simple option, but some conditions are probably only amenable to surgical excision with strict limitations. For example, nodular and small occult or verrucose sarcoids can be effectively treated by surgical excision (or cryosurgery), but there remains a high risk of recurrence. The secondary effects of surgery may be more serious even than the original disorder. While squamous cell carcinoma of the third eyelid or the cornea can often be treated by surgical excision, palpebral forms of the condition are not usually amenable to surgical removal because the defect and/or subsequent scarring may lead to clinically significant limitations of function.

In general, surgical excision is less feasible in areas where there is little 'spare skin' to allow primary closure of the defect while at the same time ensuring complete removal. The perceived limitations in such areas tend to encourage a conservative approach by the surgeon. Marginal excisions may result in a higher risk of tumour recurrence, particularly in ill-defined (and potentially malignant) tumour masses. In any case it may be very difficult to define the lesions sufficiently to be sure of complete removal.

Some classes of tumours are amenable to surgical removal with good recovery and low recurrence rates. For example:

- Lipomas and *subcutaneous* nodular sarcoids are easily removed and seldom create any untoward problem.
- Mast cell tumours can respond well to surgery even if surgical ablation is not complete.
- Melanomas have an unpredictable outcome: while many respond well to surgical ablation, some are in difficult or impossible sites and a few are highly malignant.
- Squamous cell carcinoma of the membrana nictitans (third eyelid) is frequently amenable to surgery. The availability of 'extra' mucosa permits primary closure after wide excision: it is usually possible to perform wide excision without risk of failure of closure or future cicatrization. With the possible exception of nictitans and some penile and vulval forms, squamous cell carcinomas have a high recurrence rate following surgical ablation on its own and better results are obtained when combined with cryosurgery, radiation or cytotoxic medication (see below).

The surgeon should therefore take every possible step to ensure that an appropriate choice of therapy is made and should certainly consider every possible consequence before embarking on surgical excision of tumours in particular.

There are several surgical options available to the surgeon. These include ligation by strangulating ligature, electrocautery, surgical excision, cryosurgery, hyperthermia, and laser surgery. The relative value of these options for each specific disease for which it a viable treatment option is given under the disease profiles in Part III.

Ligation by strangulating ligature

Indications

This is restricted to pedunculated, benign masses in sites where there is loose skin which allows the incorporation of a significant margin away from the mass itself that can be included in the ligature. Suitable masses include pedunculated and isolated melanomas, and certain pedunculated fibroblastic or nodular sarcoids (where it can be used in conjunction with other methods including topical cytotoxic creams).

Methods

Ligation can best be achieved by the use of Lycra in larger lesions and elastrator (castration) bands for smaller nodules (**Fig. 4.1**). Alternatives are heavy gauge elastic bands applied around the base of the lesion or the tight application of heavy suture material or string. In some cases even a hair from the tail of the horse has been used.

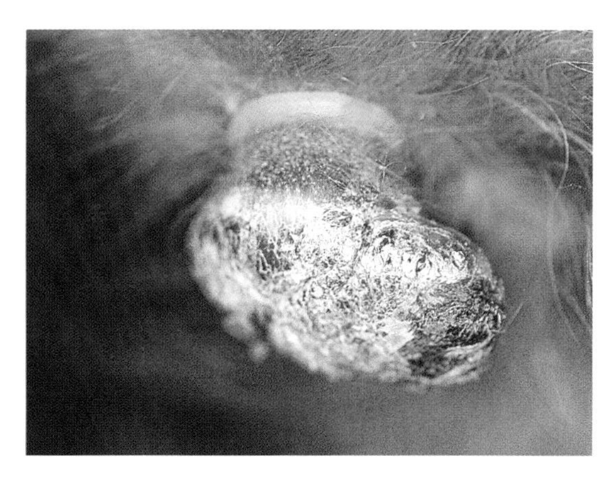

Figure 4.1 An elastic (lamb-castration) band applied below a skin nodule (sarcoid). Note the 'safe' skin margin.

Advantages

- Easy
- Cheap
- Convenient (requires little surgical skill)
- Small scar

Disadvantages

- Imprecise
- Need for 'spare' or loose skin (anatomical limitations)
- May need repeated application
- Risk of infection (tetanus in particular)
- Can be painful

Electrocautery

Indications

Where single small masses are involved, ordinary cautery is satisfactory but reoccurrence can be expected because it is again impossible to define the margins of many tumours.

Method

With large electrocautery units, both cutting and fulguration are available and should be used; the tumour should be removed with cutting current followed by treatment of the area by fulguration as far as possible, particularly the skin edges.

Advantages

- Control of haemorrhage during surgery allows precise excision.
- Electrocoagulation reduces the chance of sideways migration of tumour cells or infectious agents.

Disadvantages

- Equipment can be expensive and cumbersome.
- Treatments may require general anaesthesia.
- Large vessels may require ligation.
- Cicatrization can be problematical if large areas of skin/tumour are removed.

Thermocautery

Indications

Use is limited to small tumours or where electrocautery is not available.

Method

The technique requires a source of heat such as a gas burner to heat metal probes. Electrically heated wires can be used (tendon 'firing irons' of linear or point configurations are the main example of this and are, regrettably, sometimes used to surgically excise tumours).

Advantages

- Removal of the entire area does remove the cause.
- Haemostasis is effective.
- Necrosis of the margins limits spread of tumour cells.
- Equipment is generally available.

Disadvantages

- Lack of precision: it is difficult to control.
- Cicatrization with contraction is significant especially around eyelids or mouth.

Radiofrequency hyperthermia

Tumour cells are more sensitive to the effects of heat and this has been used in treatment of squamous cell carcinoma. Some other small tumours such as sarcoids have also been treated successfully.[24–26]

Tissue heating (to 50°C) over a 30-second period is achieved using a probe source of the radiofrequency energy. The extent of tissue damage is limited to 2–4 mm depth. Probes are usually 1 cm square and therefore overlapping and repeated applications are needed. This is a very time-consuming process for larger tumours but is more appropriate for superficial ocular/orbital masses (e.g. surface neoplasia, squamous cell carcinoma, verrucose sarcoid and limited fibroblastic sarcoids; the latter may require a more potent energy source). Treatments usually require repeated courses over 3 weeks or more.

Success rate is no better than most other modalities for both squamous cell carcinoma and sarcoids; refractory cases require further treatment by other means. The method is most successful for shallow early tumours not previously treated.

Surgical/sharp excision

Indications

This is effectively restricted to small tumours and other lesions with a well-defined margin or with sufficient skin around them to permit effective excision and primary closure after surgery. It can effectively be applied to benign or inflammatory lesions at any suitable site including dermoid cysts, inclusion cysts, eosinophillic collagen necrosis lesions and some neoplastic lesions. The latter include noninvasive squamous cell carcinoma (of the third eyelid, limbus or cornea, the penis and the vulva). Some melanomas, lipomas and mast cell tumours are effectively removed by sharp surgery, but for the most part the equine sarcoid is not amenable to this treatment as there is a high rate of recurrence. A possible exception to this is the nodular sarcoid. Those nodules, which are entirely subcutaneous, can be effectively removed using the one-cut, one-blade principle. Here, no cutting or closure instrument is reapplied to the skin for a second time and provided that the margins of the sarcoid have not been damaged during the procedure the results are usually excellent.

Where the excision is likely to leave a skin deficit which is impossible to close, alternative methods have to be employed (these may include skin grafting after surgical excision). Surgical excision is accordingly not generally applicable to ill-defined fibroblastic or occult/verrucose sarcoids or to palpebral squamous cell carcinoma.

Methods

Various surgical methods are applied in normal practice and are beyond the scope of this book.

Surgical debulking of large tumours prior to application of cryosurgery or the injection of cytotoxic or immunomodulating compounds is widely practised with variable results.

Advantages

- Easy
- Cheap
- Relatively quick
- Sometimes does not require general anaesthesia
- Convenient (requires little surgical skill)
- Small scar if primary closure can be achieved

Disadvantages

- Imprecise for ill-defined masses
- Risk of dissemination of malignant cells
- Precise surgical techniques may require general anaesthesia
- Need for 'spare' or loose skin (anatomical limitations)
- Scarring may be significant to function, e.g. eyelids

Cryosurgery/cryonecrosis therapy

Indications

This technique is useful for some types of ocular and skin squamous cell carcinoma (except most palpebral and some vulval and penile forms), melanoma and sarcoids.[27] Cryosurgical cautery of exuberant granulation tissue has also been reported. Complications arise from under- or overtreatment and injury to blood vessels, nerves, bone and tendon. Improper technique leads to loss of too much tissue or lack of kill.[28] A single freeze–thaw cycle is seldom adequate and triple freeze–thaw cycles are recommended.

Method

The best results are obtained by use of liquid nitrogen at −196°C applied by spray (**Fig. 4.2**) or probe. Modern pressurized, electrically controlled cryosurgery units have the ability to control the temperature of the probe and so provide a better means of limiting unwanted effects. Thermocouples should always be used to limit the damage and maximize the effects. Three freeze–thaw cycles with tissue temperatures of −25°C to −30°C should be applied to all tumours. Better results can sometimes be achieved by surgically debulking large tumours to allow better depth of freeze. However, excessive bleeding may create problems and significantly limit the effect. Uncontrolled freezing should be limited by surrounding protective masks created by petroleum jelly (Vaseline) and/or a polystyrene cup or cotton swabs. Extensive, and often uncontrollable, sloughing and subsequent cicatrization limit its application to areas where these are unlikely to have significant effects.

1. Select an adequate 'heat' sink (a copper rod or soldering iron can provide an adequate sink). Liquid nitrogen at −196°C provides the best coolant. Liquid nitrogen spray apparatus and electrically controlled more sophisticated machines are commercially available.
2. Insert thermocouples in adjacent tissue (unfortunately these are not commonly used).
3. Restrict circulation to the area using tourniquet if appropriate and possible.
4. Eliminate bulk by surgical trimming before freezing if indicated; this may enhance the effects of freezing but may cause extensive bleeding if a tourniquet or Esmarch bandage is not used to limit the blood supply.

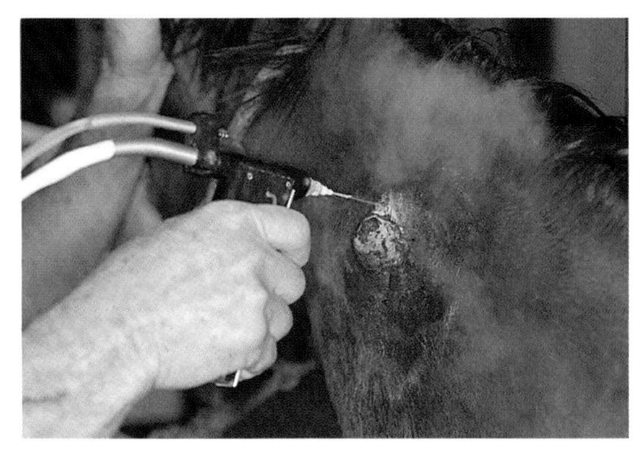

Figure 4.2 A liquid nitrogen spray apparatus being used to freeze a skin tumour on the neck of a horse.

5. Blood vessels (>1 mm) cut during debulking should be ligated prior to freezing.
6. Protect surrounding tissue with petroleum jelly (particularly if using spray methods).
7. Apply suitable cryogel to surface of mass.
8. Freeze tissues rapidly to below −20°C by applying the probe to the site.
9. Once the local temperature has fallen to below −20°C (as reflected by the thermocouples), the probe can be removed.
10. Allow to thaw slowly to body temperature (*do not* attempt to speed up the thaw by use of warm water, etc.).
11. Repeat the cycle 2–3 times.

Comments

- **Under no circumstances should liquid nitrogen be poured onto the skin – this leads to totally uncontrolled burning of tissues to arbitrary and indiscriminate depths and to 'flow' damage in adjacent normal tissue.**
- Hair follicles are destroyed by double cycle.
- Vitiligo/leukotrichia occurs with a single freeze–thaw cycle; scars occur with double or triple cycles. Always advise the owner about the likely formation of white hair and/or scarring at the site (this is the same process used to freeze-mark the skin for identification).
- Bone can become devitalized if included in freeze–thaw cycles; regeneration may take 2 years or more and sequestration can prolong healing time still further.
- Deep infiltrative tumours are seldom satisfactorily treated by cryosurgery and multiple lesions make the process very time consuming.
- Assess patient's temperament and use the correct restraint to allow the full process to be performed efficiently; many cases will require general anaesthesia, particularly if the lesion(s) are located in difficult sites or when they are numerous.
- Administer tetanus antitoxin or toxoid booster.
- Provide the owner with a full explanation of the process, the likely effects (swelling, sloughing and white skin/hair changes) and the required aftercare.

Advantages

- Convenient for small localized masses
- Cheap (limited facilities needed)
- Easily repeated if needed
- Predictable consequences (immediate and long-term)

- Can sometimes be performed under standing sedation and local anaesthesia
- Cryoantigen release into blood stream has been reported with benefits at remote sites for treatment of the equine sarcoid[29]

Disadvantages
- Tedious if multiple sites; require three cycles for each mass
- Limited applications
- Uncontrolled freezing can be very dangerous
- Need for thermocouples
- General anaesthesia if site/numbers inconvenient
- Swelling and slough of tissue
- White discoloration of hair/skin
- Scarring/cicatrization

PRINCIPLES OF IMMUNOTHERAPY IN DERMATOLOGY

Immunotherapy can be effectively divided into two categories: vaccination, and immunomodulation. Immune methods of treatment of skin disease are theoretically attractive but have strict limitations. Treatment of some viral, bacterial and fungal skin disease by these methods is currently either universally useful or actively being explored. For example, treatment of virus papillomata by the use of an autogenous vaccine has gained a considerable reputation and the possible use of vaccines to prevent dermatophytosis is being explored with some promise. However, vaccines can only be expected to be effective when the response is directed effectively at the target organism or cell. Attempts to use autogenous vaccines for treatment of the equine sarcoid (on the assumption that it is caused by a virus which can be eliminated by antibody responses) have either consistently failed or proved unreliable. There is some suggestion that they may make the condition worse.

Vaccination

Indications
Vaccination for skin disease is not currently widely used with the exception of the equine viral papilloma ('grass wart'). Autogenous vaccines may be prepared directly from tissue removed from an active lesion and after suitable precautions during preparation to ensure sterility and safety the material is injected intramuscularly.

The method works well for viral papillomata but is *contraindicated in the treatment of sarcoids.* Although some reports have suggested that a benefit can be obtained in isolated cases,[30,31] other cases may become dramatically worse with the development of multiple or miliary lesions.

Method
A small portion of a papilloma is obtained by surgical excision and placed in a sterile plastic container for delivery to the laboratory directly. If delays are anticipated, the sample should be placed on ice until it reaches the laboratory. The vaccine is prepared by homogenization of the tissue and the virus is inactivated by sterilization (usually using formalin). Adjuvants can be added. The vaccine is tested for sterility before dispatch and two (or more) injections are given 1–2 weeks apart. The responses is usually obvious by 3–6 weeks following the second injection.

Advantages
- Simple
- Cheap
- Effective for viral papilloma, particularly if multiple
- Creates long-term immunity

Disadvantages
- Only for use in the same horse (autogenous)
- Very limited efficacy range
- Unpredictable quality/efficacy

Stimulation of the immune system (immunomodulation)

These methods rely on the intense immunological response following local injection of protein cell wall extracts from mycobacterial organisms or killed or live mycobacteria, usually *Bacillus Calmette-Geurin* (BCG). Cell wall extracts can be crude (usually 'milky' in appearance) or refined and are available commercially. Viable *Bacillus Calmette-Geurin* is freeze dried and reconstitutes to a clear water solution whose concentration and volume can be varied by appropriate dilution. Simplistically, the protein material probably binds to cells directly and as it is intensely immunogenic it enables the host's immune processes to recognize the cells as foreign. Therefore, the method is restricted to individually treated lesions – there is usually no detectable effect on untreated lesions on the same animal. Furthermore, it is probably only applicable to discrete tumours – diffuse surface sarcoids of the occult and verrucose types, for example, respond poorly while nodular lesions show a good effect (particularly around the eye). Treatment of multiple lesions is therefore difficult and requires a large volume of the protein. The material has little or no effect if injected around a lesion and requires to be injected truly intralesionally. There is also a reported risk of anaphylactic reactions following repeated injections. Ideally, therefore, it should be injected intralesionally after suitable premedication has been given to prevent untoward systemic reactions.[32]

A number of commercial preparations have been developed to exploit the effect for treatment of certain cutaneous neoplasms including the equine sarcoid and squamous cell carcinoma. However, there are limitations to its use in both conditions and most of the commercial products have fallen into disuse or been withdrawn after problems with production or use.

Several protocols are commonly used. This method has a good record against periocular nodular sarcoid, somewhat less effect on fibroblastic sarcoid, and is probably impractical for verrucose or occult sarcoid. Intralesional injection seems to be vital for satisfactory results with sarcoids and it is virtually impossible to inject a significant volume of the material into the skin surface of the verrucose and occult lesions. A McClintock type (TB-Testing Automatic 0.1 ml dose) syringe can be used to spread the material into the lesion. The method has a poor record against squamous cell carcinoma in horses (whereas in cattle it has a significant if somewhat unpredictable beneficial effect). BCG and the related immunological methods are not effective against many of the other tumours including melanoma and neurofibroma. Surgical debulking of sarcoid lesions, in particular, prior to administration of BCG has been reported to improve the overall results, but in the authors' experience this is not repeatable. In general it seems unwise to use debulking with a sarcoid in particular.

Indications

Treatment of squamous cell carcinoma with BCG has a poor overall success rate, probably less than 20%. However, the method has a good reputation for treatment of nodular and fibroblastic sarcoids around the eye but, somewhat surprisingly, is much less reliable elsewhere. Indeed there is some suggestion that its use away from the head induces a more aggressive growth of the tumour mass. There is no apparent effect on lesions away from the injected ones – each lesion requires its own injection, making it tedious and expensive.

Method

Several different methods have been advocated and the chosen one will reflect the material used and the type of lesion being treated. In most protocols it is usually necessary to use up to 4–6 injections, although there are reports of single or two injections giving rapid, total resolution.[33,34] Although it has been suggested that the effect is dose related (larger tumours need more material), the proper placement of the reconstituted proteins seems equally important.

- Lesions may be injected with reconstituted BCG vaccine or purified cell wall extracts at 7–10 day intervals.
- The protocol used by Liverpool University employs intralesional injection of the reconstituted freeze-dried, live BCG organisms at intervals of 7, 14, 21, 28, 35, 42 days. Thus the second injection is administered 1 week after the first. The third injection is given after a further 2 weeks and the fourth after a further 3 weeks and so on. This protocol is described fully in **Table 4.4.**

Responses observed

- Local swellings are common.
- Repeated injections result in either exaggerated responses with further swelling or progressive shrinkage of the mass.
- Some nodular and fibroblastic sarcoids react by abscessation and discharge of purulent material.
- Anaphylaxis has been reported following repeated use of attenuated live BCG in particular. The first two injections are probably safe (provided that the method has not been used previously on this or another lesion) but thereafter appropriate precautions should be taken. This danger may be minimized either by using BCG cell wall vaccine preparations and/or premedicating with corticosteroids (e.g. dexamethasone at 0.2–0.3 mg/kg intravenously) and flunixin meglumine (at 1.1 mg/kg intravenously) at least 30 minutes before the injection is given. Antihistamines, such as tripelennamine hydrochloride (at 1 mg/kg intramuscularly), have also been used to premedicate horses prior to BCG injection. The value of the antihistamines is doubtful. True intralesional injection apparently also helps considerably.

Table 4.4 University of Liverpool protocol for periocular, nodular (and some fibroblastic) sarcoids (the method is not used for other types of sarcoid or for other neoplastic disorders)

1. Evaluate the history, size and type of tumour to be treated.

If there has been no previous exposure to this method of treatment, the patient is premedicated with corticosteroids from the third injection (e.g. dexamethasone at 0.25 mg/kg) and flunixin (at 1.1 mg/kg). An alternative method should be considered if there is a history of use of the same method, or the horse should be premedicated from the first injection. Antihistamines are of dubious value and are not used routinely. The attending veterinarian should remain with the horse for 2 hours after the injection with adrenaline at the ready!

2. Sedate and restrain the horse.
3. Perform careful surgical preparation of the site of injection.
4. Dilute one ampoule of lyophilized BCG viable bacillus[a] into an appropriate volume of water (for small tumours < 0.5 cm diameter the contents are diluted in 0.5 ml of water; for larger tumours one ampoule can be reconstituted with 1–1.5 ml) and inject intralesionally.[b] Use 1 ml tuberculin-type syringe and 24–26G needle of an appropriate length.
5. Repeat injection after 7 days (second dose after 1 week).
6. Repeat injection after 14 further days (third dose after a further 2 weeks).
7. Repeat injection after 21 further days (fourth dose given after a further 3 weeks).
8. Repeat injection after 28 further days (fifth dose after further 4 weeks), etc.
9. Up to nine injections may be required. Dosing should not stop until a suitable response is evident.

Note

- Significant reactions can develop after 3–5 injections and this should stop the treatment protocol. Localized abscessation can develop and can be alarming with a persistent discharging sinus developing for over 12 months. Total surgical excision of the abscess may be the only reliable treatment to resolve this problem. In other cases the tumour gradually shrinks with the full effect taking up to 12 months. BCG treatment of sarcoids results in a very acceptable cosmetic effect and is safe for both operator and patient. It has much to commend it but there is a significant number of failures.
- Best results are obtained in nodular sarcoids in and around the eyelids. There is no detectable effect on untreated sarcoids on a horse on which one or more individual lesions are treated with BCG.

[a] Evans Ltd, UK.

[b] It is imperative that the entire contents is injected *intralesionally*. Subcutaneous injection in the vicinity of a sarcoid is to be avoided as far as possible as there is a risk of anaphylaxis.

Advantages

- Convenient/simple and little equipment required
- Cheap (for single or few lesions)
- Can be administered to standing, sedated horse
- Effective in over 80% of palpebral nodular sarcoids

Disadvantages

- Risk of anaphylaxis[35]
- Repeated injections required
- Volume/mass-dependent (larger lesions need more material)
- No effect on lesions remote from the injected one, i.e. every lesion requires specific injection
- Must be injected intralesionally
- Limited efficacy range (not effective for squamous cell carcinoma or melanoma); little effect on sarcoids of verrucose or occult types or tumours of all types away from the periorbital region

General notes on treatment using immune methods

- Autogenous vaccines are strictly limited to the 'viral wart' or papilloma. Most of these cases will resolve spontaneously in around 8 weeks, whereas it takes about 2 months with the vaccines!
- Use of autogenous vaccines for ocular (or any other) neoplastic lesion is entirely illogical – if it were as simple as this there would be no

neoplasia! Furthermore, the use of autogenous vaccines in sarcoid therapy may be positively dangerous – it is contraindicated and should never be used.

- Freshly prepared injections of BCG must be made for each administration and the dose must be related to the size and type of tumour.
- Squamous cell carcinoma in horses is less responsive to BCG in all its forms than in cattle.
- *Corynebacterium parvum* can also be used effectively but is less predictable and is less available.

DERMATOLOGICAL RADIOTHERAPY

Ionizing radiation destroys living cells and this property is employed to treat certain types of cutaneous (and other) neoplasia. The application to cutaneous oncology is important in providing a therapeutic option for tumours which might otherwise have no chance of resolution. The techniques have significant advantages in minimizing scarring and distortion due to cicatrization in anatomical regions where normal function is of vital importance. Skin tumours involving the eyelids and periorbital skin are probably the most frequently subjected to radiation therapy but masses at other sites may also be important.

The basic principle of the technique arises because electromagnetic radiation (γ radiation) and high-energy particles (α, β radiation) ionize tissues through which they are directed.

Following a course/dose of radiation the tissues are destroyed (after a variable period) and then a process of repair needs to take place. Normal reparative tissue develops from natural stem cells to replace the destroyed tissue. It then needs to become reorganized into a natural and therefore functional organ system with restoration of blood supply and oxygenation. This process is largely similar to normal wound repair mechanisms but the slower response typical of radiation damage means that there is a greater tendency for natural tissue cells to replace the damaged cells rather than for fibrous tissue scarring. Therefore the extent of scarring is usually much less and the cosmetic results are usually very acceptable. Some cells are, however, permanently altered by the radiation rather than killed by it. This might reflect the relative resistance of the cell type or the reduced radiation dose to which it is subjected. In the skin, melanocytes along the margins of a lesion treated with radiation will often be suppressed or altered so that white skin (leukoderma) and hair (leukotrichia) may replace the normal body colour.

The procedure carries both cost and safety implications (no matter how it is applied) and therefore the technique is usually restricted to small tumours in difficult sites such as the eye and periorbital skin and over joints. There is the added advantage that radiation can be used as 'fail-safe' technique. Tumours previously treated with less-expensive techniques which have not succeeded may still be treated by this method with good prospects of success (within the inherent limitations of the method). Accurate dosimetry and careful use results in a better overall prognosis than with most other methods. It can be combined with surgical debulking (as in the treatment of corneal carcinoma *in situ*) so that less radiation needs to be applied. The full effects of radiation treatment may take several months to become apparent. Tumours treated in this way often show a progressive size reduction for up to 12 months, but in other cases considerable local necrosis occurs and abscess discharge may initially be alarming.

Radiation is delivered by brachytherapy or teletherapy, which reflect the method of generation of the radiation. There are only a few reports of the use of teletherapy for treatment of equine dermatological problems.[36]

Brachytherapy Brachytherapy is most often used in the treatment of squamous cell carcinoma, neurofibroma and nodular and fibroblastic sarcoids and other superficial tumours situated in areas which are not amenable to surgery or which have recurred after previous attempts to remove them (by whatever means). The most frequent methods for this include a number of sources of β and γ radiation which are either implanted into the tumour mass[37] or are applied directly to the surface.[38] Iridium-192 (**Fig. 4.3**) and gold-198 (**Fig. 4.4**) are γ emitters with radiation continuously emitted from the source through the target tissue. The dose of radiation can be adjusted by altering the strength of the source, the time of contact or its physical extent. For surface applications, β radiation is delivered from a strontium-90 (or similar isotope) plaque (**Fig. 4.5**). Radiation is applied in fractionated doses calculated to deliver the required 'lethal' overall dose over several days. The source is usually applied for a precalculated time once or twice daily so that the required dose is administered over a considerable period. Fractionation is more important for β radiation than for γ radiation.

The beneficial effects of radiation can be

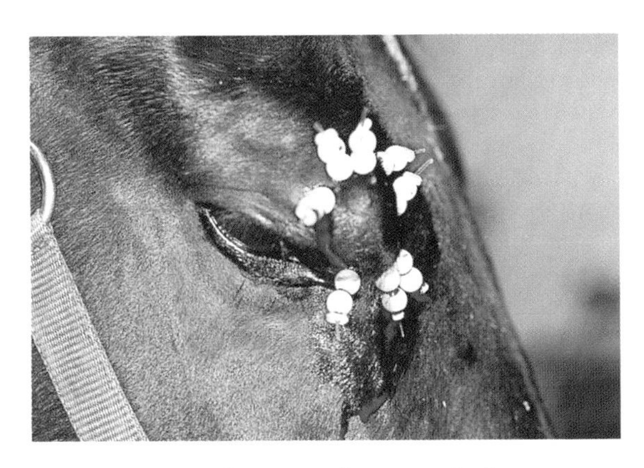

Figure 4.3 Iridium-192 linear radiation sources inserted into periocular sarcoids.

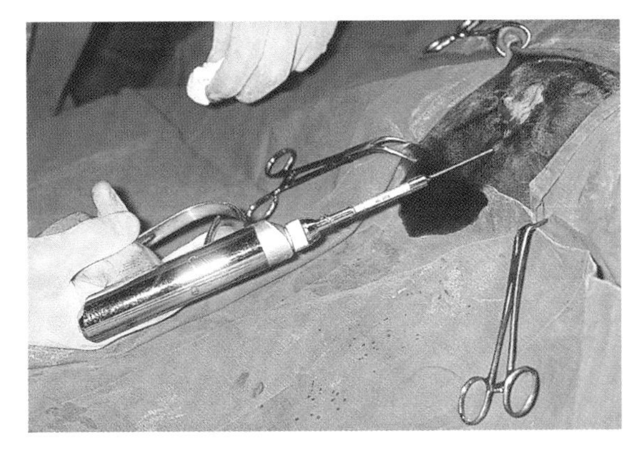

Figure 4.4 A Marston Gun being used to insert radiogold (gold-198) pellets into an anaesthetized horse to treat a palpebral squamous cell carcinoma.

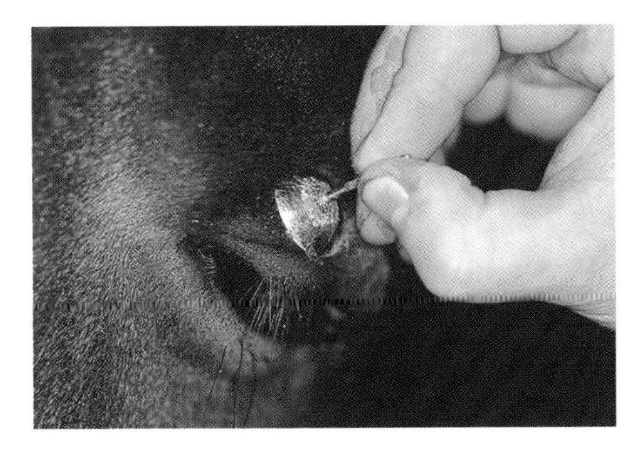

Figure 4.5 A strontium-90 plaque being applied directly to the surface of a small fibroblastic sarcoid in the upper eyelid of a 5-year-old mare.

startling, with complete resolution, and although its use has severe restrictions it is a useful fall-back where other methods fail (**Fig. 4.6a, b**).

Teletherapy A linear accelerator is used to generate radiation of specific types and power which is then beamed into the treatment area. The animal needs to be completely still and so cases subjected to this require general anaesthesia. Fractionation and multibeam technology means that deep tumours can be treated. However, it is such a specialized technique that it is very rarely available, practical or applicable.

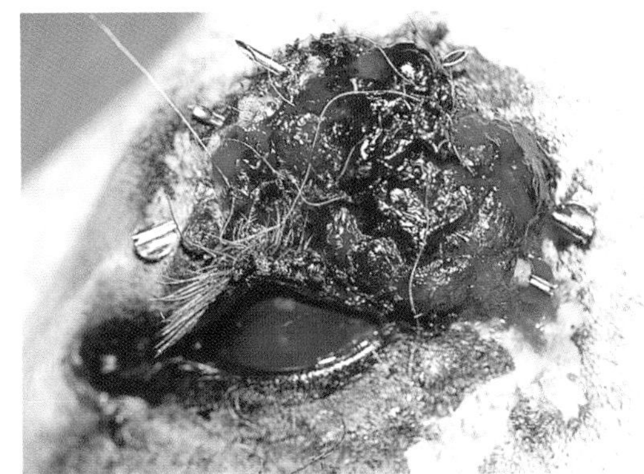

a

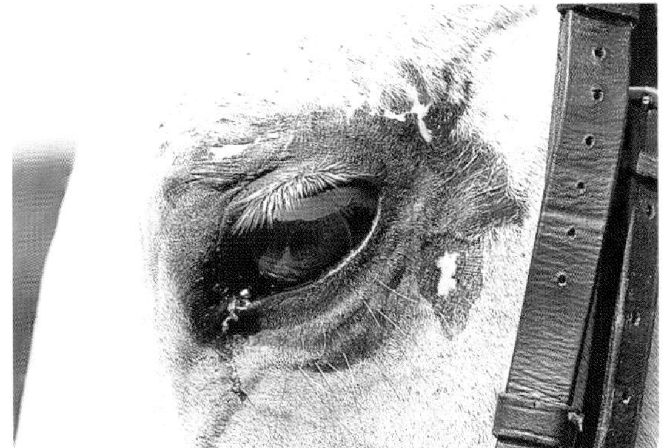

b

Figure 4.6 An aggressive fibroblastic sarcoid in the periorbital skin had been treated several times with a combination of surgery, BCG and cryosurgery without resolution. The introducers used to guide the linear iridium-192 sources are shown in (a) while the final appearance of the lesion some 12 months later is shown in (b). Note the loss of hair and the limited white-skinned area above the upper eyelid which are typical of radiation therapy. In spite of the severity of the lesion, the functional and cosmetic effects are excellent.

Advantages

- Little disfigurement and scarring.
- High primary success rate.
- Effective back-up option for other methods.
- Placement of iridium-192 wire brachytherapy can be easily achieved under sedation alone especially using after-loading techniques (this limits personal exposure).
- Strontium-90 is very safe when properly used and fractionated doses can be administered under sedation alone.
- Debulking leads to residual activity of dividing tumour cells, which are most susceptible to radiation, and to smaller treatment areas.

Disadvantages

- There is serious or potentially catastrophic personal danger to operator and staff.
- Specialist radiologist or radiophysicist is required.
- Accurate dosimetry requires detailed calculations.
- Special secure area for hospitalized horses is required.
- Cost of isotopes is very high.
- Surgical debulking may be needed to limit the radiation dose.
- Limited size/volume of tissue can be treated at a time.
- General anaesthesia is often required for placement (particularly for gold-198 seeds).
- Some extensive reactions possible with tissue necrosis – may take a long time to resolve.
- Resultant leukoderma and leukotrichia (white scars).

Hazards and effects of radiation therapy

The toxicity and hazards of radiation therapy can be divided into the acute or immediate effects and the chronic (long-standing) or permanent effects which are usually (hopefully) restricted to the treated case (rather than the operator). In the former, the skin surrounding the radiated tissue becomes inflamed (swelling, heat, pain and redness). The fastest-dividing cells in the area show the earliest effects with superficial sloughing. In the case of the eye there may be a degree of transient corneal oedema over the treated area of cornea. In the treatment of dermatological tumours the acute reactions are of little consequence but may alarm a poorly counselled owner.

Chronic effects of radiation are more obvious and remain in the long term. They may have significant implications for operators who are repeatedly exposed to radiation of any description. These changes affect slowly dividing cells, e.g. bone, cartilage and the lens. Thus damage to the lens culminating in the development of cataract can be a secondary consequence of γ radiation in and around the eye. Radiation has significant effects on melanocytes and hair follicle germ cells, leaving white skin and hair to replace the body colour (see Fig. 16.4). Only in very rare cases is there any apparent long-term effect on local cell repair and restoration of function is to be expected in almost all cases (unless the radiation dose is excessive) (see Fig. 4.6).

Systemic effects of a single course of radiation brachytherapy applied in the treatment of a skin neoplasm in the horse are seldom noticeable. There are no reports of any serious secondary effects even when repeated courses are applied, although this is a particularly unusual circumstance.

- Repeated exposure to ionizing radiation has potentially disastrous consequences for operators including the development of internal malignant neoplasia. **Any** cell can be transformed into a cancer by sufficient or inappropriate exposure to radiation.
- Unless specific reasons exist and suitable precautions can be taken, other means of treatment should be explored.
- Radiation is a dangerous 'last-ditch' resort even though it has very satisfying results for the most part! Its use **must** be very carefully considered in every case.

PART II

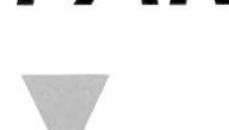

SYNDROMES IN EQUINE DERMATOLOGY

chapter 5

SYNDROMES IN EQUINE DERMATOLOGY

Pruritus (the itchy horse)	66
Alterations in hair quality and quantity (hair follicle disorders and alopecia)	68
Nodules	72
Scaling and crusting (dry dermatoses) syndrome	76
Weeping and seeping (wet dermatoses)	78
Alteration in pigmentation	80
Pastern dermatitis syndrome	82
Foot syndromes	84

PRURITUS (THE ITCHY HORSE)

Pruritus is the most common clinical sign of skin disease and is defined as 'itching'. 'It is a particular feature of allergic inflammation and parasitic infestations. Pruritus is entirely epidermal in origin and is most intense at mucocutaneous junctions.'[39] It may be a primary skin disease, usually related to insect bites, or more rarely in the horse it may be a manifestation of a systemic disease. It can also arise from hypersensitivity reactions of immediate or delayed responses. It may be related to immune-mediated diseases such as pemphigus foliaceus or to a wide variety of bacterial, fungal or parasitic diseases. It may also be due to direct irritation by chemicals or to photoactivated dermatoses.

Pruritus is not commonly associated with deep ulceration of the skin. However, ulcers may be painful and may induce self-inflicted trauma suggestive of pruritus. Pruritus can be self-perpetuating and triggered by a relatively minor episode of intense itchiness. This can be followed by rubbing, biting and self-mutilation which, in turn, causes further local inflammation and irritation. The instigating factor may not therefore be present at the time of the examination.

Pruritus arises as a result of either physical skin irritation (such as occurs with ectoparasitic infestation, e.g. *Damalinia* spp. lice) or superficial skin irritation (such as occurs with mange mites, e.g. *Chorioptes* spp./*Sarcoptes* spp.), or as result of an inflammatory response. The causes of an inflammatory response may be local or generalized, and in the former the responses can be local (restricted to the direct vicinity of the inciting cause) or can have a more widespread clinical effect. Thus an animal with a louse infestation may have no skin inflammation but severe pruritus can arise from the irritating effects of the movement of the parasites in the hair coat. Horses with chorioptic mange also itch and stamp (cardinal signs of pruritus in the horse) because of the irritation effects of parasite movement, but in this case the movement is much closer to the skin itself and the extent of movement of an individual parasite can be much more limited. Burrowing mites such as the sarcoptic mange mites have a dermal irritation effect and, while they do cause local inflammation, their movement is also responsible for the clinical responses. A single insect bite or sting may cause a prominent local inflammatory response but not all such responses are liable to induce pruritus (as opposed to pain). Even a small amount of venom may cause a serious systemic release of inflammatory mediators with systemic as well as (or without) dermatological signs including urticaria and possibly generalized pruritus. In the horse this response is somewhat less prominent than in other species. Urticaria and hypersensitivity reactions only rarely cause pruritus. However, *Culicoides* spp. hypersensitivity is probably the commonest single pruritic disease. Horses suffering from even a single (or few) bites show an extreme response in which pruritus is very significant. The response to masses of bites from the same insects in a non-sensitive horse can be very similar but is usually more transient and more restricted anatomically to the preferred regions of insect activity.

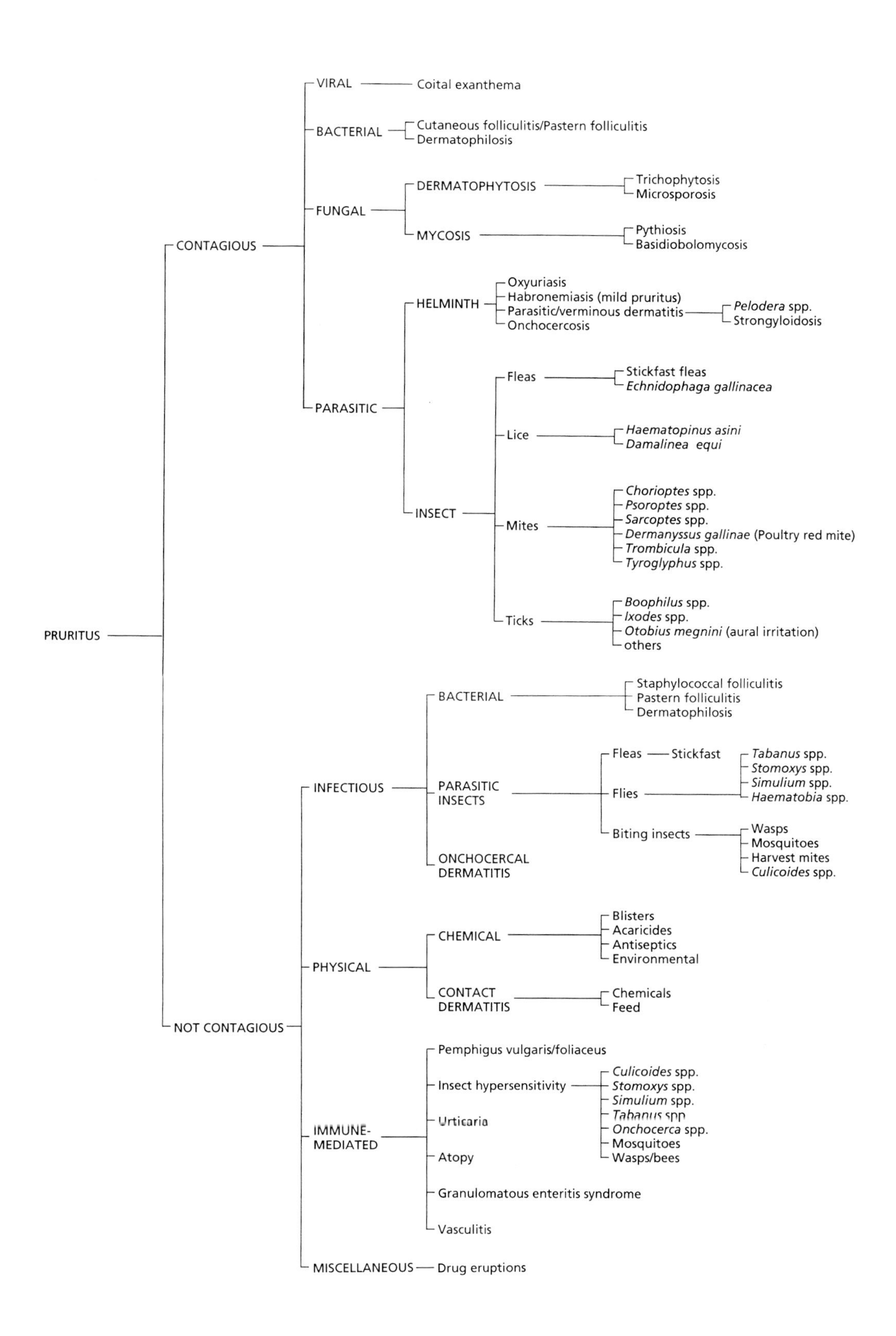
PRURITUS
CONTAGIOUS
VIRAL
Coital exanthema
BACTERIAL
Cutaneous folliculitis/Pastern folliculitis
Dermatophilosis
FUNGAL
DERMATOPHYTOSIS
Trichophytosis
Microsporosis
MYCOSIS
Pythiosis
Basidiobolomycosis
PARASITIC
HELMINTH
Oxyuriasis
Habronemiasis (mild pruritus)
Parasitic/verminous dermatitis
Onchocercosis
Pelodera spp.
Strongyloidosis
INSECT
Fleas
Stickfast fleas
Echnidophaga gallinacea
Lice
Haematopinus asini
Damalinea equi
Mites
Chorioptes spp.
Psoroptes spp.
Sarcoptes spp.
Dermanyssus gallinae (Poultry red mite)
Trombicula spp.
Tyroglyphus spp.
Ticks
Boophilus spp.
Ixodes spp.
Otobius megnini (aural irritation)
others
NOT CONTAGIOUS
INFECTIOUS
BACTERIAL
Staphylococcal folliculitis
Pastern folliculitis
Dermatophilosis
PARASITIC INSECTS
Fleas
Stickfast
Flies
Tabanus spp.
Stomoxys spp.
Simulium spp.
Haematobia spp.
Biting insects
Wasps
Mosquitoes
Harvest mites
Culicoides spp.
ONCHOCERCAL DERMATITIS
PHYSICAL
CHEMICAL
Blisters
Acaricides
Antiseptics
Environmental
CONTACT DERMATITIS
Chemicals
Feed
IMMUNE-MEDIATED
Pemphigus vulgaris/foliaceus
Insect hypersensitivity
Culicoides spp.
Stomoxys spp.
Simulium spp.
Tabanus spp.
Onchocerca spp.
Mosquitoes
Wasps/bees
Urticaria
Atopy
Granulomatous enteritis syndrome
Vasculitis
MISCELLANEOUS
Drug eruptions

ALTERATIONS IN HAIR QUALITY AND QUANTITY (HAIR FOLLICLE DISORDERS AND ALOPECIA)

Alopecia can arise from a variety of primary and secondary diseases and is defined as a 'deficiency of the hair coat'. It may be due to hair growth failure or to loss of hair. There is a significant difference between hair loss involving fracture of the shaft (stumps of hair fibres remain) and hair which is shed from the follicle, i.e. when the whole hair is shed.

Loss of hair without any other accompanying clinical signs such as pruritus, scaling, crusting, erosion or ulceration occurs in relatively few conditions. However, as these other clinical signs very frequently occur with loss of hair, they should always be considered as part of the hair loss syndrome.

For all practical purposes the only disease which is characterized by hirsutism (overgrowth of hair) is pituitary adenoma (equine Cushing's disease).

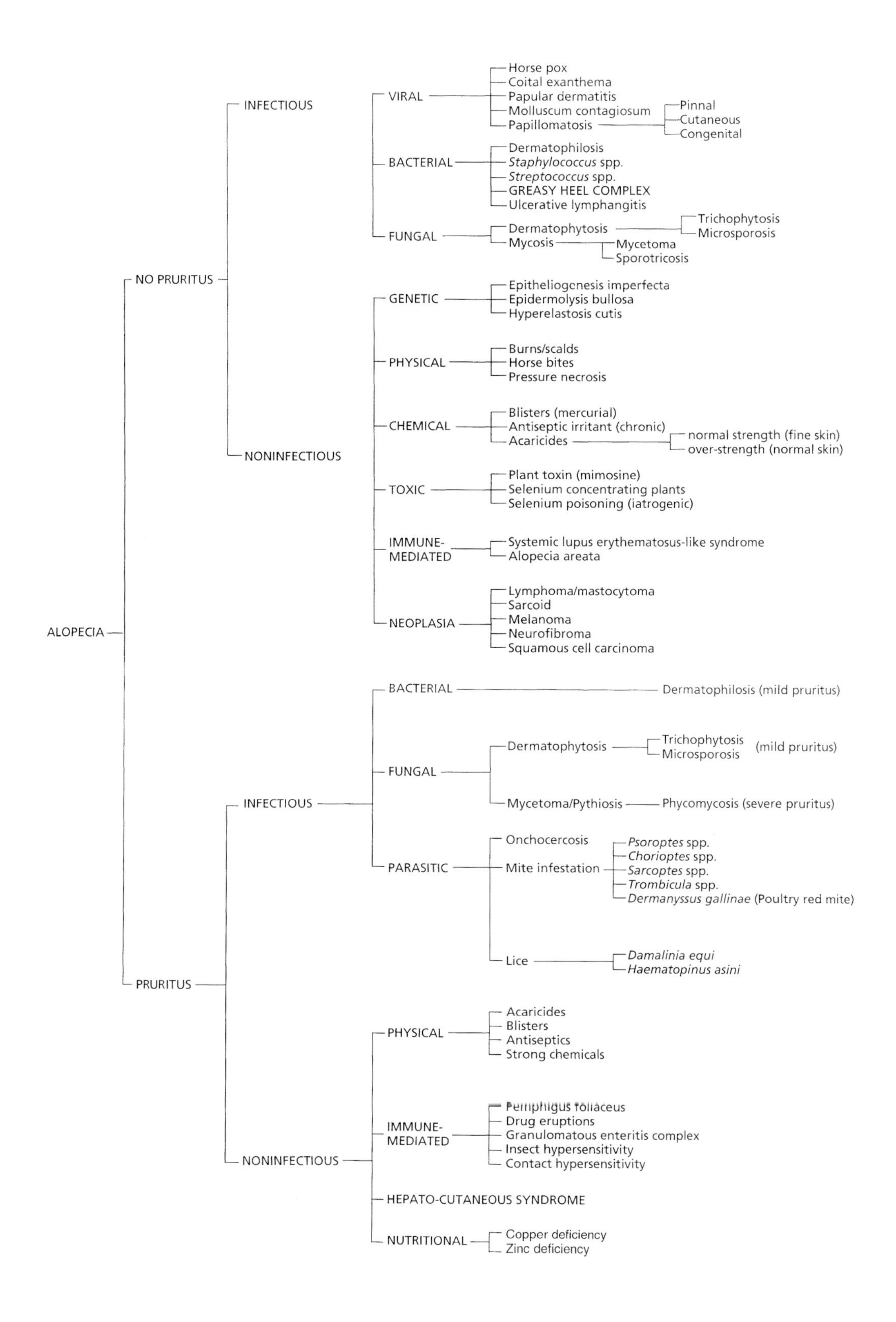
ALOPECIA
NO PRURITUS
INFECTIOUS
VIRAL
Horse pox
Coital exanthema
Papular dermatitis
Molluscum contagiosum
Papillomatosis
Pinnal
Cutaneous
Congenital
BACTERIAL
Dermatophilosis
Staphylococcus spp.
Streptococcus spp.
GREASY HEEL COMPLEX
Ulcerative lymphangitis
FUNGAL
Dermatophytosis
Trichophytosis
Microsporosis
Mycosis
Mycetoma
Sporotricosis
NONINFECTIOUS
GENETIC
Epitheliogenesis imperfecta
Epidermolysis bullosa
Hyperelastosis cutis
PHYSICAL
Burns/scalds
Horse bites
Pressure necrosis
CHEMICAL
Blisters (mercurial)
Antiseptic irritant (chronic)
Acaricides
normal strength (fine skin)
over-strength (normal skin)
TOXIC
Plant toxin (mimosine)
Selenium concentrating plants
Selenium poisoning (iatrogenic)
IMMUNE-MEDIATED
Systemic lupus erythematosus-like syndrome
Alopecia areata
NEOPLASIA
Lymphoma/mastocytoma
Sarcoid
Melanoma
Neurofibroma
Squamous cell carcinoma
PRURITUS
INFECTIOUS
BACTERIAL
Dermatophilosis (mild pruritus)
FUNGAL
Dermatophytosis
Trichophytosis
Microsporosis
(mild pruritus)
Mycetoma/Pythiosis
Phycomycosis (severe pruritus)
PARASITIC
Onchocercosis
Mite infestation
Psoroptes spp.
Chorioptes spp.
Sarcoptes spp.
Trombicula spp.
Dermanyssus gallinae (Poultry red mite)
Lice
Damalinia equi
Haematopinus asini
NONINFECTIOUS
PHYSICAL
Acaricides
Blisters
Antiseptics
Strong chemicals
IMMUNE-MEDIATED
Pemphigus foliaceus
Drug eruptions
Granulomatous enteritis complex
Insect hypersensitivity
Contact hypersensitivity
HEPATO-CUTANEOUS SYNDROME
NUTRITIONAL
Copper deficiency
Zinc deficiency

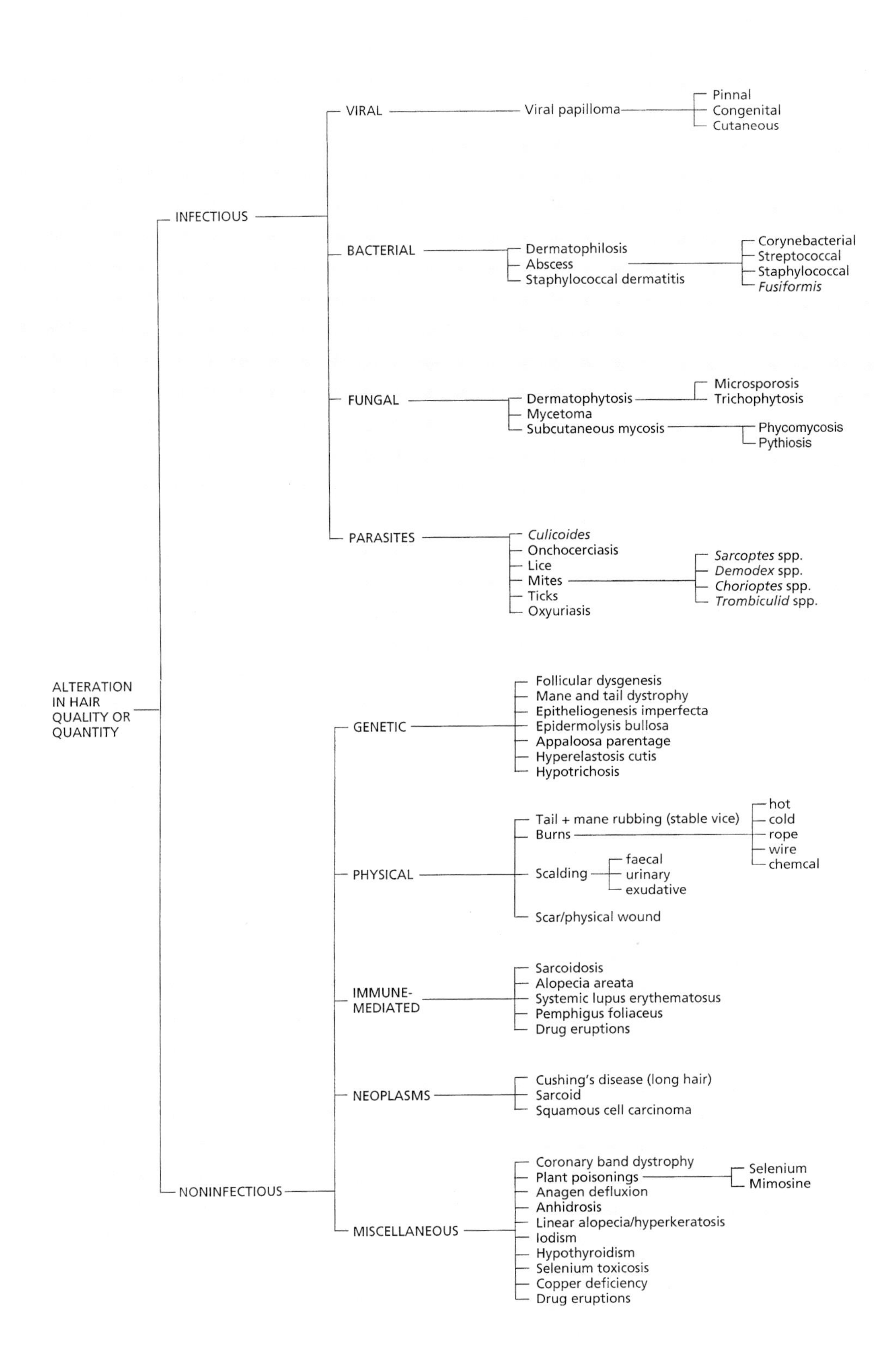
ALTERATION IN HAIR QUALITY OR QUANTITY
INFECTIOUS
VIRAL
Viral papilloma
Pinnal
Congenital
Cutaneous
BACTERIAL
Dermatophilosis
Abscess
Staphylococcal dermatitis
Corynebacterial
Streptococcal
Staphylococcal
Fusiformis
FUNGAL
Dermatophytosis
Mycetoma
Subcutaneous mycosis
Microsporosis
Trichophytosis
Phycomycosis
Pythiosis
PARASITES
Culicoides
Onchocerciasis
Lice
Mites
Ticks
Oxyuriasis
Sarcoptes spp.
Demodex spp.
Chorioptes spp.
Trombiculid spp.
NONINFECTIOUS
GENETIC
Follicular dysgenesis
Mane and tail dystrophy
Epitheliogenesis imperfecta
Epidermolysis bullosa
Appaloosa parentage
Hyperelastosis cutis
Hypotrichosis
PHYSICAL
Tail + mane rubbing (stable vice)
Burns
hot
cold
rope
wire
chemcal
Scalding
faecal
urinary
exudative
Scar/physical wound
IMMUNE-MEDIATED
Sarcoidosis
Alopecia areata
Systemic lupus erythematosus
Pemphigus foliaceus
Drug eruptions
NEOPLASMS
Cushing's disease (long hair)
Sarcoid
Squamous cell carcinoma
MISCELLANEOUS
Coronary band dystrophy
Plant poisonings
Selenium
Mimosine
Anagen defluxion
Anhidrosis
Linear alopecia/hyperkeratosis
Iodism
Hypothyroidism
Selenium toxicosis
Copper deficiency
Drug eruptions

PART II
SYNDROMES IN EQUINE DERMATOLOGY

NODULES

One or more solid skin swellings greater than 1 cm diameter, which exceeds the dimensions of a papule, are included in the category of nodular skin disease. Nodules are usually elevated above the skin surface but may be dermal or subcutaneous. They may be produced by hyperplasia of the epidermal or dermal tissues, amyloid or lipid deposition, inflammation or neoplastic proliferation. Some may originate as macules or papules but progressively increase in size, either singly or in numbers, and are then justifiably included in this category. Single or multiple nodules are commonly presented in equine practice and so their differentiation is important.

Tumours, nodules and swellings tend to be primary diseases in horses and are only rarely manifestations of systemic disorders. The major disease considerations in establishing a differential diagnosis are:

- Infectious diseases
- Hypersensitivity reactions
- Sterile inflammatory diseases
- Neoplasia

Nodules can be subdivided broadly into:

- inflammatory nodules
- noninflammatory swellings
- neoplastic lesions

Inflammatory nodules

Inflammation may be due to injury or infection and the inflammatory infiltrate will reflect the different aetiologies. The response will consequently vary from blood and tissue fluid to patent inflammatory exudate containing inflammatory cells. Visible nodules can then develop as the infiltrating cells attempt to wall off the injury or the infective process. As the lesion enlarges, the dermis and subcutis become completely infiltrated by cells and the overlying epidermis becomes atrophic. This leads to erosion, ulceration and possible exudation. These inflammatory nodules include urticarial wheals and abscesses.

Abscesses are localized lesions with a fluid content of variable consistency. They are the result of inflammatory changes, usually related to trauma and/or infection and consist of dead cells, debris and liquefied local tissue components arising through proteolytic and histolytic enzymes. While most abscesses are related to infection, they can also be sterile.

Noninflammatory swellings

Body swellings such as hernias and cysts can also fall into the nodular category, although strictly they do not meet the criteria fully.

Neoplastic nodules

Most neoplasms of the skin and subcutaneous tissue initially appear as nodules. Enlargement and secondary inflammatory changes impart the typical tumour appearance of an obvious enlarged nodule. The overlying dermis and epidermis may undergo significant changes including verrucous and ulcerative changes and necrosis. Thus the overlying surface may be normal, altered or ulcerated.

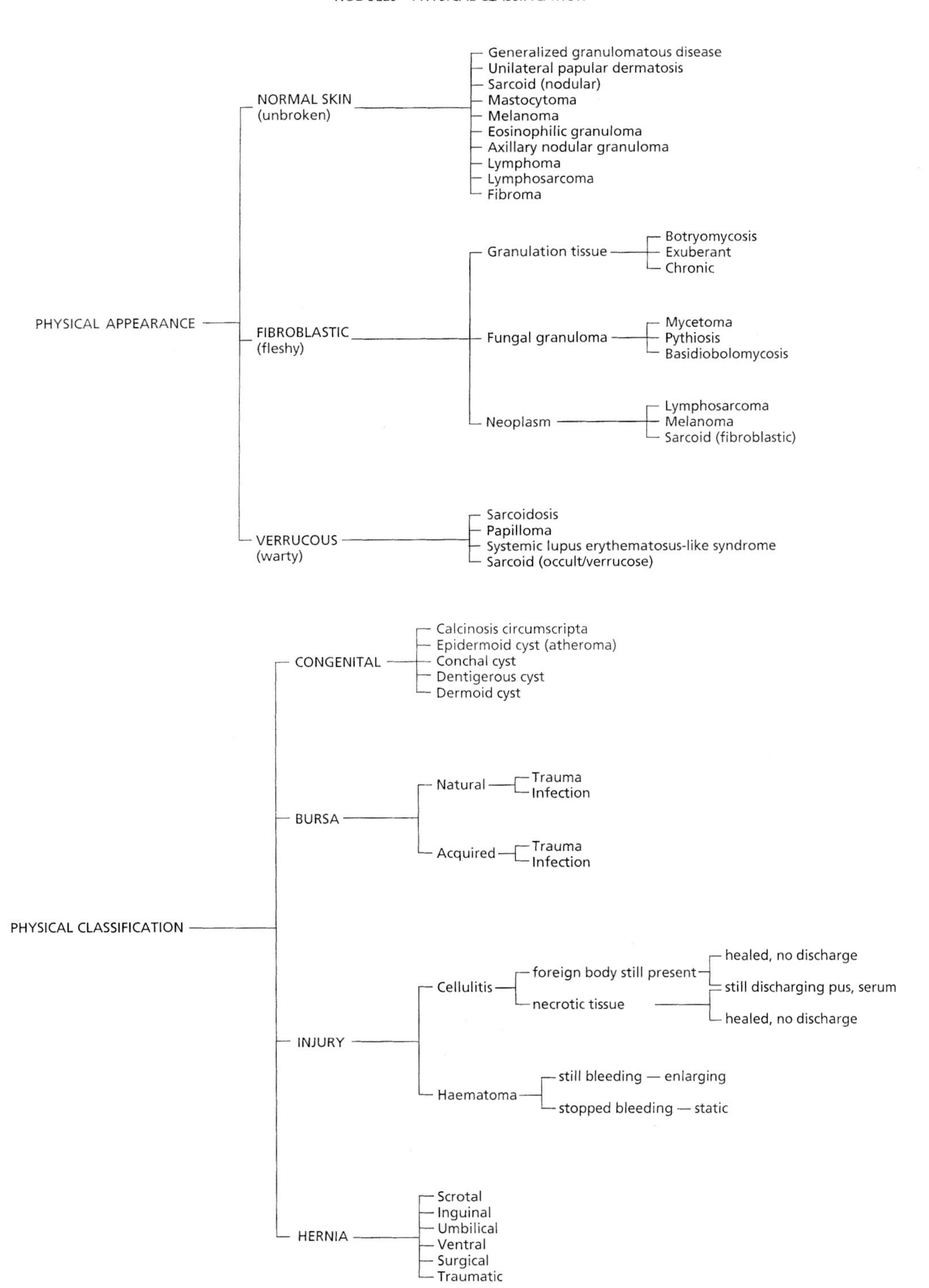
NODULES – PHYSICAL CLASSIFICATION
PHYSICAL APPEARANCE
NORMAL SKIN
(unbroken)
Generalized granulomatous disease
Unilateral papular dermatosis
Sarcoid (nodular)
Mastocytoma
Melanoma
Eosinophilic granuloma
Axillary nodular granuloma
Lymphoma
Lymphosarcoma
Fibroma
FIBROBLASTIC
(fleshy)
Granulation tissue
Botryomycosis
Exuberant
Chronic
Fungal granuloma
Mycetoma
Pythiosis
Basidiobolomycosis
Neoplasm
Lymphosarcoma
Melanoma
Sarcoid (fibroblastic)
VERRUCOUS
(warty)
Sarcoidosis
Papilloma
Systemic lupus erythematosus-like syndrome
Sarcoid (occult/verrucose)
PHYSICAL CLASSIFICATION
CONGENITAL
Calcinosis circumscripta
Epidermoid cyst (atheroma)
Conchal cyst
Dentigerous cyst
Dermoid cyst
BURSA
Natural
Trauma
Infection
Acquired
Trauma
Infection
INJURY
Cellulitis
foreign body still present
necrotic tissue
healed, no discharge
still discharging pus, serum
healed, no discharge
Haematoma
still bleeding — enlarging
stopped bleeding — static
HERNIA
Scrotal
Inguinal
Umbilical
Ventral
Surgical
Traumatic

NODULES – CLINICAL CLASSIFICATION

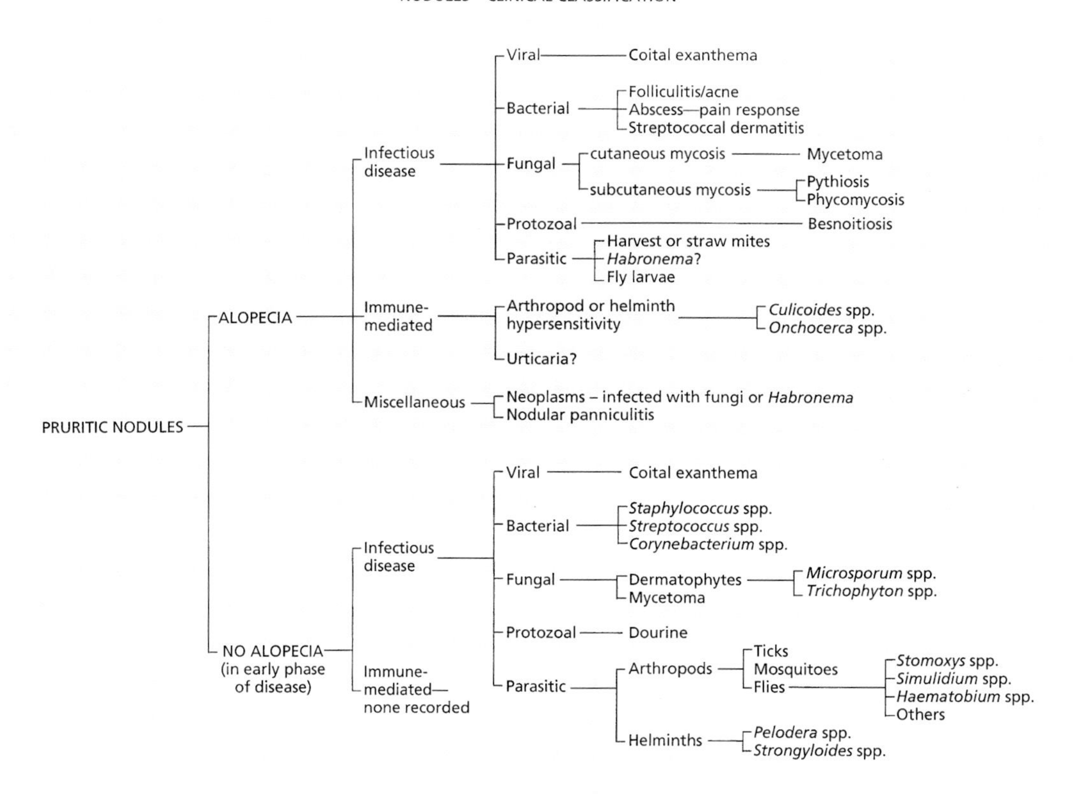

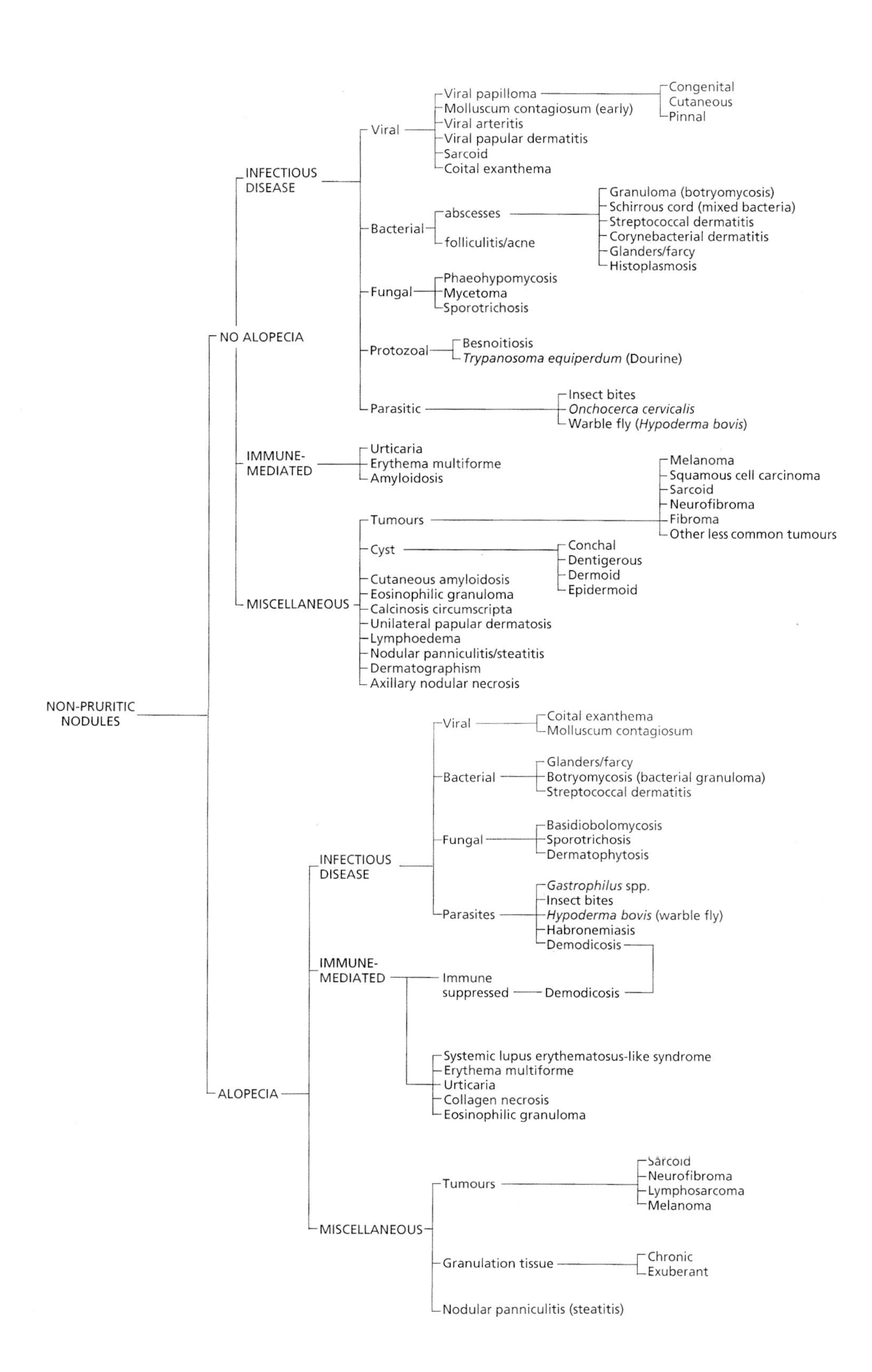

NON-PRURITIC NODULES
NO ALOPECIA
INFECTIOUS DISEASE
Viral
Viral papilloma
Congenital
Cutaneous
Pinnal
Molluscum contagiosum (early)
Viral arteritis
Viral papular dermatitis
Sarcoid
Coital exanthema
Bacterial
abscesses
folliculitis/acne
Granuloma (botryomycosis)
Schirrous cord (mixed bacteria)
Streptococcal dermatitis
Corynebacterial dermatitis
Glanders/farcy
Histoplasmosis
Fungal
Phaeohypomycosis
Mycetoma
Sporotrichosis
Protozoal
Besnoitiosis
Trypanosoma equiperdum (Dourine)
Parasitic
Insect bites
Onchocerca cervicalis
Warble fly (Hypoderma bovis)
IMMUNE-MEDIATED
Urticaria
Erythema multiforme
Amyloidosis
MISCELLANEOUS
Tumours
Melanoma
Squamous cell carcinoma
Sarcoid
Neurofibroma
Fibroma
Other less common tumours
Cyst
Conchal
Dentigerous
Dermoid
Epidermoid
Cutaneous amyloidosis
Eosinophilic granuloma
Calcinosis circumscripta
Unilateral papular dermatosis
Lymphoedema
Nodular panniculitis/steatitis
Dermatographism
Axillary nodular necrosis
ALOPECIA
INFECTIOUS DISEASE
Viral
Coital exanthema
Molluscum contagiosum
Bacterial
Glanders/farcy
Botryomycosis (bacterial granuloma)
Streptococcal dermatitis
Fungal
Basidiobolomycosis
Sporotrichosis
Dermatophytosis
Parasites
Gastrophilus spp.
Insect bites
Hypoderma bovis (warble fly)
Habronemiasis
Demodicosis
IMMUNE-MEDIATED
Immune suppressed
Demodicosis
Systemic lupus erythematosus-like syndrome
Erythema multiforme
Urticaria
Collagen necrosis
Eosinophilic granuloma
MISCELLANEOUS
Tumours
Sarcoid
Neurofibroma
Lymphosarcoma
Melanoma
Granulation tissue
Chronic
Exuberant
Nodular panniculitis (steatitis)

SCALING AND CRUSTING (DRY DERMATOSES) SYNDROME

Scaling and crusting is a common end result of skin disease of many types and aetiologies. Scale is the result of desquamated keratinocyte cells and debris from hair shafts. Any disease which induces an excessive sloughing or an excessive production of epithelial cells is characterized by scaling. For example, seborrhoeic conditions produce significant scale because of the higher rate of keratinocyte production. Scale varies in appearance from fine, almost invisible particles to extensive large, flat scales. The consistency also varies depending upon the amount of sebum included with the scale and so can be greasy in texture or very dry and dusty. The colour of the scales varies from yellow-brown to grey-white. Epidermal collarettes are not well recognized in horses but represent a circular accumulation of scale around a central focus. It usually reflects the presence of a vesicle, bulla or pustule in the superficial layers of the skin. However, many equine skin diseases have transient vesicles or other superficial dermal inflammation which result in scale formation and so scaling is a finding common to many diseases. Scaling should be differentiated from the accumulation of dust and other environmental particles such as from hay and bedding. Microscopic examination is not always conclusive.

Crusting reflects dried exudate on the surface of the skin. It will therefore vary with the character of the underlying exudate. Blood-stained exudate results in a brown or dark red crusting, while serum/plasma exudation produces yellow or pale crusts. Crusts have a tendency to aggregate around hair shafts and so can be difficult to remove. Furthermore, attempts to remove them may be painful and resented both from the underlying condition or the removal of intact growing hairs. Gross accumulations of crusts are called vegetations.

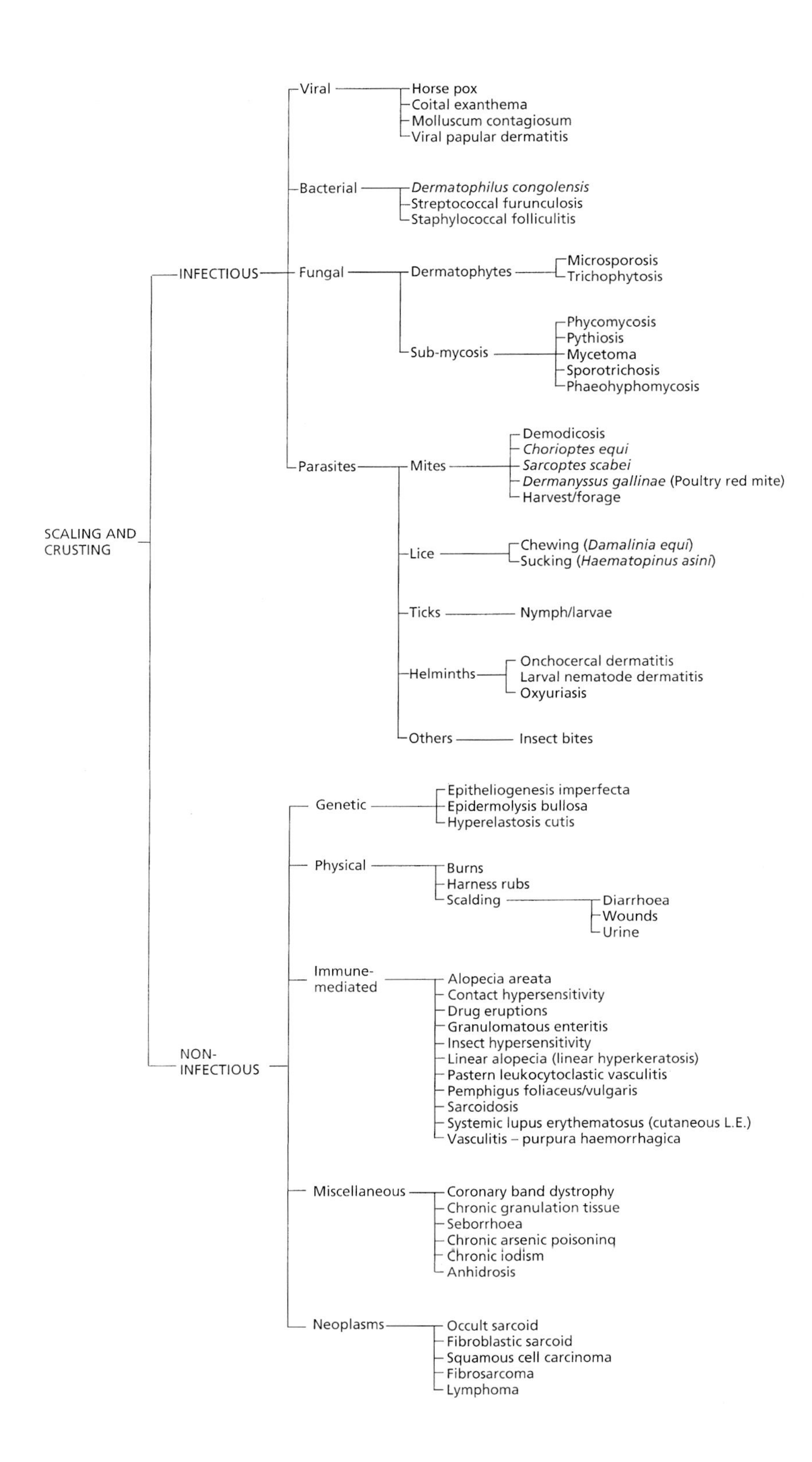
SCALING AND CRUSTING
INFECTIOUS
Viral
Horse pox
Coital exanthema
Molluscum contagiosum
Viral papular dermatitis
Bacterial
Dermatophilus congolensis
Streptococcal furunculosis
Staphylococcal folliculitis
Fungal
Dermatophytes
Microsporosis
Trichophytosis
Sub-mycosis
Phycomycosis
Pythiosis
Mycetoma
Sporotrichosis
Phaeohyphomycosis
Parasites
Mites
Demodicosis
Chorioptes equi
Sarcoptes scabei
Dermanyssus gallinae (Poultry red mite)
Harvest/forage
Lice
Chewing (Damalinia equi)
Sucking (Haematopinus asini)
Ticks
Nymph/larvae
Helminths
Onchocercal dermatitis
Larval nematode dermatitis
Oxyuriasis
Others
Insect bites
NON-INFECTIOUS
Genetic
Epitheliogenesis imperfecta
Epidermolysis bullosa
Hyperelastosis cutis
Physical
Burns
Harness rubs
Scalding
Diarrhoea
Wounds
Urine
Immune-mediated
Alopecia areata
Contact hypersensitivity
Drug eruptions
Granulomatous enteritis
Insect hypersensitivity
Linear alopecia (linear hyperkeratosis)
Pastern leukocytoclastic vasculitis
Pemphigus foliaceus/vulgaris
Sarcoidosis
Systemic lupus erythematosus (cutaneous L.E.)
Vasculitis – purpura haemorrhagica
Miscellaneous
Coronary band dystrophy
Chronic granulation tissue
Seborrhoea
Chronic arsenic poisoninq
Chronic iodism
Anhidrosis
Neoplasms
Occult sarcoid
Fibroblastic sarcoid
Squamous cell carcinoma
Fibrosarcoma
Lymphoma

WEEPING AND SEEPING (WET DERMATOSES)

Weeping and seeping is the result of exudation of inflammatory or other fluids onto the skin surface. This can be a primary event but is much more commonly the result of wetting and surface damage which results in a secondary exudative disorder. Investigation of such a case requires a very careful history taking to establish the possible primary factors. The distribution of the abnormal skin is important. For example a wet, exudative dermatosis over the dorsum of the horse might suggest that the instigating factors were related to sunlight or wetting of the skin. Exudation from white areas only might be suggestive of actinic dermatoses, or if the lesions were restricted to the pastern of a white foot the diagnoses of dermatophilosis, pastern leukoclastic vasculitis or pastern folliculitis might be suggested.

Detection of the primary condition might be very difficult because the presence of serum or more particularly infected serum and inflammatory exudate also causes skin inflammation and further exudation.

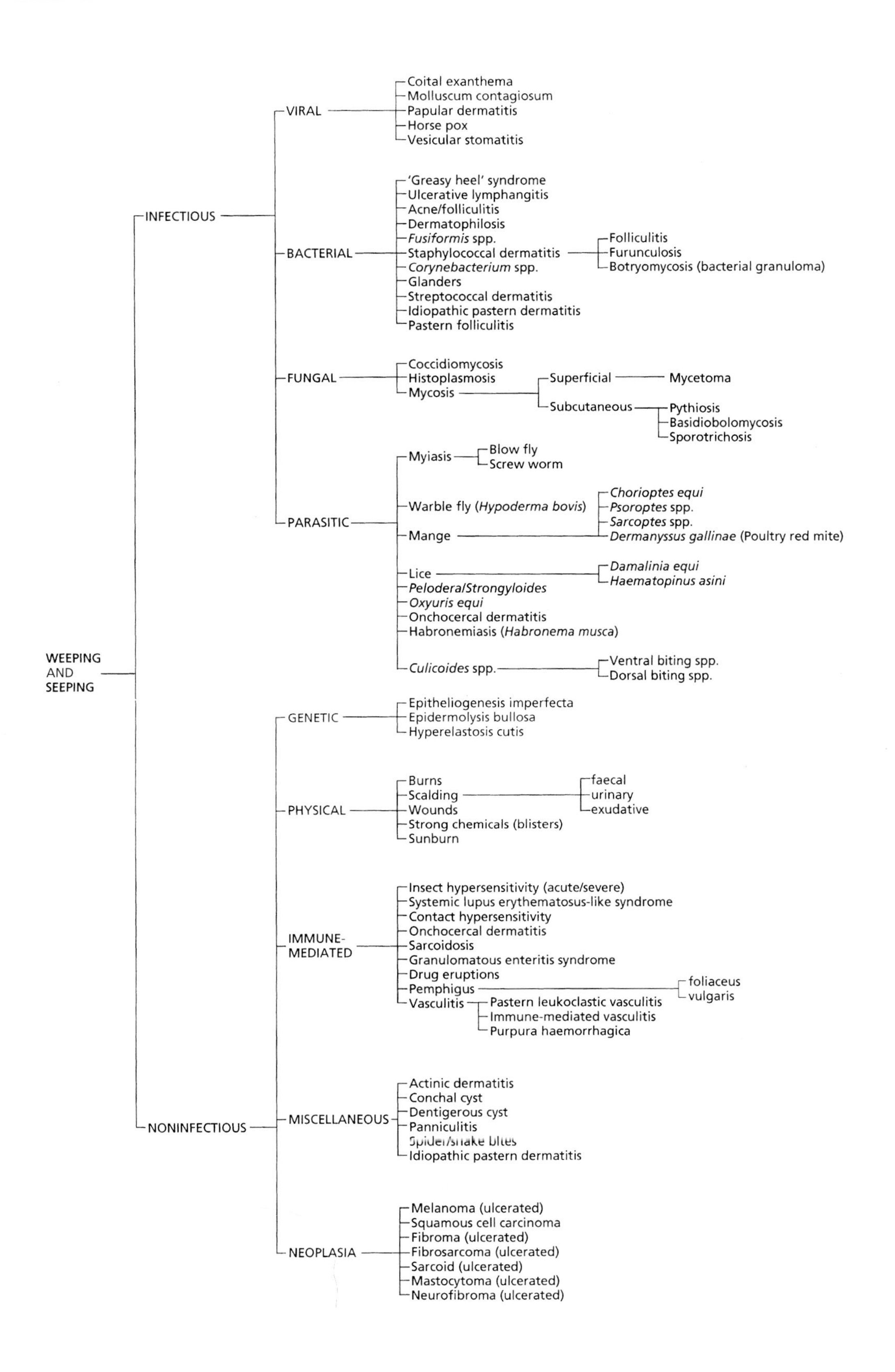
WEEPING AND SEEPING
INFECTIOUS
VIRAL
Coital exanthema
Molluscum contagiosum
Papular dermatitis
Horse pox
Vesicular stomatitis
BACTERIAL
'Greasy heel' syndrome
Ulcerative lymphangitis
Acne/folliculitis
Dermatophilosis
Fusiformis spp.
Staphylococcal dermatitis
Folliculitis
Furunculosis
Botryomycosis (bacterial granuloma)
Corynebacterium spp.
Glanders
Streptococcal dermatitis
Idiopathic pastern dermatitis
Pastern folliculitis
FUNGAL
Coccidiomycosis
Histoplasmosis
Mycosis
Superficial
Mycetoma
Subcutaneous
Pythiosis
Basidiobolomycosis
Sporotrichosis
PARASITIC
Myiasis
Blow fly
Screw worm
Warble fly (Hypoderma bovis)
Mange
Chorioptes equi
Psoroptes spp.
Sarcoptes spp.
Dermanyssus gallinae (Poultry red mite)
Lice
Damalinia equi
Haematopinus asini
Pelodera/Strongyloides
Oxyuris equi
Onchocercal dermatitis
Habronemiasis (Habronema musca)
Culicoides spp.
Ventral biting spp.
Dorsal biting spp.
NONINFECTIOUS
GENETIC
Epitheliogenesis imperfecta
Epidermolysis bullosa
Hyperelastosis cutis
PHYSICAL
Burns
Scalding
faecal
urinary
exudative
Wounds
Strong chemicals (blisters)
Sunburn
IMMUNE-MEDIATED
Insect hypersensitivity (acute/severe)
Systemic lupus erythematosus-like syndrome
Contact hypersensitivity
Onchocercal dermatitis
Sarcoidosis
Granulomatous enteritis syndrome
Drug eruptions
Pemphigus
foliaceus
vulgaris
Vasculitis
Pastern leukoclastic vasculitis
Immune-mediated vasculitis
Purpura haemorrhagica
MISCELLANEOUS
Actinic dermatitis
Conchal cyst
Dentigerous cyst
Panniculitis
Spider/snake bites
Idiopathic pastern dermatitis
NEOPLASIA
Melanoma (ulcerated)
Squamous cell carcinoma
Fibroma (ulcerated)
Fibrosarcoma (ulcerated)
Sarcoid (ulcerated)
Mastocytoma (ulcerated)
Neurofibroma (ulcerated)

ALTERATION IN PIGMENTATION

The appearance of white hairs on a previously whole-coloured horse often causes some owners serious distress, and while some cases are easily identified and for which an explanation can be offered, there are others which are difficult to identify and may even be impossible to explain with our present state of knowledge.

Cutaneous pigmentation is the result of interaction between melanocytes and keratinocytes. Melanocytes are present in many tissues but are in their highest concentrations in skin (dermis, hair follicles), mucous membranes, eye and meninges. Epidermal melanocytes are usually found in the basal cell layer and supply melanin to the keratinocytes. Melanin pigment is produced from tyrosine under the influence of the enzyme tyrosinase in the presence of copper (this being one possible explanation for the poor pigmentation of skin and hair when copper is deficient). This interaction occurs within melanosomes within the melanocyte and once fully laden with melanin the pigment is transferred to the keratinocytes in the dermis and epidermis.

Hyperpigmentation is caused by an increased amount of melanin in the epidermis and/or the dermis. It is uncommon in horses as for the most part they already have darkly pigmented skin. However, where stimuli from excessive friction or trauma from harness occurs, hyperpigmentation or melanotrichia (conversion of natural body colour hair to black) can occur (see Figure 16.6).

Melanocytes in the epidermis and melanocytes in the hair bulbs are frequently affected independently of each other. Where the melanocytes in the epidermis are affected, the skin loses pigment and the condition is referred to as leukoderma. Where pigment is lost from the hair bulb, it leads to white hairs or leukotrichia. The independent relationship between hair and skin is easily demonstrated by shaving the area and noting the discrepancy between the location of the original white hairs and the underlying white-skinned area.

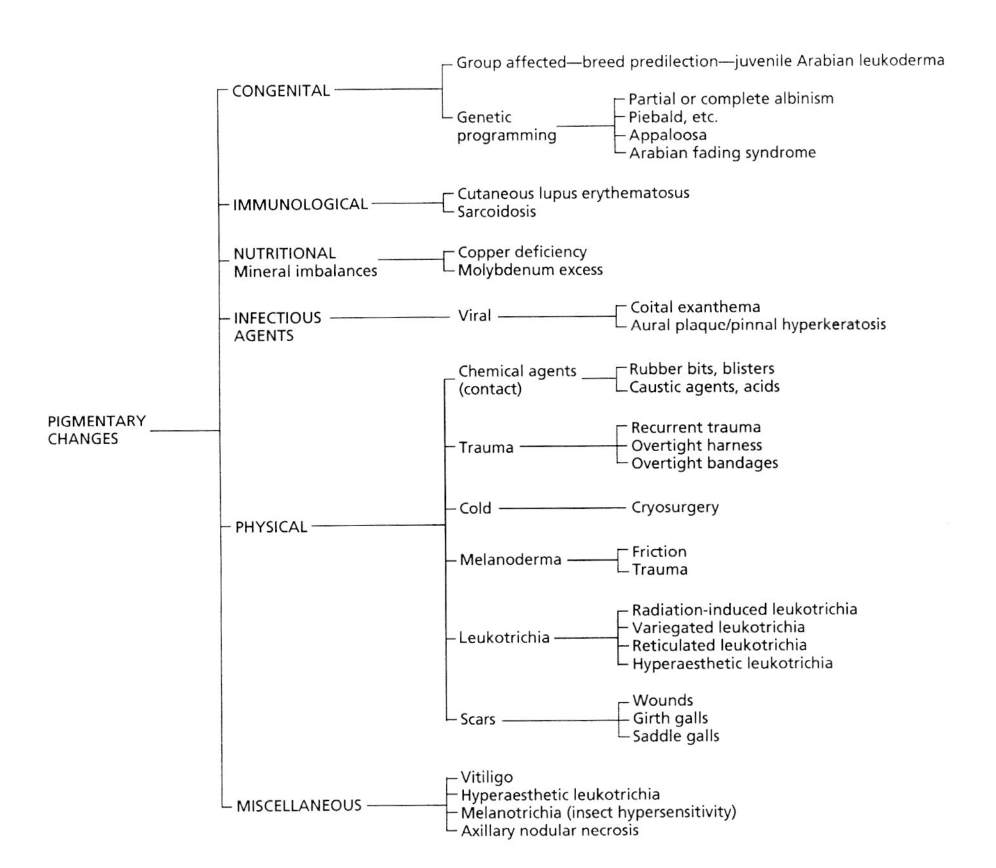
PIGMENTARY CHANGES
CONGENITAL
Group affected—breed predilection—juvenile Arabian leukoderma
Genetic programming
Partial or complete albinism
Piebald, etc.
Appaloosa
Arabian fading syndrome
IMMUNOLOGICAL
Cutaneous lupus erythematosus
Sarcoidosis
NUTRITIONAL Mineral imbalances
Copper deficiency
Molybdenum excess
INFECTIOUS AGENTS
Viral
Coital exanthema
Aural plaque/pinnal hyperkeratosis
PHYSICAL
Chemical agents (contact)
Rubber bits, blisters
Caustic agents, acids
Trauma
Recurrent trauma
Overtight harness
Overtight bandages
Cold
Cryosurgery
Melanoderma
Friction
Trauma
Leukotrichia
Radiation-induced leukotrichia
Variegated leukotrichia
Reticulated leukotrichia
Hyperaesthetic leukotrichia
Scars
Wounds
Girth galls
Saddle galls
MISCELLANEOUS
Vitiligo
Hyperaesthetic leukotrichia
Melanotrichia (insect hypersensitivity)
Axillary nodular necrosis

PASTERN DERMATITIS SYNDROME

Diseases of the pastern and coronet may be related to or linked to disease processes elsewhere on the horse, or they may be confined to the coronet and pastern alone. Combined, they represent a set of diseases which are both difficult to manage and difficult to explain to owners when they fail to respond to medication. Proximity to the ground inflicts significant challenges to the skin of the lower limb due to changeable conditions (from dry stables to unhygienic stables, to normal paddock, to dried-out hard, spiked, clay soil, etc.). Almost every case will have had a great array of 'ointments', 'salves' and 'cures' applied before veterinary attention is sought, and it is little wonder that some horses develop serious lameness and unremitting chronic dermatoses.

It is often difficult to identify the primary problem and treat it satisfactorily. Some lower-limb problems are found as part of a general disease pattern such as dermatophilosis, occasionally dermatophytosis and less commonly vasculitis. Others, such as pastern and cannon leukocytoclastic vasculitis have, as yet, unidentified causes and require further investigation. Many of the latter diseases can justifiably be included in the 'greasy heel syndrome' (see page 202).

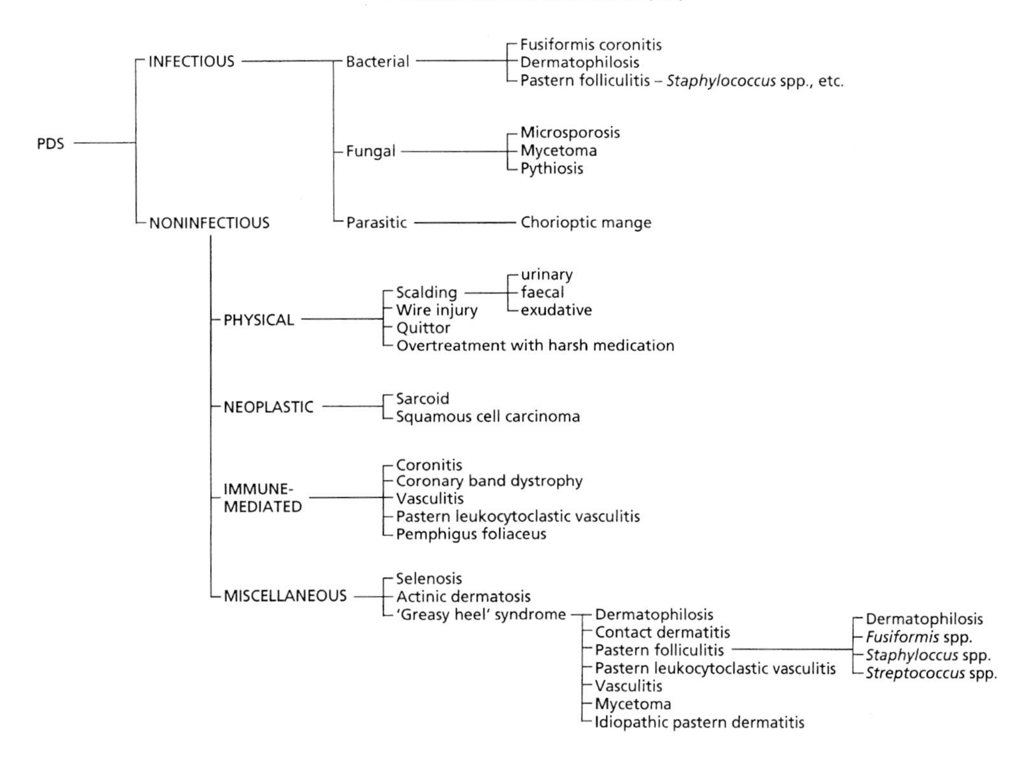
PASTERN DERMATITIS SYNDROME (PDS)
PDS
INFECTIOUS
Bacterial
Fusiformis coronitis
Dermatophilosis
Pastern folliculitis – *Staphylococcus* spp., etc.
Fungal
Microsporosis
Mycetoma
Pythiosis
Parasitic
Chorioptic mange
NONINFECTIOUS
PHYSICAL
Scalding
urinary
faecal
exudative
Wire injury
Quittor
Overtreatment with harsh medication
NEOPLASTIC
Sarcoid
Squamous cell carcinoma
IMMUNE-MEDIATED
Coronitis
Coronary band dystrophy
Vasculitis
Pastern leukocytoclastic vasculitis
Pemphigus foliaceus
MISCELLANEOUS
Selenosis
Actinic dermatosis
'Greasy heel' syndrome
Dermatophilosis
Contact dermatitis
Pastern folliculitis
Dermatophilosis
Fusiformis spp.
Staphyloccus spp.
Streptococcus spp.
Pastern leukocytoclastic vasculitis
Vasculitis
Mycetoma
Idiopathic pastern dermatitis

FOOT SYNDROMES

The outer structures of the foot are of dermal origin. Although they are commonly grouped together and then may be regarded as a unique structure, the conditions that affect them are often of dermatological relevance. The hoof can be divided for practical purposes into:

- the coronet
- the hoof wall
- the sole (including the frog and digital cushion)

In spite of the common origin of the tissues, the pathological conditions are significantly different for each of these structural parts. However, their health or otherwise is intimately inter-related. For example, conditions affecting the coronet such as coronary band dysplasia or pemphigus foliaceus can cause significant pathology in the hoof wall. Wall abnormalities can result directly in sole disorders, for example a keratoma originating high in the wall will cause significant distortion of the wall and the sole. A solar penetration can manifest as a discharging sinus at the coronary band but this could easily be mistaken for lateral cartilage necrosis (quittor). Also, the general health of the horse and its management can have a significant bearing on the condition of the hoof. Certain cracks in the hoof wall may be due to management factors or genetic factors or both. The health of the keratin producing tissues and the periople (the thin waterproof outer layer of the hoof wall) are strongly dependent on the health of the animal and the health of the foot. Errors or changes in nutritional status or the health of the horn-producing tissue will soon reflect in obvious changes in the hoof wall. Laminitic episodes provide perhaps the most obvious changes to hoof growth; the 'laminitic rings' are characteristic but not pathognomonic. Accurate diagnosis of the primary underlying problem is essential if effective therapeutic measures are to be taken.

The formation and maintenance of the sole is somewhat different from that of the wall and so repair mechanisms are also different. The sole has a complex arrangement of tissues and is subjected to direct concussive axial forces that are not duplicated in any other tissue. There are few tissues that have to withstand the focal forces created, for example, when a horse stands on a sharp stone. Furthermore the sole is in contact with much organic matter – often heavily contaminated with bacteria – and so damage is often accompanied by infection. The natural elastic nature of the frog and digital cushion also adds some complicating factors – tracts left by foreign bodies such as nails may close tightly after removal of the object and the tract may be almost invisible. The consequences of this can be very serious. Treatment should take account of the need to protect the integrity of the sole to avoid the introduction of foreign matter and infection. Trauma, including penetration of the sole, is common and the inter-relationship with the underlying synovial and tendon structures is vitally important. Even minor sole disorders can have life threatening implications.

Damage to the wall of the hoof can arise from failure of normal production of horn or from direct trauma. The close proximity of the horn to the sensitive laminae of the hoof means that damage is likely to cause lameness. Healing relies heavily on repair originating in the coronary band; growth is usually slow even in the healthy foot and so repair of hoof disorders is likely to be protracted and suitable supportive measures may need to be taken to permit the tissues to heal at all. Both the sole and the wall are subjected to significant pressure forces at every weight-bearing step. The frog and underlying digital cushion are compressed and the heels are forced outward. Under normal conditions the natural flexibility of the structures permits this without any damage or stress. Outward flexion of the heels is a major natural shock-absorbing mechanism. When the hoof capsule is damaged by trauma or disease this movement can be detrimental to the healing process. The slow repair of hoof wall disorders means that special attention must be paid both to the primary aetiology of the condition and to any secondary consequences on the hoof itself. Treatment of wall disease therefore has an important temporal aspect and so early diagnosis is essential.

The coronary band is a particularly interesting anatomical feature in the horse. It sometimes provides important information on underlying systemic or generalized disease processes. Thus several autoimmune disorders are manifest by inflammation or changes in the function of the coronary band. In some cases the condition may then only become manifest when the hoof wall shows abnormal growth patterns. Traumatic damage to the coronary band almost always affects the hoof growth in that region. Distorted or altered hoof growth or in some cases a complete failure of hoof wall production may have serious implications for the horse. It is important to realize that similar tissues are present around the ergots and chestnuts and so whenever coronary band disease is suspected these structures should also be examined carefully.

The cutaneous hoof structures are also liable to some specific neoplastic changes. Some of these are significant challenges to the veterinary surgeon but most are benign and if correctly diagnosed and managed carry a good or reasonable prognosis. A good outcome following treatment of these conditions is very satisfying but a good understanding of the anatomical relationships and appropriate aftercare are vital if this is to be achieved.

Inevitably some disorders of the hoof have profound implications for the welfare and health of the animal itself. The use of the horse may be severely restricted if damage or disease of the hoof affects its ability to work safely and soundly. The underlying structures are critical and the interrelationship between the coronary band, the hoof capsule and the sole with the soft tissues and the synovial structures and tendons of the foot, make an accurate and early diagnosis particularly important. Failure to address the primary problem can lead to frustrating failures and possibly even a fatal outcome. The value of a skilled farrier when dealing with hoof disorders cannot be overstated.

FOOT DISORDERS SYNDROME – SOLE, FROG

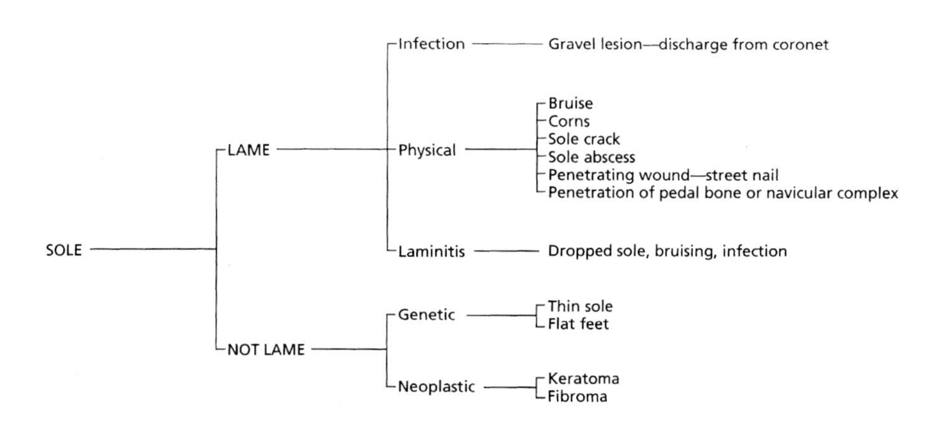

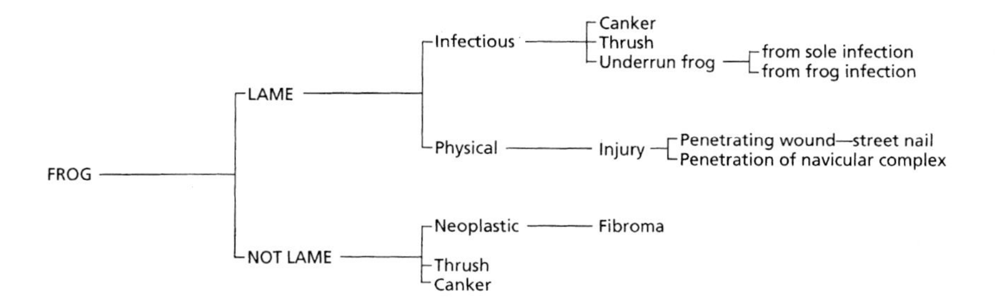

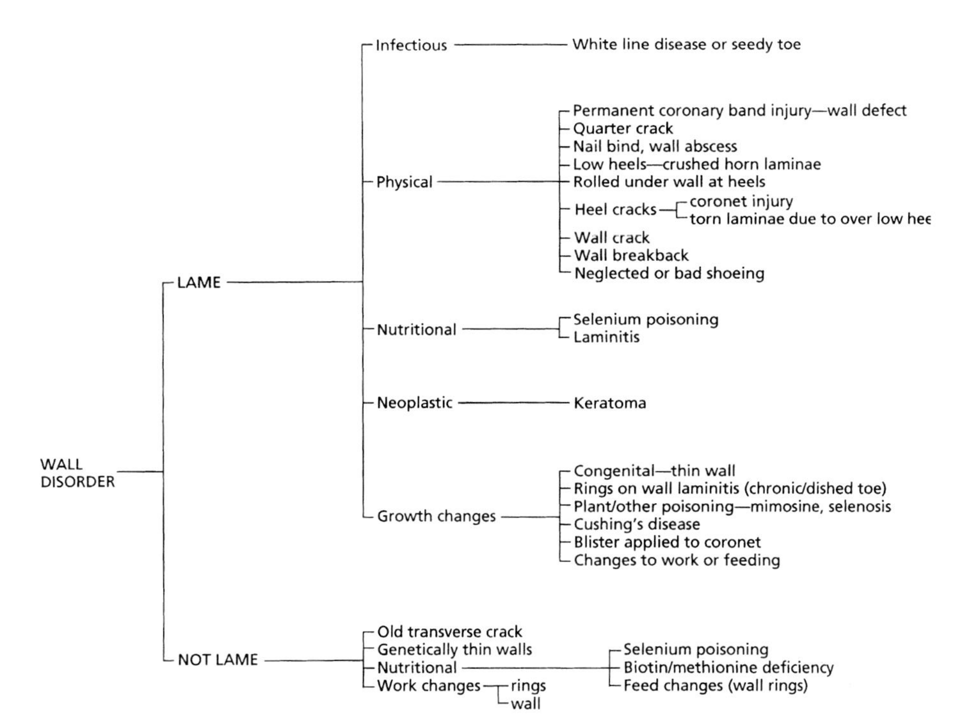
FOOT DISORDERS SYNDROME – WALL
WALL DISORDER
LAME
Infectious
White line disease or seedy toe
Physical
Permanent coronary band injury—wall defect
Quarter crack
Nail bind, wall abscess
Low heels—crushed horn laminae
Rolled under wall at heels
Heel cracks
coronet injury
torn laminae due to over low hee
Wall crack
Wall breakback
Neglected or bad shoeing
Nutritional
Selenium poisoning
Laminitis
Neoplastic
Keratoma
Growth changes
Congenital—thin wall
Rings on wall laminitis (chronic/dished toe)
Plant/other poisoning—mimosine, selenosis
Cushing's disease
Blister applied to coronet
Changes to work or feeding
NOT LAME
Old transverse crack
Genetically thin walls
Nutritional
Work changes
rings
wall
Selenium poisoning
Biotin/methionine deficiency
Feed changes (wall rings)

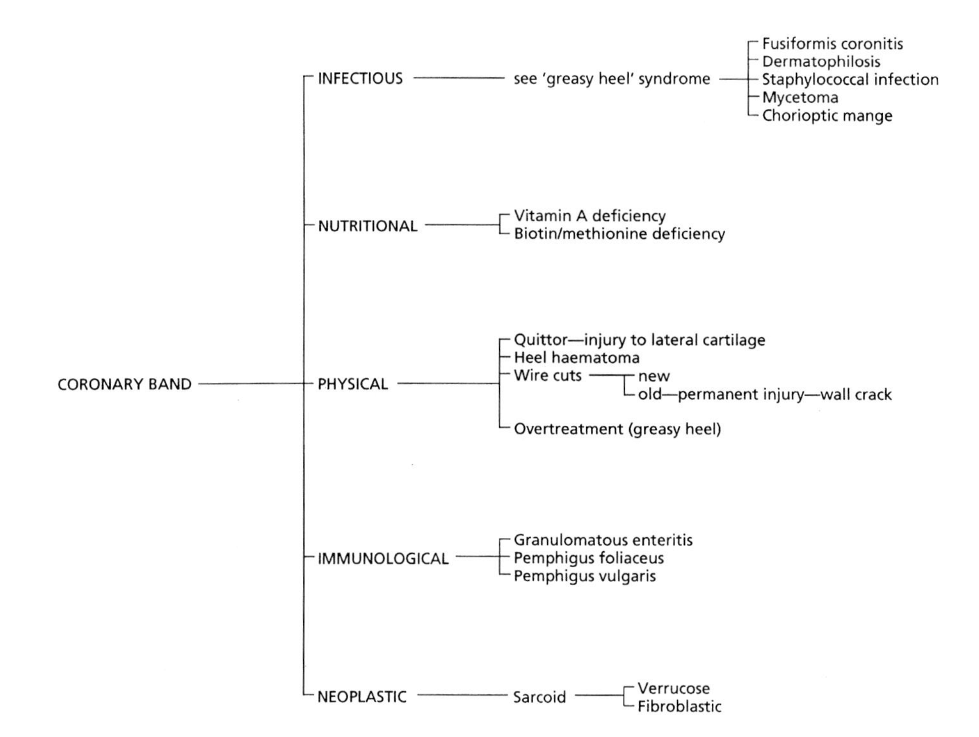
FOOT DISORDERS SYNDROME – CORONARY BAND
CORONARY BAND
INFECTIOUS
see 'greasy heel' syndrome
Fusiformis coronitis
Dermatophilosis
Staphylococcal infection
Mycetoma
Chorioptic mange
NUTRITIONAL
Vitamin A deficiency
Biotin/methionine deficiency
PHYSICAL
Quittor—injury to lateral cartilage
Heel haematoma
Wire cuts
new
old—permanent injury—wall crack
Overtreatment (greasy heel)
IMMUNOLOGICAL
Granulomatous enteritis
Pemphigus foliaceus
Pemphigus vulgaris
NEOPLASTIC
Sarcoid
Verrucose
Fibroblastic

PART III

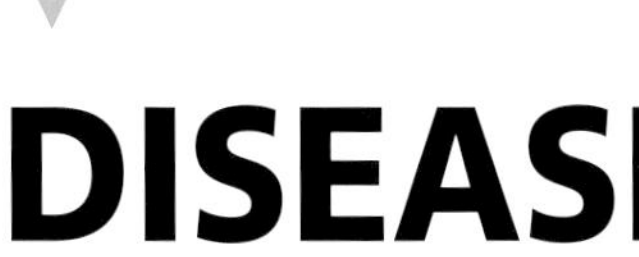

DISEASE PROFILES

section A
INFECTIOUS DISEASES

chapter 6
Viral diseases 91

chapter 7
Bacterial diseases 97

chapter 8
Fungal diseases 111

chapter 9
Protozoal diseases 121

chapter 10
Metazoan/parasitic diseases 123

section B
NONINFECTIOUS DISEASES

chapter 11
Congenital/developmental diseases 145

chapter 12
Immune-mediated/allergic diseases 155

chapter 13
Chemical and toxic dermatoses 183

chapter 14
Endocrine disorders 189

chapter 15
Nutritional disorders 191

chapter 16
Iatrogenic and idiopathic disorders 195

chapter 17
Physical and traumatic disorders 205

chapter 18
Injuries and diseases of the hoof 227

chapter 19
Neoplastic conditions 241

Key to abbreviations

- Geographical distribution

Eur	Europe
NAm	North America
SAm	South America
Afr	Africa
Aus	Australasia
Asi	Asia
MidEast	Middle East
Ind	India

Where no mention is made, the condition is universal

Cont	Contagious
Cont. bov	Contagious to cattle
(human figure symbol)	Zoonosis

REP	Reportable/notifiable in some parts of the world

section A

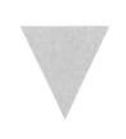

INFECTIOUS DISEASES

chapter 6

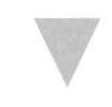

VIRAL DISEASES

Horse pox	91
Vesicular stomatitis	92
Molluscum contagiosum	92
Equine viral arteritis (EVA)	93
Equine viral papular dermatitis (Uasin Gishu disease)	93
Congenital papillomatosis (neonatal wart)	94
Papillomatosis	95
Equine coital exanthema (ECE)	95

HORSE POX

USA; Aus; Eur – Cont

Profile

Rare, benign, mildly contagious, cutaneous infection due to a pox virus as yet unclassified. The virus is similar to the cowpox virus.

Clinical signs

Oral lesions (buccal horse pox/contagious pustular stomatitis) (**Fig. 6.1**). Pastern/fetlock lesions (leg pox). Vulval lesions (genital pox). Vesicles rapidly develop and burst to become pustules with surface crusts and exudate. Mild systemic signs (pyrexia and depression) may be seen.

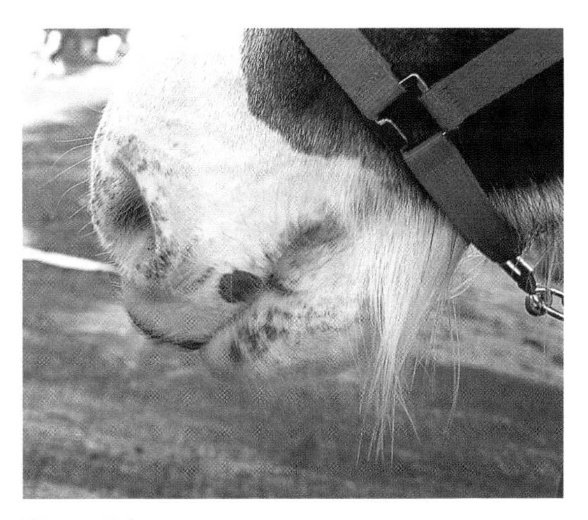

Figure 6.1
Typical ulcerative, vesicular and scabby lesions of horse pox on the lips and nasal margin.

Differential diagnosis

- Molluscum contagiosum
- Papillomatosis
- Immune-mediated disease
- Viral papular dermatitis
- Dermatophytosis (ringworm)
- Coital exanthema

Diagnostic confirmation

- Clinical signs
- Biopsy
- Virus isolation
- Electron microscopy

Treatment

No specific treatment is available. Spontaneous

remission with long-standing, solid immunity is usual after about 4 weeks.

VESICULAR STOMATITIS

NAm; SAm – Cont – REP

Profile

Contagious viral disease of limited geographical distribution.

Clinical signs

Inflammation and vesicle formation in mouth and tongue and to a lesser extent the skin of the mammary gland and prepuce. Coronet and digital skin are also sometimes affected. Vesicles rupture leaving a very painful small ulcerated lesion. Major signs include inappetance, fever, depression and lameness. Extensive oral ulceration causes drooling of saliva and intense rubbing of the mouth and lips on mangers or doors. Lesions resolve over 3–7 days with solid immunity.

Differential diagnosis

- Viral papular dermatitis
- Molluscum contagiosum
- Horse pox
- Bullous pemphigoid/pemphigus vulgaris
- Other genital infections

Diagnostic confirmation

- Characteristic clinical features and history
- Serology
- Virus isolation possible

Treatment

None is possible or required. Isolation and, if relevant, reporting of cases to the disease regulatory body (in view of possible transmissibility to cattle and confusion with foot and mouth disease).

MOLLUSCUM CONTAGIOSUM

Afr – Cont

Profile

A mildly contagious cutaneous infection caused by an unclassified pox virus. Restricted geographically at present to South Africa.

Clinical signs

Multiple, raised, well-defined grey/white papules with a waxy surface (1–2 mm) primarily in hairless or sparsely haired areas such as the penis, prepuce, scrotum, mammary glands, thighs (**Fig. 6.2**), axilla and muzzle. Other body areas can also be affected. Individual lesions may coalesce and form larger aggregations closely resembling papillomata.[40]

Older lesions become smaller and umbilicated. They may develop a central pore from which a caseous plug is extruded.

In areas where hair is thicker, nodules are covered with powdery scabs which, when detached, remove the hairs.

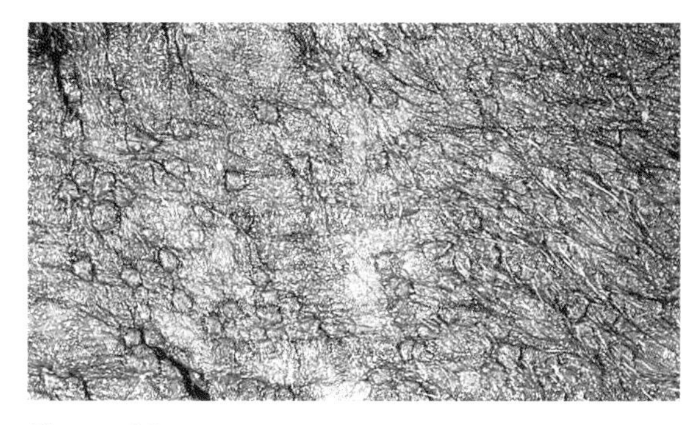

Figure 6.2
Molluscum contagiosum lesions showing the typical waxy, raised papules.

Differential diagnosis

- Papillomatosis
- Immune-mediated disease
- Occult/verrucose sarcoid
- Viral papular dermatitis
- Dermatophytosis (ringworm)
- Horse pox
- Coital exanthema

Diagnostic confirmation

- Characteristic histopathology showing epidermal hyperplasia and hypertrophy. Individual keratinocytes are swollen and contain large intracytoplasmic inclusion (molluscum) bodies.

Treatment

No specific treatment is available. Spontaneous remission with new hair growth has been reported to take up to 2–3 years.

EQUINE VIRAL ARTERITIS (EVA)

NAm; Aus; Eur; Asia – Cont – REP

Profile

Caused by a togavirus which causes abortion, infertility and skin disease; some strains are relatively less virulent and infection may go unnoticed. Incubation period 3–14 days. Transmission is through the respiratory tract (by droplet and microaerosol) or urogenital tract (urine or semen). Carrier status of stallions is an important aspect of the epidemiology.

Clinical signs

Skin signs Rash resulting from vasculitis with skin papules and plaques closely resembling urticarial lesions.

Systemic signs Variable, pyrexia and depression. Increased respiratory rate. Oedema of limbs and less frequently, head, ventral abdomen, scrotum, prepuce and conjunctiva ('red eye'). Coughing may or may not be associated with the disease. Reduced exercise tolerance in horses showing clinical disease. Abortion occurs in affected pregnant mares during or just after the febrile phase.

Differential diagnosis

- Urticaria/allergy (including food/contact allergy)
- Purpura haemorrhagica
- Insect bites/stings
- Viral and bacterial respiratory infections

Diagnostic confirmation

- Virus isolation from respiratory (upper respiratory tract swabs) or reproductive tracts (semen from 'shedder' stallions). Virus can also be isolated or identified in the buffy coat of blood and in urine as well as the placenta of aborted mares.
- Paired sera 14 days apart are necessary for the serum neutralization test (titre >1:4 is regarded as positive).
- Laboratory findings include a leukopenia.
- Histopathology: Necrosis of the media of small arteries and neutrophilic infiltration and thrombosis of smaller submucosal vessels.

Treatment

No treatment is available. Vaccinations are effective and can be used to control the spread of the disease. Castration of carrier stallions is the only means of elimination of the carrier state in the stallion.

EQUINE VIRAL PAPULAR DERMATITIS (Uasin Gishu disease)

NAm; Aus; Afr – Cont

Profile

Infectious skin disease caused by an unspecified pox virus. Spread is direct or indirect by vectors such as flies. Incubation period is about 7 days with a course of 2–3 weeks.

Clinical signs

Sudden appearance of many annular papular lesions which quickly develop crusts with hair loss primarily over the trunk and scrotal skin (**Fig. 6.3**). Lesions are not pruritic or painful and become scaly after about 2 weeks. There are no systemic signs and most cases resolve within 4–6 weeks.

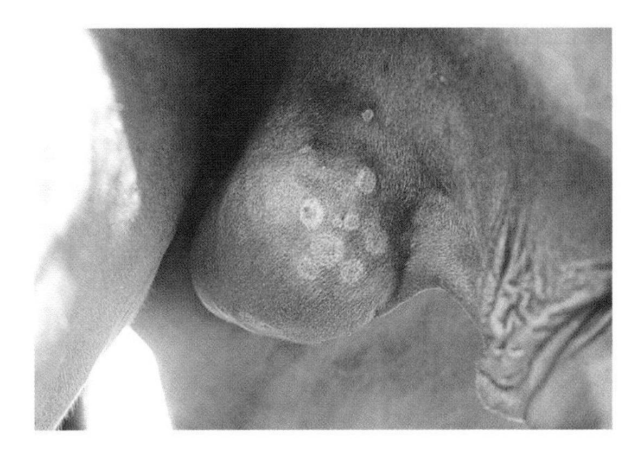

Figure 6.3
Unilateral viral papular dermatitis lesions on the scrotum of a stallion.

Differential diagnosis

- Dermatophytosis (ringworm)
- Sarcoid (occult)
- Horse pox
- Pemphigus foliaceus
- Molluscum contagiosum
- Urticaria/Insect bites
- Coital exanthema

Diagnostic confirmation

- Virus isolation from papular lesions.
- Biopsy shows hyperplasia, superficial and deep dermatitis with ballooning degeneration and eosinophilic intracytoplasmic inclusion bodies.

Treatment
No specific treatment is needed. The disease has no systemic implications and resolves spontaneously. Isolation of affected horses is wise and disinfection of premises may help limit spread.

CONGENITAL PAPILLOMATOSIS (neonatal wart)

Profile
Papilloma virus apparently has the ability to pass across the mare's placenta. Viral papillomata are not an uncommon finding on the skin of newborn foals.

Clinical signs
Cauliflower-like, flattened warts from 5 mm to 20 cm on the skin of a newborn foal at any site on head, neck or trunk[41] (**Fig. 6.4**). They are usually single and no other signs are usually present.

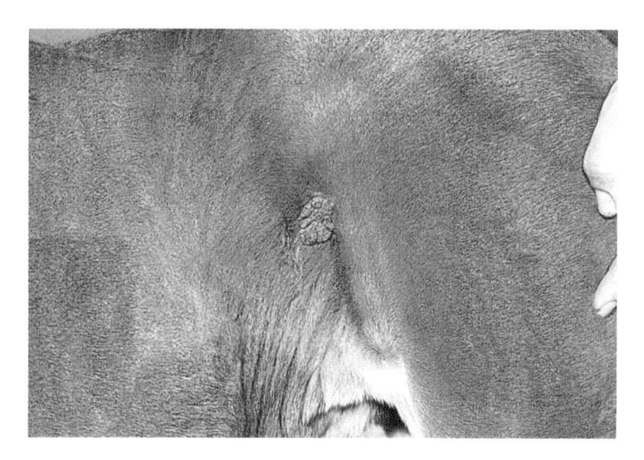

Figure 6.4
Congenital (viral) papilloma on a foal.

Differential diagnosis
- No other condition really resembles this.

Diagnostic confirmation
- Simple diagnosis based on clinical appearance
- Histopathology
- Virus isolation on fresh unpreserved samples

Treatment
Easily treated by ligation or surgical removal. Podophyllin paste (50%) applied daily for 20 days may also be effective. Rarely, spontaneous resolution occurs.

PAPILLOMATOSIS

Cont

Profile
Viral skin disease caused by a host-specific papovavirus (equine papilloma virus) affecting basal cell layers of the epithelium. Usually only younger horses (6 months to 4 years). Occasionally seen in aged horses (over 25 years). Incubation period of approximately 60–70 days. Moderately contagious by direct and indirect contact between co-grazing horses (hence the name 'grass warts').

A clinically distinct papillary acanthosis (pinnal hyperkeratosis/aural plaque) is probably a form of papilloma[42] caused by a different virus of the papilloma group. It seems likely that the papilloma virus is transmitted by black flies (*Simulium* spp.).

Clinical signs
Multiple (often many) single or coalescent pink or grey vegetative lesions most often on muzzle

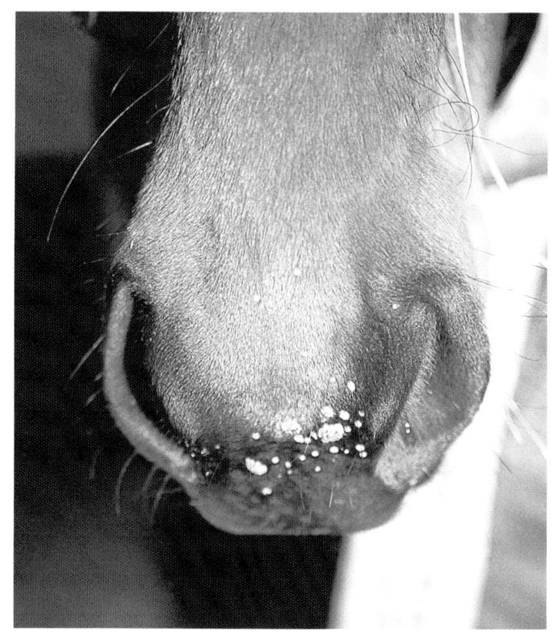

Figure 6.5
Viral papillomas on the muzzle of a grazing yearling thoroughbred. Notice that some of the lesions have coalesced.

(**Fig. 6.5**), lips, face (**Fig. 6.6**), distal limbs and genitalia. Usually increase in number rather than size of individual lesions. Single large lesions can be found on the vulval lips or on the preputial skin or the free portion of the penis. Lesions on older horses may be persistent and a few may remain static for many years.

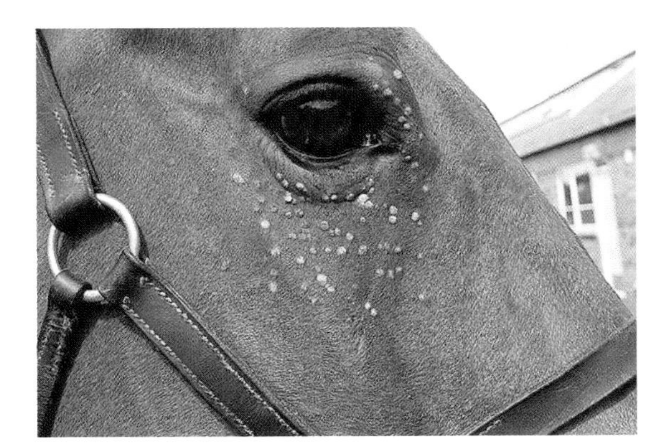

Figure 6.6
Healing discrete viral papillomas on the face of a yearling.

Pinnal papilloma or papillary acanthosis (also known as aural plaque) presents as a flat hyperkeratotic, flaking pink or pink-grey proliferative area on the inner skin of the pinna (**Fig. 6.7**). A few cases develop extensive involvement of the inner skin of the pinna. It can extend into the ear canal itself where accumulations of scales and wax may create problems. Although some cases of head-shaking and handling resentment have been attributed to it, few cases show obvious pain or inflammation unless the lesions are interfered with or handled. In contrast to the cutaneous form, spontaneous regression does not seem to occur. Owners often refer to the disease as 'ear fungus' or 'fungal plaques' but there is no clinical or pathological suggestion that these are of fungal origin.

Differential diagnosis

- Verrucose sarcoid
- Squamous cell carcinoma (especially facial and vulval proliferative forms)
- Molluscum contagiosum

Diagnostic confirmation

- Characteristic clinical appearance and history in young horses
- Contagion (others of the same age affected)
- Biopsy for histopathology

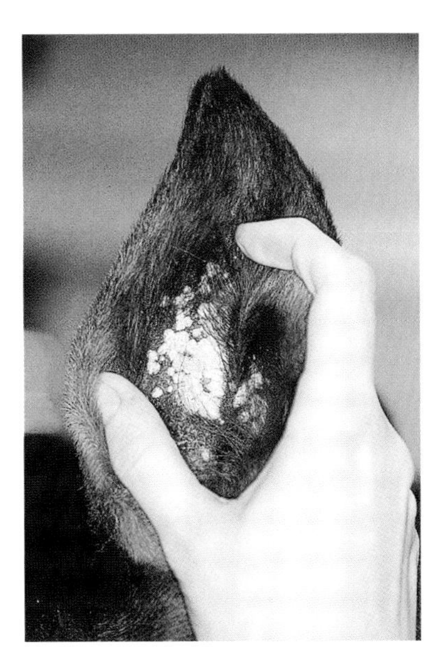

Figure 6.7
Papillary acanthosis (pinnal hyperkeratosis/aural plaque) on the inner skin surface of the ear.

Treatment

No treatment is usually required. Most lesions on young horses will resolve spontaneously after 3–4 months.

Autogenous vaccines have a fairly good reputation but take some weeks to prepare and complete the course. It is uncertain whether there is definite clinical advantage from this method.

Surgical removal from around the eyes and commissure of the mouth is needed very occasionally. Unsightly lesions respond well to cryosurgery, radiofrequency hyperthermia or surgical removal.

May be little or no spontaneous regression in the aged horse.

Note: Pinnal papilloma (aural plaque) seldom resolves and is best regarded as a minor blemish. It should not be subjected to treatment attempts (the cure is frequently worse than the disease).

EQUINE COITAL EXANTHEMA

Cont

Profile

A contagious, venereal, viral skin disease caused by equine herpes virus (EHV-3).[43] Transmission may also occur by indirect contact (fomites, inhalation of virus-laden droplets). Incubation period of 5–7 days.

Clinical signs

Multiple, rapidly developing papules (1–5 mm diameter) which quickly develop necrotic tops and become obvious pustule-like lesions on the penis – principally in the area of the junction of parietal and visceral folds of the prepuce on the dorsal surface (the site of the most prolonged contact with the vulva during coitus) (**Fig. 6.8**). Some horses may also develop lesions around the nose and mouth.

In mares similar lesions develop on the mucosal surface of the vulva and often extend to the skin of the vulva and perineum (**Fig. 6.9**); severe cases can also affect the anus and tail skin. Perineal swelling and oedema of the vulval lips develop by the fourth day.

The lesions may be mildly pruritic but are not painful. The developing lesions closely resemble pustules but they do not produce identifiable liquid pus. It would seem that the initial cell necrosis is not followed by liquefaction. Healing lesions become covered with serum-encrusted scabs. Over 3–5 days oedema regresses and healthy granulation occurs by 10–14 days. Healing lesions may leave permanently depigmented areas (leukoderma).

Typically of latent herpesviruses, individual horses may show recurrent recrudescence during periods of stress (including transport, disease or pregnancy).

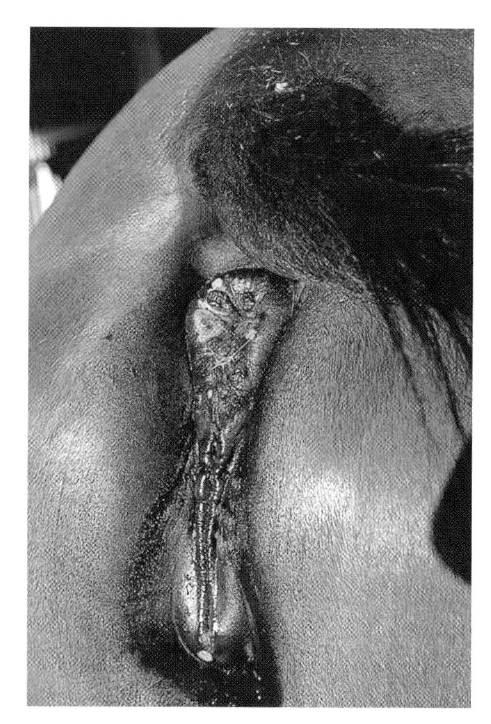

Figure 6.9
Equine coital exanthema on the vulval lips and perineal skin of a mare.

Differential diagnosis

- Papular dermatitis
- Molluscum contagiosum
- Horse pox (genital form)
- Bullous pemphigoid
- Other genital infections (including dourine)
- Vesicular stomatitis
- Squamous cell carcinoma (precancerous stages)

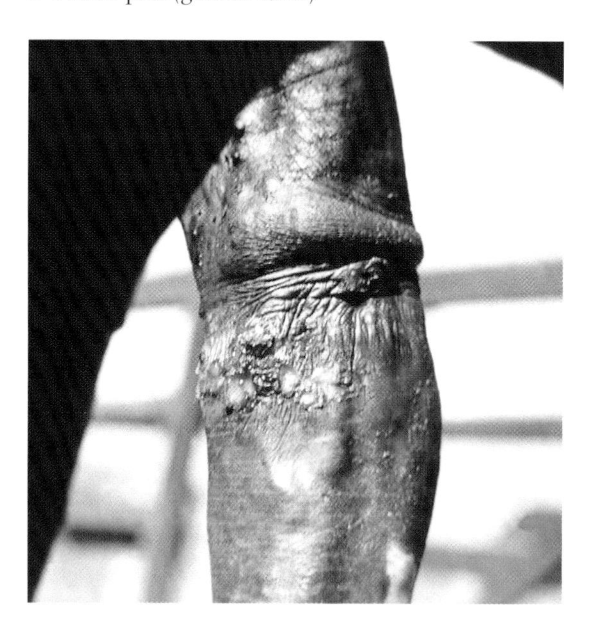

Figure 6.8
Equine coital exanthema on a stallion's penis.

Diagnostic confirmation

- Clinical signs
- History
- Virus isolation: only successful when samples are taken early in the course of disease (fresh lesions are essential).
- Paired sera 14–28 days apart can be used for serum neutralization test (SNT) and complement fixation test (CFT).

Treatment

Do not breed affected animals until completely cleared of active lesions. Clean off scabs with diluted hydrogen peroxide and carefully medicate individual lesions with strong iodine solution. Then apply a daily treatment with a cotton bud dipped in a soothing, antibiotic/antiseptic ointment. The value of parenteral corticosteroids is doubtful in the management of any latent herpesvirus infection but topical applications can be helpful. There is no vaccine at present.

chapter 7

BACTERIAL DISEASES

Abscess	97
Cheek abscess	98
Bacterial folliculitis and furunculosis (acne)	99
Pastern folliculitis	100
Bacterial granuloma (botriomycosis/ staphylococcal pseudomycetoma)	101
Dermatophilosis	102
Staphylococcal dermatitis	106
Streptococcal dermatitis/folliculitis	107
Glanders ('farcy')	108
Ulcerative lymphangitis	109

ABSCESS

Profile

A circumscribed collection of inflammatory debris (pus) developing in acute or chronic localized infection and/or tissue destruction. Frequently accompanied by pain, heat, swelling and perilesional inflammation. Dermal abscesses may be infected or sterile. Infected abscesses can be caused by a variety of organisms but more common organisms involved are *Streptococcus equi* and *Corynebacterium pseudotuberculosis*. Systemic (haematogenous) dissemination of infective emboli (septicaemia/pyaemia) is common in severe infections with *Streptococcus equi equi* (bastard strangles) and *Rhodococcus equi* and cutaneous abscess can be found with both infections. Abscess due to *Clostridium* spp. are often associated with intramuscular injections and particularly with non-antibiotic and mildly irritant drugs.

The infecting organism usually gains access through wounds but can be disseminated into the skin through the blood and/or the lymphatic system or as extensions from infected foci in adjacent subdermal tissues. Ectoparasites may be responsible for some cutaneous abscesses in the pectoral and chest regions (particularly those due to *Corynebacterium pseudotuberculosis*).[44]

In immunocompromised horses (such as Cushing's disease cases) oral abscesses are particularly common from even minor infections of small abrasions.

Sterile abscess usually develops in response to noninfective tissue necrosis. It can also develop if infection is controlled but inflammation and inflammatory debris persist.

Clinical signs

Characteristic progression from a hard, painful nodule surrounded by an area of acute inflammation with heat and swelling which develops a softer centre. The fluid may fluctuate on palpation. The overlying skin becomes thinner and eventually bursts (**Fig. 7.1**). The accumulated debris/pus is usually fluid in consistency and if in a suitable site it may drain under gravity.

Oral and facial abscesses are common in horses suffering from Cushing's disease (hyperadrenocorticism).

Clostridial abscess is characteristically associated with gas formation and has a less localized character. Pain and local swelling are often severe and there may be extensive sloughing of the skin

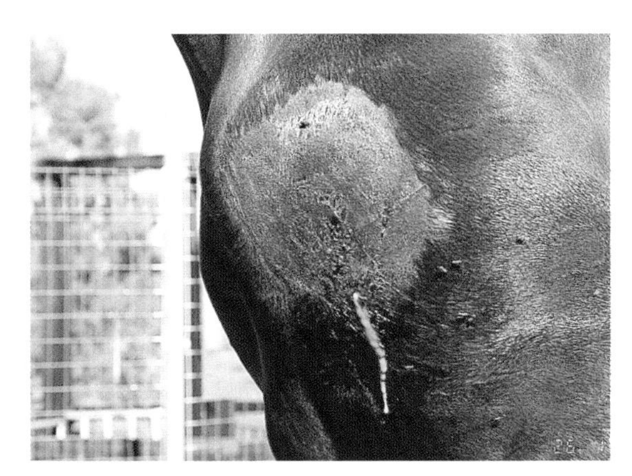

Figure 7.1 A large abscess on the chest of a horse. The abscess is discharging from a small tract which developed at softer skin. A pure growth of *Streptococcus equi* was isolated from the pus.

and underlying necrotic muscle, etc. (**Fig. 7.2**). The affected horse is invariably very ill until the infection is controlled.

Chronic (cold) and sterile abscesses are usually well walled-off and may or may not be attached to the skin.

Differential diagnosis

- Haematoma
- Cyst
- Acute eosinophilic granuloma
- Hernia
- Nodular neoplastic lesions (e.g. sarcoid/lymphosarcoma)

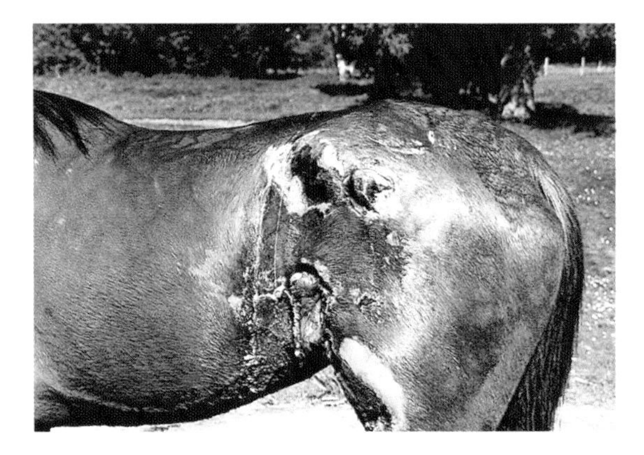

Figure 7.2 Clostridial infection of an injection site resulted in extensive skin necrosis and a prolonged recovery time with extensive scarring.

Diagnostic confirmation

- Characteristic appearance and ultrasonographic features (fluid filled, hypoechoic central portion with typical 'snow-storm' appearance).
- Aspiration of contents usually allows identification of the nature of the pus and the bacterial species involved.

Treatment

Poulticing and hot compresses can be used to speed up the development of the mature abscess. There is no advantage in opening an abscess in the early (hard) stages except in the case of clostridial infection when oxygenation/aeration of affected tissues is important. The value of antibiotics is dubious in most cases. Early administration of appropriate drugs may markedly delay final healing and in some cases apparently results in exacerbation after withdrawal of the drugs. However, antibiotics can sometimes cure the condition before bursting without further complication or treatment. Drainage of the mature abscess is probably the most important aspect of management, but the infecting organism will have a significant bearing on the value and choice of antibiotics (systemically or locally).

Purpura haemorrhagica (see p. 181) can be a sequel to prolonged abscessation (particularly that due to *Streptococcus equi equi*, *S. equi zooepidemicus*) whether or not the abscesses are satisfactorily treated and/or drained.

Note: Horses suspected of either strangles or Wyoming strangles should be isolated before and after abscesses are surgically drained. In many cases rapid improvement in the horse's demeanour follows surgical drainage.

CHEEK ABSCESS

Profile

Acute abscess formation at or around the lateral commissures of the mouth. Possibly caused by dirty bits, dental damage to internal mucosa of the cheek or penetrating wounds due to barley or oat awns.

Clinical signs

Acute, painful swelling of commissure of the mouth or adjacent cheek area. Small area of exudation over pointing abscess (**Fig. 7.3**). Hair loss (alopecia) on skin overlying the abscess is common. Although oral lesions heal well for the

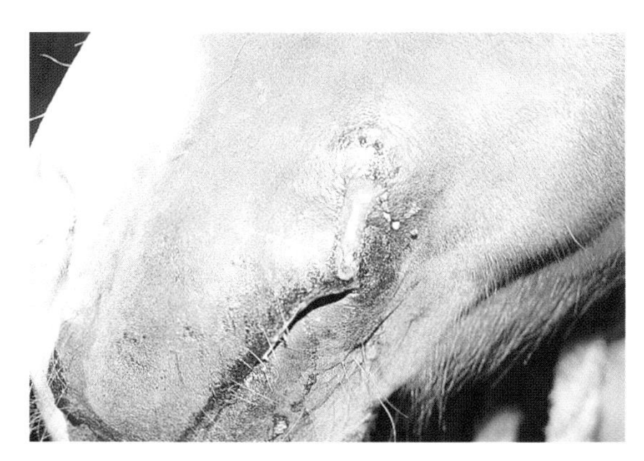

Figure 7.3 Cheek abscess. Note hair loss overlying the abscess.

most part, chronic ulceration at the site of cheek abscesses is common.

Oral abscessation is a common secondary feature of Cushing's disease (pituitary-based hyperadrenocorticism) in horses over 15 years of age.

Differential diagnosis

- Bit injury in the mouth
- Buccal laceration from teeth inside the commissure
- Foreign bodies
- Tumours (ulcerated melanoma, squamous cell carcinoma or sarcoid in particular)

Diagnostic confirmation

- Cuts or wounds inside the mouth adjacent to the abscess
- Typical clinical features

Treatment

Alternating hot and cold fomentation will hasten development of the abscess, but it may be impossible to apply these principles to the lesion. Surgical lancing and drainage when the abscess points sufficiently is the treatment of choice. Early use of antibiotics should be avoided.

BACTERIAL FOLLICULITIS AND FURUNCULOSIS (ACNE)

Profile

Folliculitis is inflammation of the hair follicle with accumulation of inflammatory cells within the follicle lumen. It can be caused by bacteria (staphylococcal and streptococcal species are commonest) or (much more rarely) fungi. As the infective process proceeds, degeneration of the hair follicle leads to infection of the surrounding dermis and subcutis. This is called furunculosis. Usually related to area of rubbing due to dirty or ill-fitting harness, rugs or saddle cloths. Most cases occur in late spring or early summer coincidental with hair shedding, humidity and increasing work with dirty or poorly maintained tack. Poorly groomed horses have a higher tendency to develop the condition.

Clinical signs

Rapid development of small (2–5 mm diameter) painful papules which may be more easily felt than seen unless the hair is closely clipped (**Fig. 7.4**). The first sign may be the presence of areas of erect hairs. The papules develop an ulcerated central area with extensive local oedema and exudation. Palpation is usually resented and pain is usually marked. There is seldom pruritus and in uncomplicated cases there are no systemic signs of illness.

Healing lesions become flat and alopecic and may develop leukoderma and leukotrichia (white saddle or girth marks may arise from this as well as other causes including persistent trauma).

Some superficial lesions fail to heal and these may become deeply infected (furunculosis) with sinus tracts and discharging sinuses. Chronic granulation tissue diffusely infiltrated with microabscesses and sinus tracts is often classified as botriomycosis on the skin, see Fig. 7.7, or as scirrhous cord at the site of non-healing castration wounds).

Where multiple infections coalesce, it becomes a carbuncle or boil; these occur in horses with saddle rash/scab (*Staphylococcus aureus*, *S. intermedius*), heat rash, cheek abscess (see Fig. 7.3) and 'pigeon-

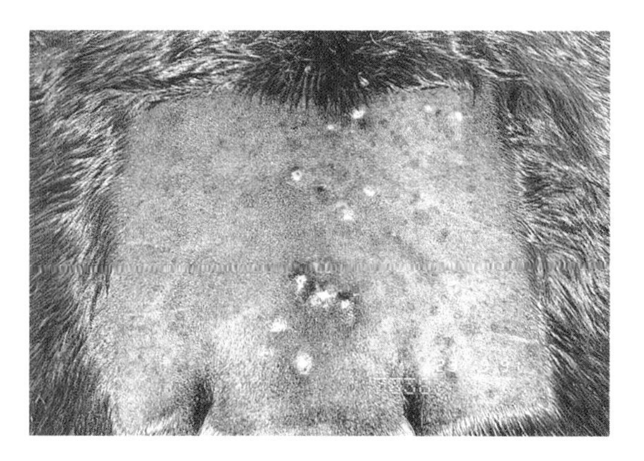

Figure 7.4 Bacterial folliculitis due to *Staphylococcus intermedius* infection.

breast' (Wyoming strangles due to *Corynebacterium pseudotuberculosis*).

Differential diagnosis
- Fungal folliculitis
- Dermatophytosis
- Onchocerciasis
- Dermatophilosis
- Generalized granulomatous disease (enteritis/sarcoidosis)
- Pemphigus foliaceus
- Other bacterial pyoderma (e.g. *Streptococcus equi equi* – strangles)
- Greasy heel syndrome

Diagnostic confirmation
- Clinical features and pain are characteristic.
- Bacteriological culture and sensitivity are important but deep biopsy may be needed for significant culture.
- Biopsy is usually avoided if possible but a fine biopsy punch (3 mm) may be useful particularly for culture.

Treatment
All tack and rug contact with the affected skin should be prevented. Skin washes with chlorhexidine or povidone-iodine surgical scrub solutions are useful in controlling the spread of the organisms responsible. Proprietary antiseptic shampoos are available (usually containing chlorhexidine, povidone-iodine or hexachlorophene) but human equivalents should probably not be used. Parenteral antibiotics such as penicillin (parenterally) or potentiated sulphonamides (parenterally and orally) for up to 2 weeks[45] may be advisable. Recurrences are nevertheless common.

Wash and sterilize all tack, grooming equipment, rugs, etc. Tertiary amine disinfectants have strong antibacterial properties without much risk of damage to tack or other equipment.

Fumigation of all tack with formaldehyde gas is often the best approach to sterilization of the equipment but is more difficult (see p. 37). Severe outbreaks have been controlled with autogenous vaccine.

PASTERN FOLLICULITIS

Profile
A bacterial folliculitis and pyoderma of the pastern and coronet caused by *Staphylococcus aureus*, *S. hyicus* and possibly *S. intermedius*. The disease is a component of the 'greasy heel' syndrome (see p. 202).

Clinical signs
Usually limited to posterior of pastern and bulbs of the heels on one or more limbs (**Fig. 7.5**). Very early cases consist of papules which coalesce and produce large areas of ulceration and suppuration. Matting hair and oedema of the skin produce a swollen, painful exudative limb. Oedema may extend up the limb and deep spread of the infection can cause extensive cellulitis (diffuse, pyogenic infection of the connective tissues). The horse may exhibit lameness but systemic effects are usually absent.

Differential diagnosis
- Other forms of 'greasy heel' including:
  - Dermatophilosis
  - Mycetoma (deep dermal mycosis)
- *Fusobacterium* spp. cannon dermatitis
- Coronary band dystrophy/vitamin A deficiency
- Vasculitis (immune mediated or photoactivated)
- Pemphigus foliaceus
- Chorioptic mange (with self-trauma)
- Contact/irritant dermatitis

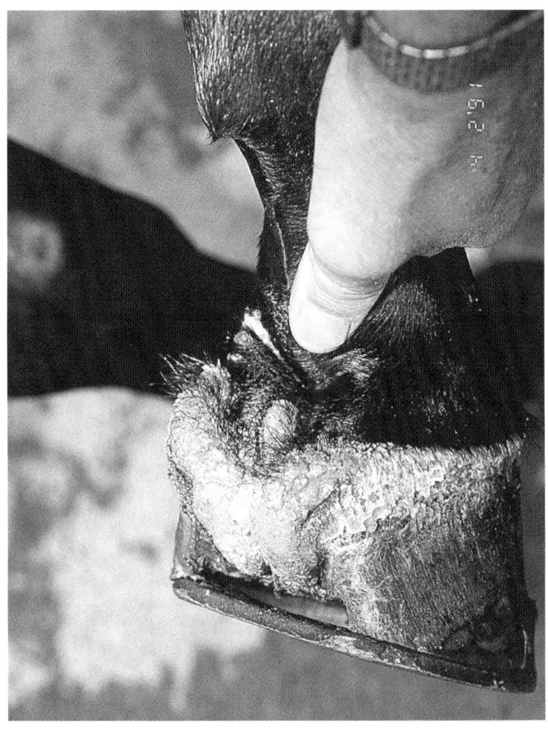

Figure 7.5 Pastern folliculitis. A mixed culture of *Staphylococcus aureus* and *S. hyicus* was obtained from swabs taken from biopsy specimens.

Diagnostic confirmation

- Typical clinical appearance
- Smears or culture of organism usually definitive but often produce mixed cultures of facultative pathogens and commensals.

Treatment

Effective treatment is usually a painful process – sedatives and analgesia may be needed in severe cases involving more than one limb. General anaesthesia may be worthwhile if the condition is extensive, very painful or involves more than one limb. The affected areas must be close-clipped, cleaned and scrubbed with chlorhexidine or povidone-iodine antiseptic soaps. Topical antibiotic creams can be useful but on their own are almost useless. Severe cases may need parenteral antibiotics based on sensitivity tests, but antibiotic delivery and penetration are unpredictable. Recovery is usually slow and difficult.

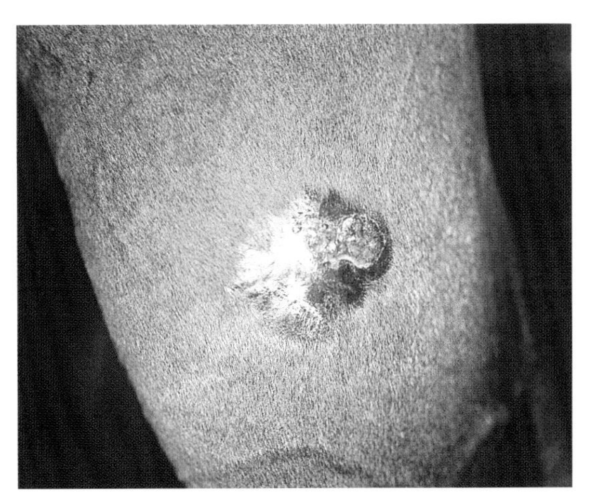

Figure 7.6 Bacterial granuloma (botryomycosis/staphylococcal pseudomycetoma) showing the typical non-healing indurated margins. The lesion showed an intermittent slight purulent discharge.

BACTERIAL GRANULOMA (BOTRYOMYCOSIS/STAPHYLOCOCCAL PSEUDOMYCETOMA

Profile

A pyogranulomatous disease most often associated with skin injury such as laceration, puncture or surgery. Most lesions occur on the limb or lip/chin regions. The clinical appearance is due to the formation of miliary interlinking microabscesses from *Staphylococcus* spp. infection. In spite of the name botryo*mycosis* there is no evidence of a fungal aetiology.

Clinical signs

A slow or non-healing wound with induration of the wound margins (**Fig. 7.6**) is typical. Chronic purulent discharge from one or more sinuses within the wound site is common.

Exuberant granulation tissue forming rosettes of complex granulation tissue and multiple microabscesses with sinuses may develop (hence the derivation *botryo-* meaning grape-like) (**Fig. 7.7**). Small yellow-white granules/grains may be visible in the purulent discharge. Tracking along lymphatic vessels sometimes occurs. It can reach large (or even enormous) proportions. The condition is seldom painful or pruritic. Affected horses do not often show systemic illness, but very large lesions can be debilitating.

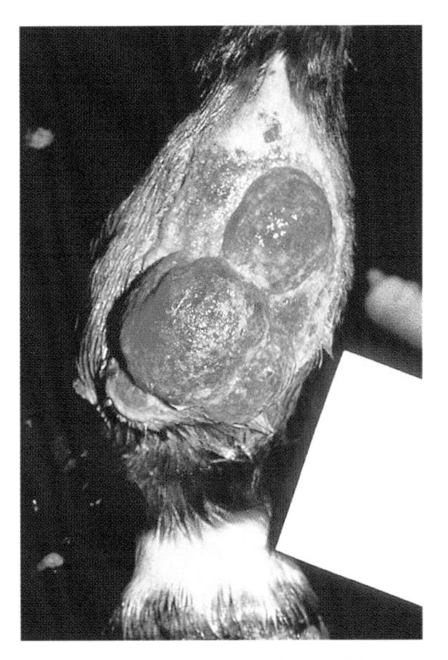

Figure 7.7 Bacterial granuloma (botryomycosis/staphylococcal pseudomycetoma) with multiple rosettes of pyogranuloma. *Staphylococcus aureus* was isolated from the multiple tracts and microabscesses which were found when the lesion was surgically removed.

Differential diagnosis

- Exuberant granulation tissue (from any other cause) (see Chapter 17, p. 217).
- Fibroblastic (and mixed) sarcoid at distal limb sites can be *very* similar.
- Foreign body/sequestrum resulting in a sinus tract and chronic inflammation.

- *Habronema musca* infestation of a wound.
- Bacterial fibrogranuloma.
- Pythiosis/deep fungal infections/fungal granuloma.
- Squamous cell carcinoma (of the face).

Diagnostic confirmation

- History of injury and failure of healing
- No response to normal therapeutic procedures
- Histopathology characteristic
- Culture from deep tissue biopsy samples

Treatment

Careful surgical excision with debridement of all affected tissue is always the preferred option. Other possible reasons for a non-healing wound must be established and if indicated these must be addressed (see p. 207). Oral potassium iodide or prolonged courses of antibiotics can provide useful assistance but cannot be relied upon solely. Relapses or recurrences following sufficiently aggressive initial treatment are unusual. Consideration should be given to early grafting of the resulting granulating wound to encourage rapid wound closure.

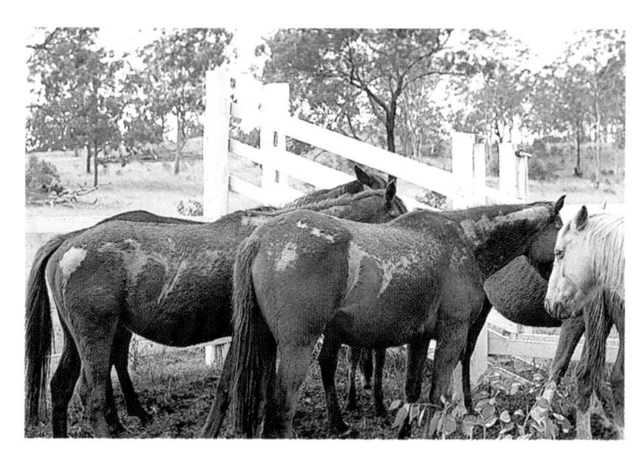

Figure 7.8 Dermatophilosis infection (*Dermatophilus congolensis*). The picture shows several horses with the lesions restricted to those areas which would be wetted by rain ('rain scald').

DERMATOPHILOSIS

Cont

Profile

One of the most important and commonest skin infections of the horse. Dermatitis caused by *Dermatophilus congolensis* characterized by exudation, matted hair with excessive scab formation and alopecia. Usually but not exclusively associated with prolonged moist conditions.[46]

Clinical signs

Two distinct syndromes are described but there is a marked overlap and there are many variations. The distribution of the lesions reflects the areas which are subjected to moistening or wetting by rain (**Fig. 7.8**) or by sweating under rugs, etc. The head, neck, dorsum and sides of the abdomen and thorax are most often affected. The condition can also be more localized to limited areas of the body such as the dorsum (**Fig. 7.9**) and the cannon region of the hind limbs in race horses.

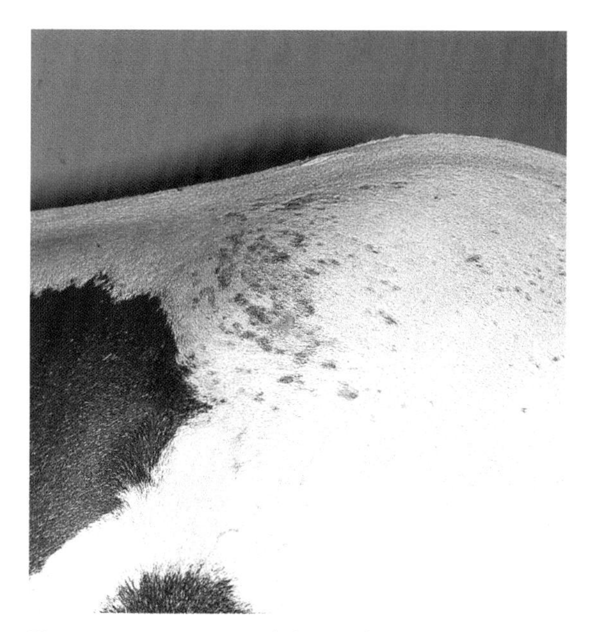

Figure 7.9 Dermatophilosis infection restricted to a limited area of the dorsum of a coloured horse.

General signs

Mild or severe, localized or generalized alopecia and crusting with little or no pruritus is typical. Severely affected horses may be lethargic and depressed with a poor appetite, weight loss, fever and enlarged lymph nodes.

Lesions on head and legs occur more prominently on white skin areas and can have severe erythema exacerbated by a type of photodermatitis associated with *D. congolensis* infection (**Fig. 7.10**).

Winter (long-coat) form Coat hair becomes matted with an underlying purulent exudate. Skin

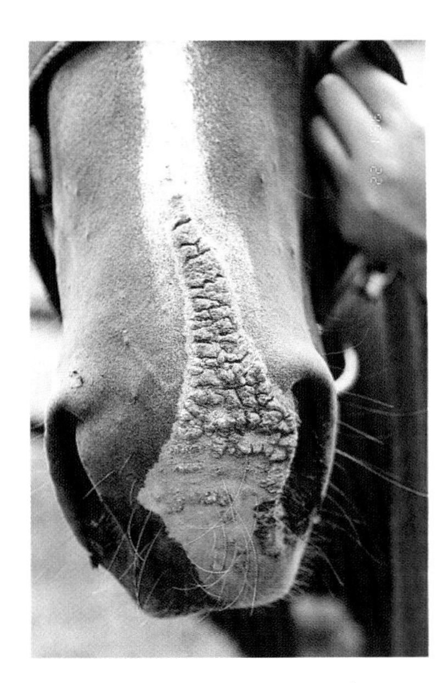

Figure 7.10 Dermatophilosis infection exacerbated by a type of photosensitization. Note that the damage is restricted and does not involve all of the nonpigmented skin. In such cases liver function must always be assessed carefully.

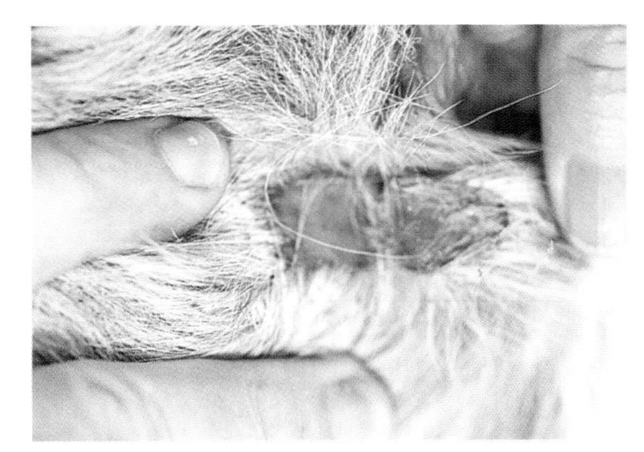

Figure 7.11 Dermatophilosis infection. Removal of a fresh scab reveals a 'pool' of pus and underlying silvery, hairless skin. The organism can easily be identified in the purulent material.

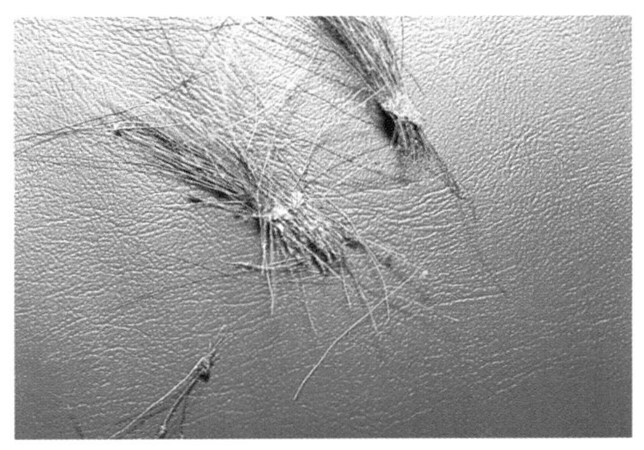

Figure 7.12 Dermatophilosis infection (chronic) showing typical 'paint-brush' dried exudate some way up the shaft of the hairs.

crusting and flaking occurs – the crusts are often better felt than seen and removal often removes hair as well. Most active lesions show a thick, glutinous, creamy, white-yellow or greenish pus adhering between the skin and the overlying scab. Removal of the scab reveals an eroded, ulcerated or bleeding purulent skin, typically with an ovoid shape and the base of the scab has a moist purulent appearance (**Fig. 7.11**). The undersurface of the plucked scab is often concave and has the hair roots protruding through the scab giving a characteristic 'paint brush' appearance (**Fig. 7.12**).

Moist eczematous lesions occur on foals kept in wet unhygienic stables and on the back of the pastern of older horses (part of the greasy heel syndrome) (**Fig. 7.13**).

Summer (short-coat) form Lesions tend to be smaller than the winter form with scabs comprising a few hairs embedded in a dried exudate which is often fixed some way up the hair shafts (see **Fig. 7.12**). Scabs are palpable as small 'shot-like' lumps (1–2 mm diameter) in the hair coat. Extensive superficial shedding of the hair coat is common imparting a 'moth-eaten' appearance. The coat is easily dislodged by grooming (even rubbing with a hand). Extensive areas can be involved. The palmar pastern area can also be affected by a dry scabbing and scaling dermatitis (**Fig. 7.14**) with firmly adherent scabs and crusts.

A distinctive clinical entity caused by the same bacterium occurs on the hind cannon of racehorses. The lesions are typical of the summer type dermatophilosis with closely placed small matted hair patches down the front of both hind cannons (**Fig. 7.15**). It is likely that this arises from exercise-induced trauma during training rather than racing as the grass is usually dry by the afternoon. It can also follow trauma through cinder or sand damage acquired during training or racing.

Differential diagnosis

- Papular dermatitis
- Dermatophytosis
- Larval nematode dermatitis

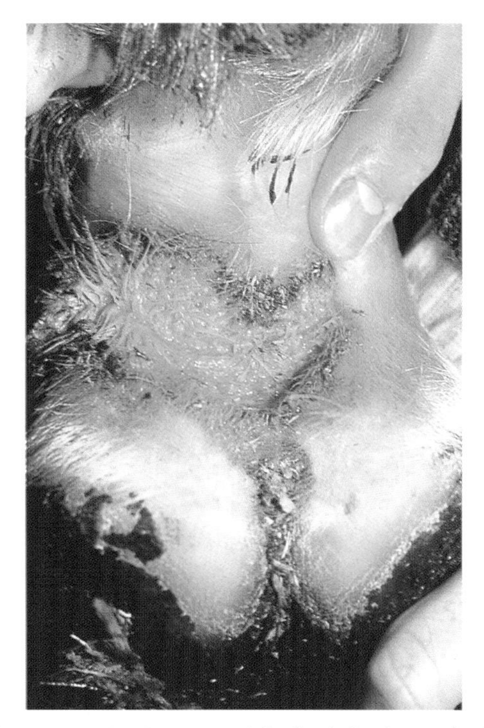

Figure 7.13 Dermatophilosis infection of the pastern region which is commonly known as 'mud rash'. Notice the marked inflammation and exudation associated with the most severe areas. The organism can readily be identified in direct smears from the area, but mixed infections (with *Staphylococcus* spp. and *Streptococcal* spp.) are common.

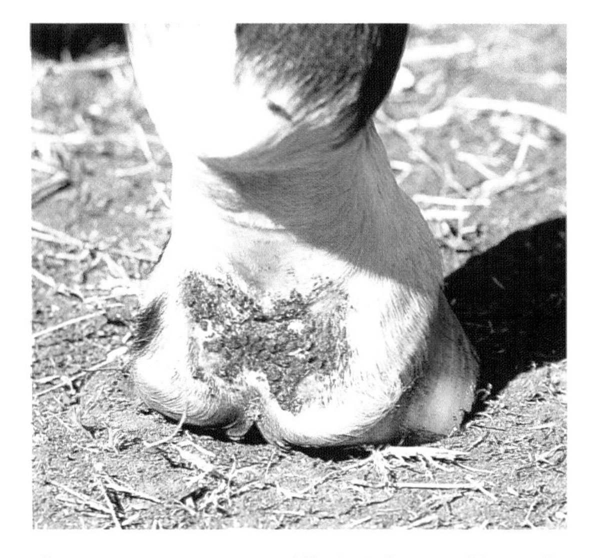

Figure 7.14 Dermatophilosis infection (chronic). Dried, matted and scabbed lesion over the bulbs of the heel and pastern.

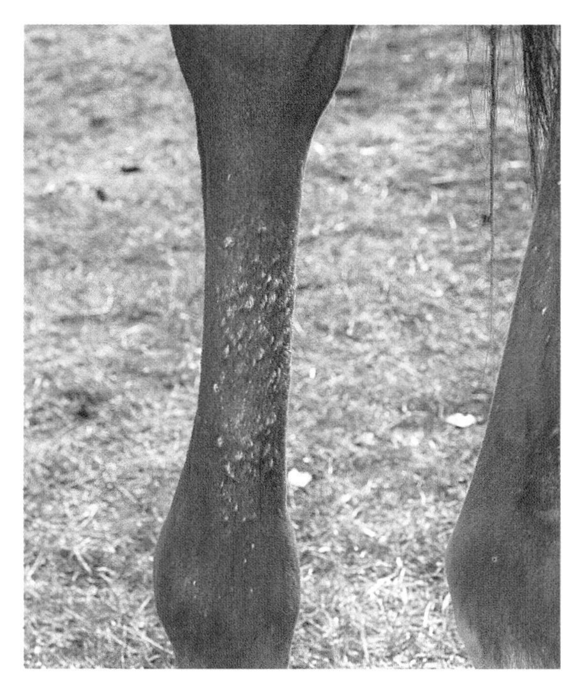

Figure 7.15 Dermatophilosis infection affecting only the dorsal aspects of the hind cannon skin which was attributed to traumatic damage from cinder track and wetting through long grass on the gallops.

- Chorioptic mange
- Sunburn/actinic dermatosis (facial and pastern forms)
- Rope/wire injury or other direct trauma (pastern forms)
- Pemphigus foliaceus
- Food allergy
- Alopecia areata
- Linear keratosis
- Sarcoidosis
- Pastern leukocytoclastic vasculitis
- Contact dermatitis
- Generalized granulomatous disease (enteritis)
- Pastern folliculitis
- Coronary band dystrophy
- Mercurial poisoning
- Scalding of skin (wound exudate, urine, (foal) diarrhoea)
- Anhidrosis

Diagnostic confirmation

- Clinical appearance of matted hair encased with exudate and protrusion of hairs is almost

pathognomonic. Lesions usually have well-defined anatomical distributions along the dorsum, lower limbs, face, back of the pastern and front of the hind cannons.
- Microscopic examination of a smear made from a fresh scab or fresh pus shows the typical branching 'rail-road' organism. The smears can be effectively stained with any of the commoner stains including Wright–Giemsa (Dif-Qik), Giemsa, methylene blue or Gram's stain (**Fig. 7.16**).
- Culture may require specialized treatment (see p. 26).

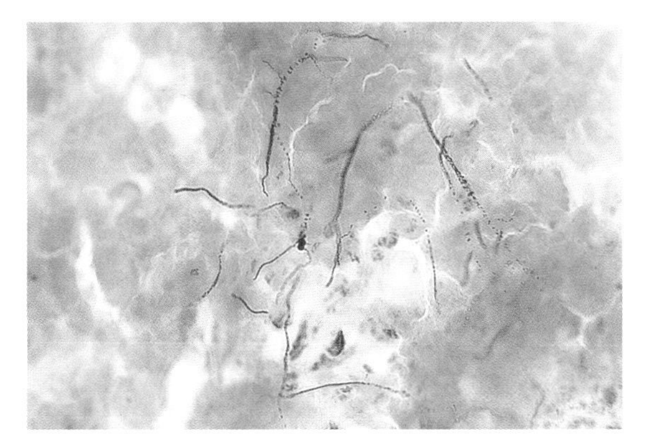

Figure 7.16 *Dermatophilosis congolensis*. Identified by Gram's stain on a smear taken from the purulent material under a scab. Higher magnification will reveal the railway-line appearance of the branching mycelial chains.

Local treatment

Affected areas on the body should be gently but thoroughly washed with chlorhexidine or povidone-iodine-based antiseptic washes (surgical scrub for example). Gentle soaking of the skin will allow removal of most of the crusts and scabs and infected debris. The skin should be dried very carefully (possibly with the help of hair dryers set at lower temperatures). *Following washing the skin must be kept dry.* Localized areas of dermatitis which may crack or exude serum can be treated with emollients containing antibiotics and (possibly) corticosteroids. White Lotion (zinc sulphate and lead acetate solution BPC) can be helpful for cracked and inflamed areas.

Daily application of 5% potassium permanganate in 0.5% brilliant green solution for 5 days is an effective and relatively cheap treatment for large areas. The solution can easily be dispensed in large volumes. It is safe, easy to use and has no irritant properties.

Alternative treatments for large areas include:

- Surgical scrub antiseptic soaps/scrub solutions (povidone-iodine, tertiary amine or chlorhexidine)
- 0.1% chloramine (a halamide disinfectant)
- 4% polyvinylpyrrolidine-iodine solution
- 4% povidone-iodine solution

Infections on white-skinned areas of the nose and legs may be associated with secondary photodermatitis and despite antibiotic treatment may continue to exhibit dermatitis due to sunlight exposure; stabling or protection of the area from sunlight is required and in many cases this is a significant benefit in reducing the wetting of the coat and limbs. A sunblock (factor 15 or higher) can be used on white skin in horses which have to be turned out.

Fetlock lesions Protective bandaging of the fetlock and cannon regions should not be used if possible except during exercise itself. Bandaging *must* be used with caution: it may increase the severity of the disease by keeping the skin moist and may also cut into the inflamed skin and induce even more exudation. Contact with wet bedding should be avoided. Chronic scarring occurs with prolonged infections. The skin weakens and becomes increasingly prone to re-infection. Secondary lameness can occur.

Systemic treatment

Parenteral penicillin administered daily for 3–5 days is sometimes helpful.

Systemic or local treatment of generalized infection in large groups of horses is not usually feasible. Under these conditions the horses should be housed to prevent skin wetting and most cases will gradually resolve over 3–6 weeks. Sunlight may hasten resolution in these provided that the skin can be kept dry. Further rain or wetting usually causes a recurrence of the disease. In severe cases, individual treatment becomes necessary. Individual treatments can be very difficult without facilities to prevent skin-wetting. Overtreatment with harsh antiseptics can lead to physical and chemical dermatitis as a complication of the original infection and must therefore be avoided.

Note: Infections on white-skinned areas of the nose and legs may be associated with a secondary photodermatitis and, despite antibiotic treatment, may continue to exhibit dermatitis due to exposure to sunlight. Stabling or protection of the affected area from sunlight is essential. Furthermore, primary or secondary exudative (photo- or other) dermatitis may act as a focus for replication of *Dermatophilus congolensis*.

All horses showing dermatitis limited to the white areas *must* be investigated for possible hepatic involvement or plant poisoning.

Control

Remove horse(s) from contact with wet grass and wet stables. Ensure that bedding is clean, nonirritating and dry. Keep the horse out of the rain. Avoid overgrooming of mildly affected horses and isolate cases. Clean/sterilize all grooming equipment and tack (consider formaldehyde fumigation or scrubbing/soaking with a tertiary amine disinfectant). Individual grooming kits are advisable, in any case, in stable yards.

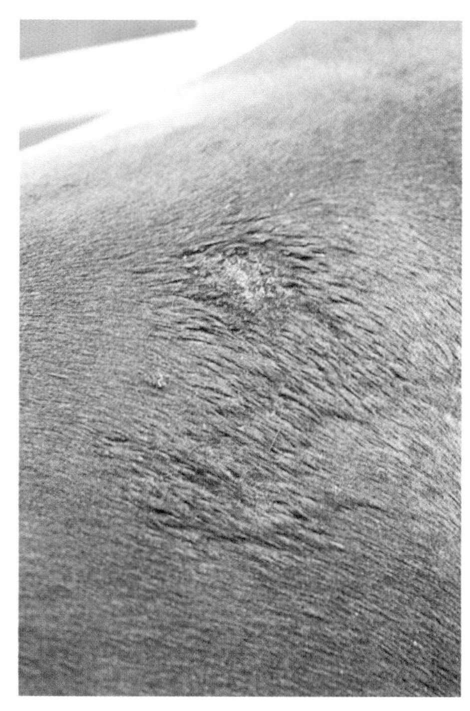

Figure 7.17 Staphylococcal dermatitis ('saddle rash') due to *Staphylococcus aureus* infection. The affected area of the saddle was extremely painful to the touch.

STAPHYLOCOCCAL DERMATITIS

Cont

Profile

A contagious bacterial disease which causes acute folliculitis, furunculosis and scab formation associated with painful skin lesions distributed primarily in areas of close tack or harness contact. Most cases occur in spring and early summer, possibly related to hair shedding, higher ambient temperatures and increasing work with dirty tack. *Staphylococcus aureus* and *S. intermedius* are the most frequent isolates from lesions.[47] *S. hyicus* has been isolated from some 'greasy heel'-type lesions of the pastern and coronet.

Clinical signs

Rapidly developing, localized, inflammatory, purulent skin lesion associated with severe pain rather than pruritus. Examination of the affected area is often markedly resented with avoiding behaviour (ducking, moving away or kicking/biting).

Small (1–2 mm) painful lesions rapidly coalesce to produce large areas of exudative dermatitis with surrounding oedema. Surface scabs and hair matting develop but little pus is present.

Lesions are principally associated with harness areas and saddle cloths and most commonly affect the skin of the back, saddle (**Fig. 7.17**), loins and chest and occasionally the distal limb regions.

Differential diagnosis

- Streptococcal folliculitis
- Dermatophilosis
- Dermatophytosis (*Trichophyton* spp.)
- *Corynebacterium pseudotuberculosis* infection
- Chemical/medicant (overstrength or inappropriate) irritation or burns
- Other causes of 'greasy heel' syndrome

Diagnostic confirmation

- History of unhygienic conditions, dirty tack and dusty stables
- Typical distribution of lesions
- Pain often marked
- Direct smear and culture from fresh lesions

Treatment

Close clipping and thorough cleaning of affected area with chlorhexidine (or povidone-iodine) soapy solutions (may be very painful and require sedative and analgesia). Washing with tertiary amine antiseptic (surgical scrub) solution is probably sensible. Autogenous vaccines may be useful if many horses are involved simultaneously but this has not been universally accepted as being effective.

Systemic or topical antibiotics have little effect. Thorough cleansing of all equipment and rugs, etc. is advisable.

Control

Isolate cases and avoid all indirect contact (grooming equipment and harness, etc.). Wash all equipment in tertiary amine disinfectant or fumigate with formaldehyde gas (see p. 37).

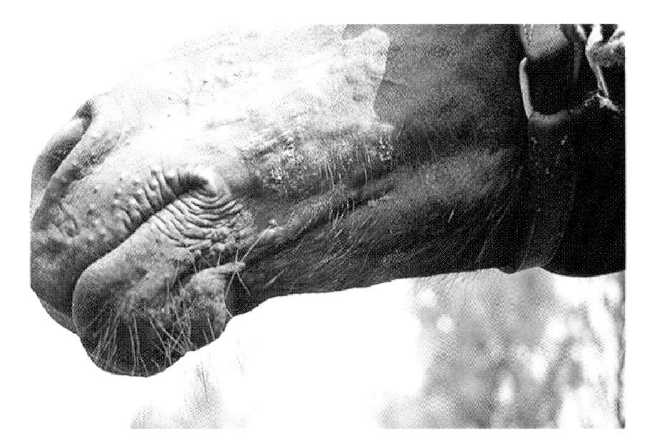

Figure 7.18 Streptococcal folliculitis (*Streptococcus equi* var. *equi*). The small pustular lesions were painful and there was little or no exudate.

STREPTOCOCCAL DERMATITIS/FOLLICULITIS

Cont

Profile

A highly contagious skin disease, particularly if caused by *Streptococcus equi equi* (strangles). Other cases may be caused by *Streptococcus equi zooepidemicus* or other streptococcal species. The typical lesions are folliculitis, furunculosis and ulcerative lymphangitis.

Clinical signs

Small, painful follicular infections around mouth (**Fig. 7.18**), vulva and wounds. May become generalized in cases of strangles (bastard strangles) and cause lymphadenopathy, abscess formation and very painful localized swellings with discharging abscesses along lymphatic vessels (**Fig. 7.19**). Loss of hair and serum exudation precede rupture of abscess.

Differential diagnosis

- Staphylococcal folliculitis
- Dermatophilosis
- Cellulitis (diffuse pyogenic infection of connective tissue)
- *Corynebacterium pseudotuberculosis* infection
- Glanders

Diagnostic confirmation

- Needle aspirate derived smear shows Gram-positive cocci. (Note that direct impression smears may be misleading with mixed commensal and opportunistic pathogens being detected.)
- Culture for *Streptococcus* spp. is characteristic.

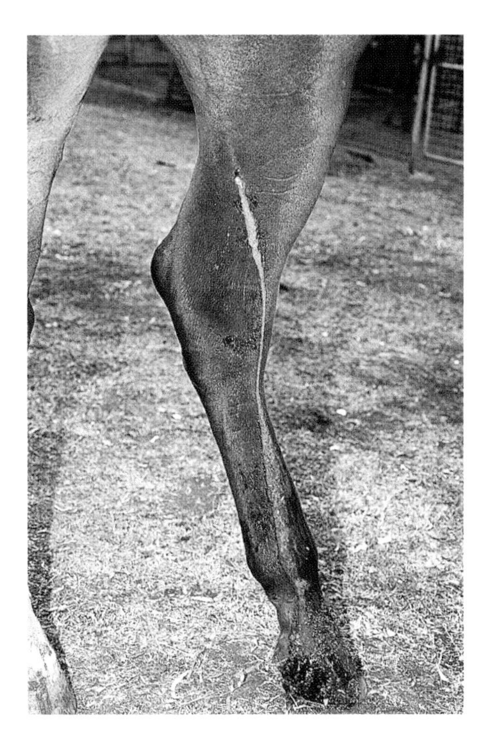

Figure 7.19 Streptococcal septicaemia (*Streptococcus equi* var. *equi*) was isolated in pure culture from this purulent material which drained from a small abscess associated with localized lymphangitis.

Treatment

Clip out area affected and clean with chlorhexidine (or povidone-iodine or tertiary amine) antiseptic (surgical) scrub solution. Lance and drain abscesses when mature (i.e. when overlying skin is thin and contents are fluid). Affected horses should be isolated until the infection has totally resolved. Value of prolonged treatment with intramuscular penicillin is controversial: 7–28 days is often required.

Note: Horses may develop an immune-mediated vasculitis and purpura haemorrhagica (see p. 180) or immune-mediated thrombocytopenic purpura or haemolytic anaemia some weeks later (particularly if challenged by a second infection cycle).[48,49] The secondary effects can be extremely serious and sometimes cannot be differentiated from drug eruptions and reactions.

GLANDERS ('Farcy')

Asi; Ind; Afr; MidEast – Cont; – REP

Profile

Glanders is a highly contagious frequently fatal disease of equidae (and others, including man) caused by *Pseudomonas* (*Malleomyces*) *mallei*. Man can be affected by direct contact or indirectly by contact with specimens or cultures of the organism. Mules and donkeys show more severe signs with a more acute course. The disease is characterized by formation of ulcerating nodules in the mucous membranes of the respiratory tract and internal organs. Nodules and ulcerating, discharging skin lesions which result from cutaneous lymphatic involvement is known as 'farcy'. The disease has been eradicated from large areas of the world by aggressive slaughter policies. Movement of animals from endemic areas is invariably strictly controlled.

Clinical signs

Skin lesions can occur at any site but are most common at sites of trauma such as the lateral aspect of the hind limbs and the neck (**Fig. 7.20**). Lesions start as subcutaneous nodules which ulcerate and discharge a characteristic honey-like secretion. Granulation, healing and cicatrization follow. Progressive spread up lymphatics causes cording, lymphangitis and regional lymphadenopathy. Draining lymph nodes and lymphatic nodules may abscessate, producing deep sinus tracts. Gross thickening of the limb(s) may occur.

Systemic signs of respiratory tract infections with mucopurulent (honey-like) nasal discharge with stellate nasal mucosal ulceration, cough, epistaxis and fever are present in most cases at some time or another.

General signs include malaise, poor exercise tolerance and weight loss.

The disease is invariably fatal eventually (often after a prolonged illness).

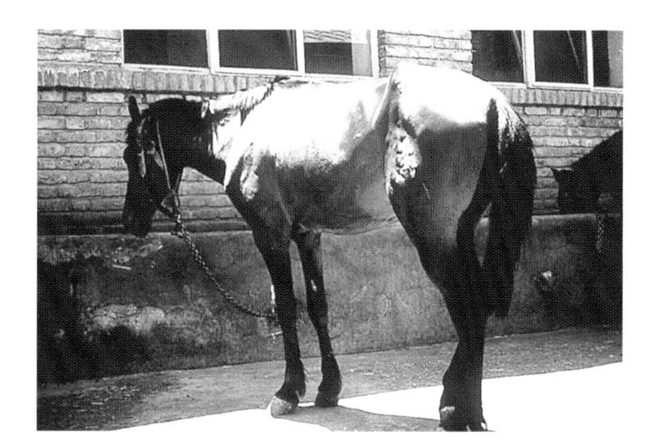

Figure 7.20 Glanders. Note the extensive ulcerative lymphangitis over the harness contact areas and the weight loss.

Differential diagnosis

- Sporotrichosis (*Sporothrix schenchii*)
- Epizootic lymphangitis (*Histoplasma farciminosum*)
- Ulcerative lymphangitis (*Corynebacterium paratuberculosis*)
- Respiratory tract infections (*Streptococcus equi equi*, etc.)
- Septicaemic (bastard) strangles (*Streptococcus equi equi*)
- Malevolent sarcoid
- Cutaneous histiocytic and generalized lymphosarcoma

Diagnostic confirmation

- Geographical region.
- Characteristic debility, nasal discharge and inability to work.
- Culture of Gram-negative, facultative anaerobic rods.
- Mallein (intradermo-palpebral) test is currently the best means of diagnosis in the living horse. Mallein (a purified protein derivative of killed *Pseudomonas mallei*) is injected intradermally into the lower eyelid about 1 cm from its margin. A marked painful swelling at the site after 24 and 48 hours, fever and an ocular discharge develop in affected horses. The test reflects the marked hypersensitivity of affected horses but some severely affected and debilitated horses may not show a clear positive test result.
- Complement fixation.
- Bacterial isolation.

The disease can be fatal to humans and extreme care must be taken in sampling suspect cases. The laboratory must also be warned of the special nature of the specimens so that appropriate precautions can be taken.

Treatment

None. The reportable nature of the disease makes treatment irrelevant. Death is almost inevitable but can take several months or even some years, during which suffering is considerable. No vaccines have been developed which are uniformly or acceptably effective. The disease remains a potential disaster for susceptible populations of horses and so movement from endemic areas is strictly controlled or forbidden.

ULCERATIVE LYMPHANGITIS

Cont

Profile

A mildly contagious disease characterized by lymphangitis of the lower limbs due to *Corynebacterium paratuberculosis*. The disease can affect horses of any age.

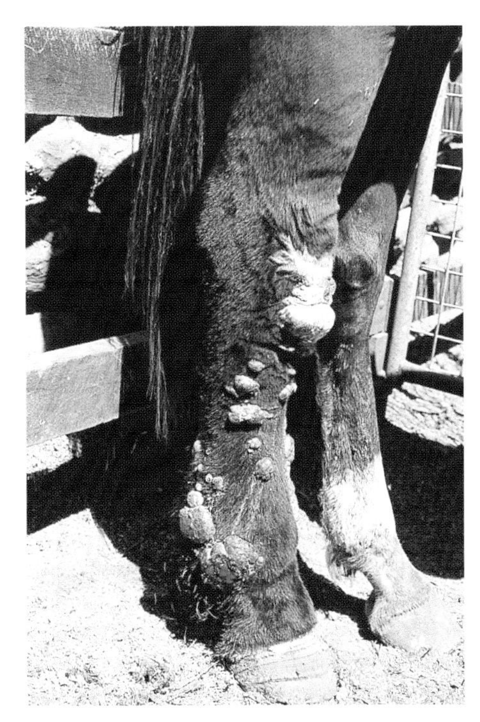

Figure 7.21 Ulcerative lymphangitis (chronic form). Extensive thickened and scarred lymphatic vessels and numerous ulcerative lesions. Note that the other limb is normal.

Clinical signs

Sudden onset of moderate to severe oedema of lower limb with swelling extending to elbow or stifle. Most often in hind legs and usually only one leg affected. Leg is painful but pain responses can be masked by the extensive limb bulk as a result of the oedema. Recurrences of the oedema are common. Serum exudate over the distal limb may occur with cording of the lymphatics of the proximal limb region. Ulceration and discharge of creamy, greenish pus occurs only occasionally. Multiple small, draining sores are characteristic of the disease especially in the United States (**Fig. 7.21**).

Differential diagnosis

- Sporotrichosis
- Mycetoma (deep mycosis)
- Systemic mycosis
- Enzootic lymphangitis
- Glanders
- Purpura haemorrhagica
- Staphylococcal abscess/cellulitis
- Wound healing failure/recurrent trauma
- Foreign body punctures, e.g. thistle and awns
- Cutaneous forms of lymphosarcoma
- Malevolent sarcoid

Diagnostic confirmation

- Clinical appearance is characteristic.
- Culture from exudate may give positive culture of *Corynebacterium pseudotuberculosis*, *Rhodococcus equi*, *Streptococcus* spp. or *Staphylococcus* spp.

Treatment

Depending on culture results, treat with appropriate antibiotics plus intravenous medication with 5 g sodium iodide daily for 7 or more days until signs of iodism occur (lacrimation and skin scaling). Repeated courses may be required. Chronic lymphatic nodules can be removed with elastic ligatures around the base of the swelling. The prognosis is very guarded as recurrences are common and treatment is difficult and rather nonspecific.

chapter 8

FUNGAL DISEASES

Trichophytosis	111
Microsporosis	113
Mycetoma	114
Phaeohyphomycosis	115
Sporotrichosis	116
Histoplasmosis (epizootic lymphangitis)	117
Fungal granuloma/pythiosis (phycomycosis)/basidiobolomycosis	117

TRICHOPHYTOSIS

Cont; Cont.bov;

Profile

Ringworm due to *Trichophyton* spp. is a highly contagious disease which affects horses of all ages. Younger horses are naturally less resistant and take longer to recover than older ones. Transmission is by direct or indirect contact with a source of infection.

The most common species are *Trichophyton equinum* var. *equinum* (TEVE), *T. equinum* var. *autotrophicum* (TEVA), and less commonly *T. verrucosum* (most often from cattle contact) and *T. mentagrophytes*[50, 51] (most often from rodent and cat contact). The spores are highly resistant to environmental destruction and may persist in stables and on tack, etc. for years. Most cases occur in winter months when horses are closely grouped and groomed heavily. Wet, warm weather has also been associated with outbreaks.

Infection relies upon the presence of active (live) spores and skin abrasion (even if very mild) and this is the reason for most lesions developing on girths and saddle friction areas.

Clinical signs

Early lesions appear as erect hairs in circular areas of 5–20 mm diameter (**Fig. 8.1**). Hair can easily be plucked from the site 10–12 days post-infection (**Fig. 8.2**). Hair loss also occurs naturally with prominent silvery scaling of the underlying healing skin (**Fig. 8.3**). The lesions expand centrifugally but may lose the circular appearance, becoming diffuse and ill-defined. Girth and shoulder/chest

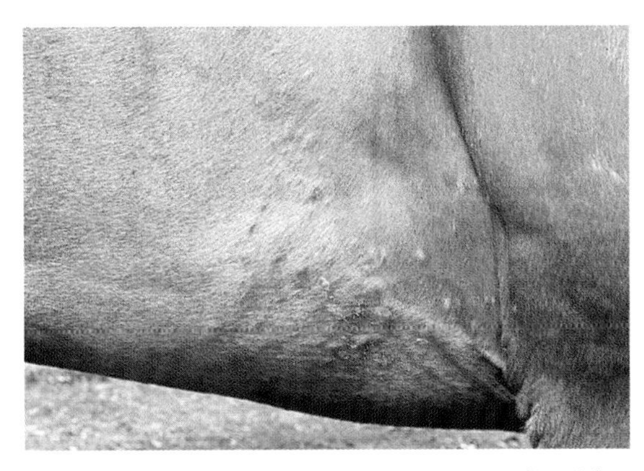

Figure 8.1 Ringworm. Early lesions of *Trichophyton equinum* var. *equinum* infection in the girth area (attributed to a contaminated girth some 5–7 days previously).

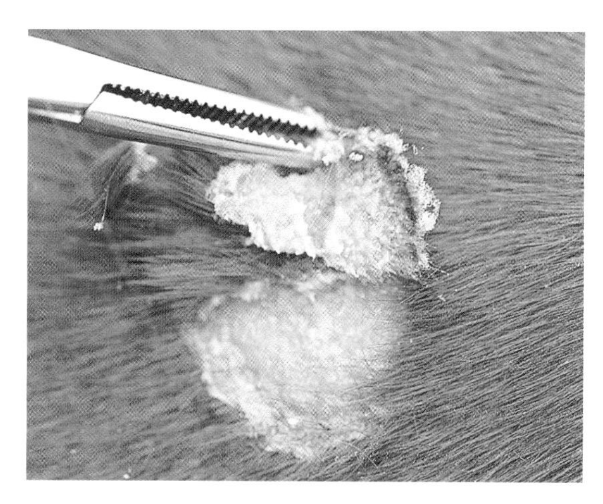

Figure 8.2 Ringworm. Removal of the hair in a mat at 10 days after natural infection with *Trichophyton equinum* var. *equinum*.

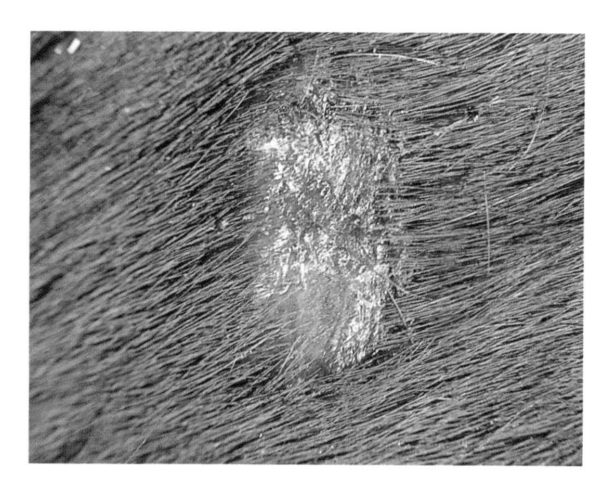

Figure 8.3 Ringworm. The typical silvery, slightly scaly appearance of a lesion due to *Trichophyton equinum* var. *autotrophicum* infection. The hair loss in this case occurred naturally and infection was considered to have arisen some 14 days previously.

wall areas are common sites owing to infection from contaminated girths, riding boots, etc. (**Fig. 8.4**). Generalized infections are also common, particularly in younger horses (**Fig. 8.5**).

Lesions are pruritic only in the early stages of infection; however, the horse can be irritable if lesions are 'picked' with a fingernail (when performing this test, due hygiene precautions must be taken for self-protection). This response persists even 5–10 days after treatment if the lesion is still infected and is a useful aid to diagnosis when the

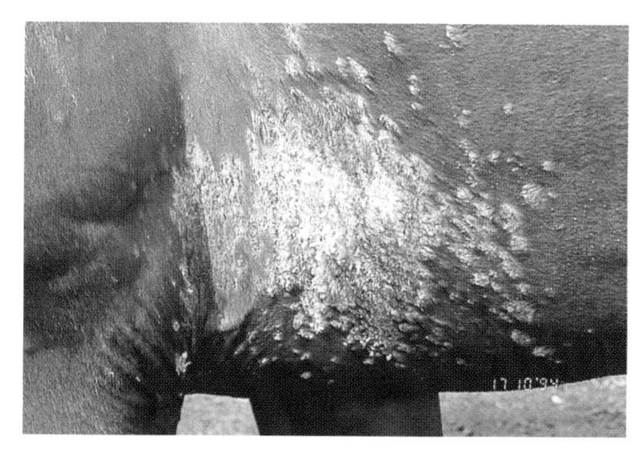

Figure 8.4 Ringworm. Diffuse infection with *Trichophyton equinum* var. *autotrophicum* in the girth and chest wall areas due to infection from contaminated girths and riding boots.

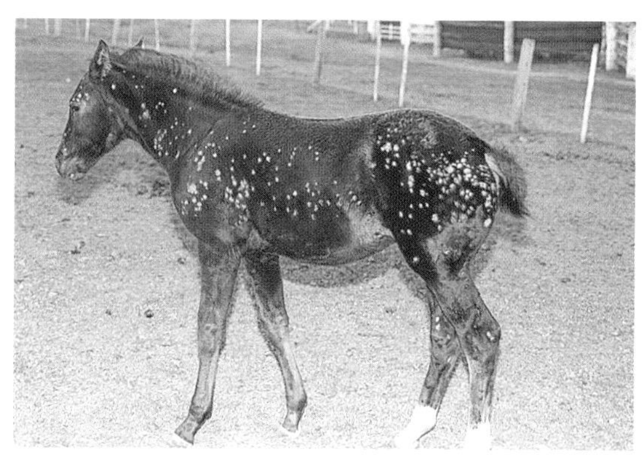

Figure 8.5 Ringworm. Generalized infection with *Trichophyton equinum* var. *autotrophicum* in a 6 month Warmblood foal.

hair has been shed and scale and scab are still present on the lesion. The healing lesions are usually markedly alopecic, smooth and silvery in colour. There may be secondary infection under the shedding scab with accumulation of purulent material.

Differential diagnosis

- *Microsporum gypseum* infection
- Dermatophilosis (*Dermatophilus congolensis*)
- Culicoides allergy/hypersensitivity (sweet itch)
- Insect bites and hypersensitivity
- Mite or louse infestation
- Sarcoidosis
- Granulomatous enteritis syndrome
- Alopecia areata
- Anhidrosis
- Actinic dermatitis

- Mercurial poisoning
- Wound/exudate/lachrymal scalding

Diagnostic confirmation

- Characteristic clinical signs and history of contact with infected horses (or other species).
- Hair plucking from fresh lesions examined microscopically after clearing with chlorolactophenol or 10% potassium hydroxide solution. Hyphae and relatively large endothrix spores will be seen. Staining with lactophenol cotton blue can assist the recognition of the hyphae.

It is not easy to be certain of the species of fungus involved without culture. Cultures of hair plucking on commercially prepared Sabouraud's agar at 25°C show characteristic colonies and change in colour of medium. For TEVE vitamin enrichment is important and this can be achieved by the addition of two drops of injectable vitamin B complex to the medium. The species can be confirmed from the colony and conidial spore characteristics.

Infected hairs do *not* fluoresce under ultraviolet light.

Treatment

Most cases will resolve spontaneously after 6–12 weeks (particularly if the horses are in sunshine).[52] Treatment does not shorten the course but may limit the spread of infection. Subsequent immunity can last for an extended period.

Treatment is directed at the use of fungicidal treatment of the horse and sporocidal treatment of the environment. The infected areas should be clipped (taking care to disinfect the clippers at regular intervals and particularly thoroughly after each horse). All horses in contact should be considered for treatment at the same time and access to sunlight should be encouraged. The horse(s) may be washed with a fungicidal wash such as enilconazole, natamycin or benzuldasic acid. Proprietary washes of these compounds are widely available. A 2% miconazole–2% chlorhexidine shampoo applied twice weekly has been shown to be effective in reducing the infectivity and so limiting an outbreak.[13] Some tertiary amine surgical scrub solutions have a strong antifungal (but limited sporocidal) effect. Spot treatment of lesions (with the above solutions or miconazole) is probably not very useful in the horse in view of the rapid spread across the horse. Individual lesions and the immediate surrounding hair may also be scrubbed for 1–2 minutes daily for 7–10 days with one of the following treatments:

10% povidone iodine solution
2.5% lime sulphur in water
10% thiabendazole in water
2.5–10% tincture of iodine (painted on, not scrubbed)
0.3% halamid
tertiary amine disinfectant scrub solution

Oral griseofulvin may be administered daily for 15–60 days[53] but the results of this alone are very variable and, in any case, it probably does not reduce the infectivity of the spores and fungus-laden hairs. It should therefore not be used alone except perhaps in grazing horses. The drug is teratogenic and must not be used in pregnant mares. There are no reports of its efficacy.

Control

Prevention of spread between horses is important. All scabs and infected hairs should be carefully removed and burned.

Appropriately diluted washes of antifungal drugs such as natamycin, potassium monopersulphate and enilconazole are particularly useful as a spray (or fumigant) for the environment and infected equipment – most have strong sporocidal effects and this will reduce the chances of re-infection or infection of unaffected horses. A number of modern disinfectants, including in particular the halogenated tertiary amines and inorganic peroxygen compounds, have potent antifungal effects and some are sporocidal. These should probably not be used on the horse unless appropriate instructions from the manufacturer are available.

The stable environment can be effectively disinfected by 'fogging' with potassium monopersulphate (using an industrial or horticultural fogging machine) or enilconazole distributed in the same fashion.[54]

Contaminated tack and other equipment may be washed in suitable fungicidal disinfectants, but these can be unreliable. Preferably, all tack and equipment should be fumigated with formaldehyde gas (see p. 37).

MICROSPOROSIS

Cont;

Profile

Ringworm due to *Microsporum gypseum*, *M. equinum* or *M. canis* (microsporosis) is less common than trichophytosis. The disease is highly contagious, being spread by direct and indirect contact with infected horses or contaminated equipment or environment. It can also be spread by biting insects and skin abrasion.[55] The organism can frequently be isolated from the soil or bedding over 6–12 weeks after infected horses have had access to it. The spores are probably very resistant to environmental conditions and may survive for years.

Clinical signs

Small hairless areas (alopecia), most commonly on the face and legs, but lesions may also follow the distribution of insect bites elsewhere (**Fig. 8.6**). Not

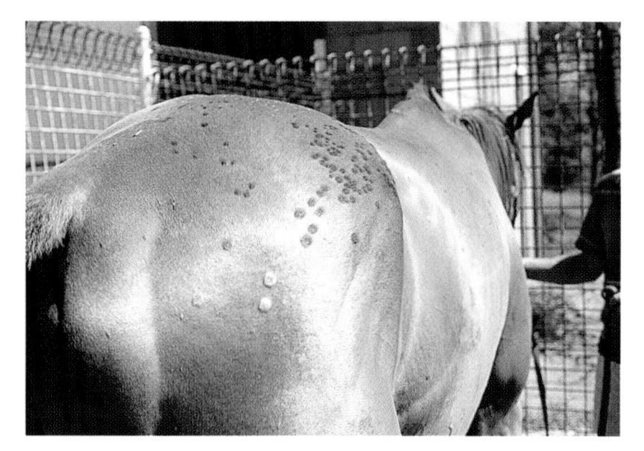

Figure 8.6 Ringworm. *Microsporum gypseum*-infected insect bites over the rump. Note that the pattern is consistent with biting flies. It was not possible to pluck the infected hairs easily.

all the hairs in a particular area will be equally affected and so, when a lesion is plucked, not all the hairs are shed. Plucking of the lesion is therefore often resented by the horse and plucking is often difficult. This effect is characteristic of microsporosis and is quite different from trichophytosis.

Some lesions are exudative and may even be overtly purulent as a result of secondary bacterial folliculitis. Lesions are not pruritic but are positive to a scratch test (i.e. the horse will respond to gentle scratching of the area) (when performing this test, due hygiene precautions must be taken for self-protection).

Differential diagnosis

- Trichophytosis
- *Stomoxys calcitrans* (stable fly) bites
- *Culicoides* spp. hypersensitivity (sweet itch)
- Mange mites
- Nymphal tick infestation
- Lice infestation (biting or sucking species)
- Onchocercal dermatitis
- Occult sarcoid
- Chemical irritation
- Alopecia areata

Diagnostic confirmation

- Clinical appearance of lesions in patterns according to the transmission method.
- *M. equinum* and some *M. canis* isolates may fluoresce under ultraviolet light (Wood's lamp). *M. gypseum* does *not* fluoresce.
- Hair samples should be examined after clearing with warm chlorolactophenol or 10% potassium hydroxide. Single or chains of ectothrix spores and hyphae may be seen.
- Culture of hair plucking on commercially prepared indicator Sabouraud's agar show characteristic colonies and conidial spores with characteristic colour change.

Treatment

Treatment is as for trichophytosis (above) but the response to both systemic (oral) griseofulvin and topical antifungal/fungicidal washes is significantly slower and more variable. However, again the disease will ultimately resolve spontaneously (usually after 4–12 weeks).

Control

As for trichophytosis (above). Removal of affected horses from contaminated yards after treatment is probably advisable, but the organism appears to have less resistance to environmental factors and so, by contrast to trichophytosis, may not appear annually.

Disinfection of the stable and all equipment and tack is important and again formaldehyde gas is probably the most reliable method.

MYCETOMA

NAm; Aus; Eur(Spain); Afr

Profile

True eumycotic mycetomas are caused by fungal contamination of wounds by free-living (soil and plant) fungi. The fungi cause chronic subcutaneous infections characterized by tumour-like lesions with extensive sinus tracts and fistulae. They commonly have granular components (so-called 'kunkers'). The most common fungi are *Curvularia geniculata* and *Pseudoallescheria boydii*. The former produces a very dark lesion known as a black-grained mycetoma,[56,57] while the latter produces a white-grained mycetoma. *Altenaria* spp. are also liable to produce small granulomas at the sites of contaminated skin injuries.

Actinomycotic mycetomas are due to such bacteria as *Actinobacillus* spp., *Nocardia* spp. *and Actinomyces* spp. and so are not strictly mycetomas.

Clinical signs

Ulcerating nodules on limbs, head or ventral abdomen with cording of lymphatic vessels. Lesions show a chronic seropurulent discharge from granulating ulcers. The condition is accompanied by mild pruritus. Some asymptomatic nodules, similar in appearance to papilloma but black or dark in colour, covered by ulcerated hairless skin may be present.[58] Biopsy of the excised lesion readily identifies the unusual but characteristic colour and consistency of the lesions (**Fig. 8.7**).

Differential diagnosis

- Pythiosis (*Pythium* spp.)
- Basidiobolus infection (*Basiodiobolus haptosporus*)
- Sporotrichosis (*Sporothrix schenkii*)
- Glanders/farcy (*Pseudomonas mallei*)
- Ulcerative lymphangitis
- Pastern folliculitis
- Nodular and malevolent sarcoid
- Melanoma

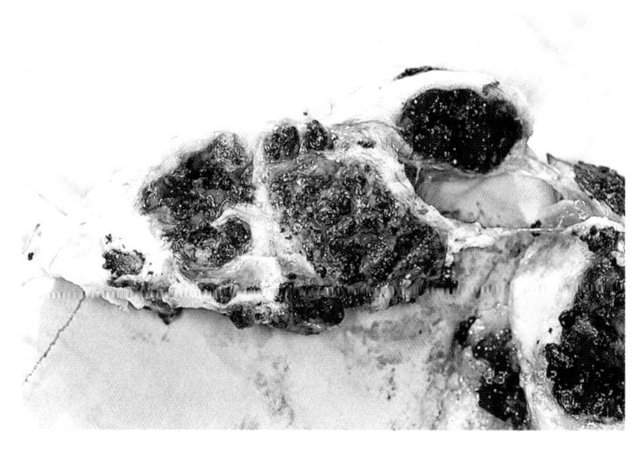

Figure 8.7 Black-grained mycetoma (due to *Curvularia geniculata*). Surgically removed from the skin of a horse in northern Australia.

Diagnostic confirmation

- Restricted geographical area.
- Physical examination is suggestive.
- Biopsy is required for confirmation.
- Isolation and culture of *Curvularia geniculata* or *Pseudoallescheria boydii* from deep within nodules or from biopsy.

Treatment

Some response to aggressive surgical removal of affected nodules, but recurrence is common. Oral potassium iodide (5–10 g twice daily by mouth) for 3–6 weeks may improve the condition. Antibiotics are largely ineffective and systemic antifungal drugs are prohibitively expensive and only marginally effective.

PHAEOHYPHOMYCOSIS

Asia; Aus; NAm; Eur

Profile

A chronic subcutaneous and systemic fungal disease with small, multiple subcutaneous nodules, caused in tropical countries by *Drechslera spicifera*.[59] It differs from mycetoma (above) in that the hyphae remain discrete and do not aggregate into nodules. The fungus gains access to the skin via wounds. In temperate climates a similar condition (which may be indistinguishable from phaeohyphomyocosis can occur (most often on the head and ears) from deep and chronic infection with a variety of less pathogenic fungi including *Alternaria* spp.

Clinical signs

Small, black or darkly coloured, denuded plaques and nodules primarily containing papules and pustules or multiple fibrotic subcutaneous nodules on the sides of the neck, body (**Fig. 8.8**) and limbs. The lesions can, however, occur at any site.

Differential diagnosis

- Eosinophilic granuloma
- Cutaneous collagen necrosis complex
- Molluscum contagiosum
- Mixed and nodular sarcoid
- Cutaneous lymphosarcoma
- Melanoma
- Insect bite reactions

Diagnostic confirmation

- Biopsy is essential (fungal elements may be identified directly on sections).

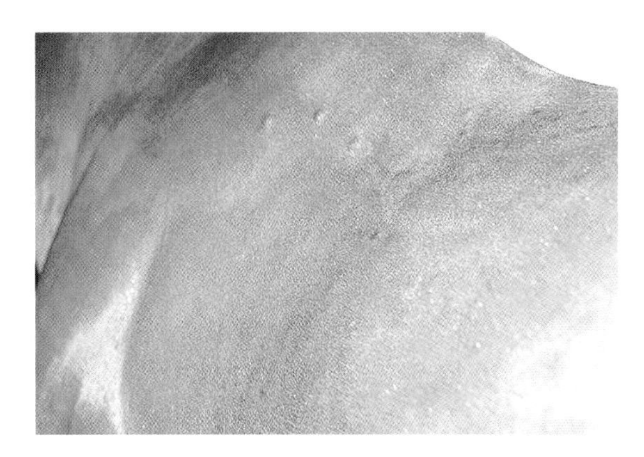

Figure 8.8 Phaeohyphomycosis. Multiple fibrotic subcutaneous nodules on the sides of the body. *Drechslera spicifera* was isolated from an excised lesion.

- Culture and identification of *Drechslera spicifera* from the deepest regions of the biopsy specimen on Sabouraud's dextrose agar (without anti-biotic additions). Initially the colony grows rapidly and is white-grey but soon changes to a brown-black colour.

Treatment
Treatment is likely to be prolonged and even in mild cases only marginally effective. Systemic iodide therapy (sodium iodide at 40 mg/kg as a 20% solution by slow intravenous injection once daily for 3–5 days then orally until cured or 5–10 g twice daily of potassium iodide by mouth until signs of iodism appear or a cure is achieved) may be partially effective. Amphotericin B or ketoconazole therapy may also be useful. Topical application of etisazole in dimethyl sulphoxide (DMSO) can be effective.[60]

SPOROTRICHOSIS

Eur; Ind; NAm –

Profile
A chronic, progressive, sporadic infection of skin and subcutaneous/lymphatic tissue caused by *Sporothrix schenckii*. Infection is usually introduced through small skin wounds.[60]

Clinical signs
Firm, well-demarcated, painless, subcutaneous nodules (1–5 cm diameter) associated with 'corded hardened lymphatics' most commonly on the lower limb regions (fetlock particularly). Ulceration of surface of nodules with creamy, white-grey, purulent discharge and surface encrustation and scabbing (**Fig. 8.9**). Remarkably, the regional lymph nodes are seldom involved. Repeated episodes over some months result in lymphatic cording (lymphangitis) in some cases only.

Differential diagnosis
- Ulcerative (bacterial) lymphangitis *(Corynebacterium paratuberculosis)*
- Epizootic lymphangitis (*Histoplasma farciminosum)*
- Glanders (*Pseudomonas mallei*)
- Mycetoma
- Malevolent sarcoid
- Cutaneous histiocytic lymphosarcoma and lymphoma

Diagnostic confirmation
- Characteristic cording and nodules on lymphatic vessels.
- Gram stain of exudate from impression smear.
- Culture on Sabouraud's agar.
- Biopsy is not usually diagnostic.

Treatment
Systemic iodide therapy (sodium iodide at 40 mg/kg as a 20% solution by slow intravenous injection once daily for 3–5 days then orally until cured or 10 g of potassium iodide daily by mouth until signs of iodism appear). Topical iodine applied to ulcerated lesions has also been used.

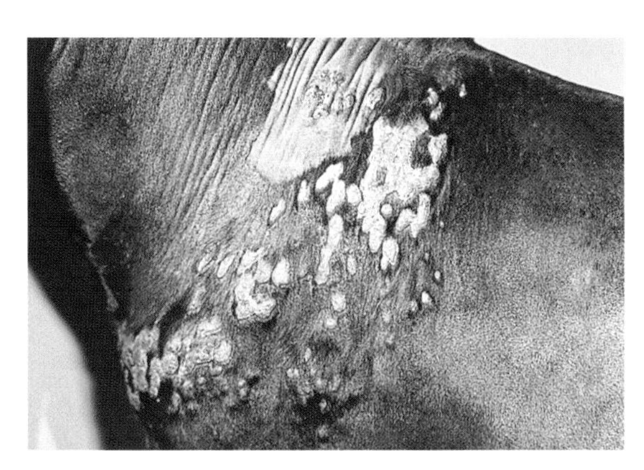

Figure 8.9 Sporotrichosis. Note the skin and subcutaneous/lymphatic nodules caused by *Sporothrix schenckii* infection of small wounds at sites of skin abrasion from harness.

Iodine therapy is the only available and useful medical approach. The value of amphotericin B is uncertain. Surgical removal of affected nodules can be performed and can be effective in limiting the disease.

HISTOPLASMOSIS (epizootic lymphangitis)

Afr; Asia; Eur – Cont;

Profile

A rare, chronic contagious disease due to *Histoplasma farciminosum* characterized by suppurative lymphangitis primarily affecting the hind legs and neck, lips and other areas where harness abrasions occur. It is also known as African farcy, pseudoglanders or equine cryptococcosis. Its geographical distribution is very restricted to limited areas in a few countries.

Clinical signs

Gross enlargement and inflammation of cutaneous (and other) lymphatic vessels with lymphadenitis. Skin ulceration along corded lymphatics with a 'mouldy' odour from lesions (**Fig. 8.10**). Most cases have no systemic signs, but the disease can affect the nasal cavity, lungs, pleural cavity, eyes and joints, which makes it clinically very similar to glanders. However, the absence of significant systemic signs readily differentiates this from glanders. Ocular histoplasmosis affects the conjunctiva and skin of the periorbital region; it is commoner in donkeys than horses.

Differential diagnosis

- Glanders
- Ulcerative lymphangitis
- Sporotrichosis
- Malevolent sarcoid
- Cutaneous lymphosarcoma

Diagnostic confirmation

- Direct impression smears from discharging lesions
- Biopsy and culture from biopsy on Sabouraud's agar with very slow growth over 2–3 weeks

Treatment

Not usually attempted with slaughter policies in force to control the spread of the condition. Some horses recover spontaneously and are then solidly immune.

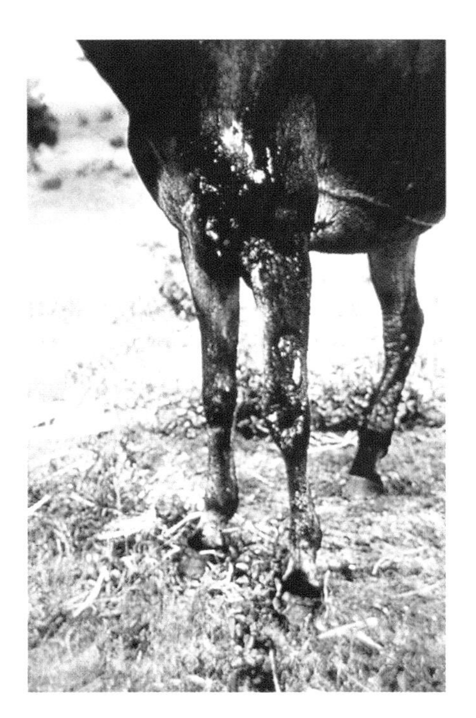

Figure 8.10 Histoplasmosis (epizootic lymphangitis) due to *Histoplasma farciminosum.*

FUNGAL GRANULOMA/PYTHIOSIS (phycomycosis)/basidiobolomycosis

Aus; NAm; SAm – Cont

Profile

A chronic subcutaneous fungal, ulcerative granulomatous skin disease caused by *Pythium insidiosum* occurring in subtropical and tropical areas and affecting horses of all types and ages and both sexes. Also called bursatti, Florida horse leeches and swamp cancer. The fungi are actively drawn to sites of tissue damage and wetting. Lesions most commonly occur on the limbs, abdomen, neck, lips and nasal margins and cases rarely show systemic involvement.

Basidiobolus haptosporus causes a similar disease to pythiosis but is confined to head and abdomen; no leg lesions have been recorded.

Clinical signs

Pythiosis Ulceration of skin or wound with pruritus manifest as biting and kicking at affected area(s). Dense granulation tissue containing masses of yellow-grey necrotic tissue which is sometimes calcified (known as 'kunkers'). The lesions (which are most often single and unilateral) may expand

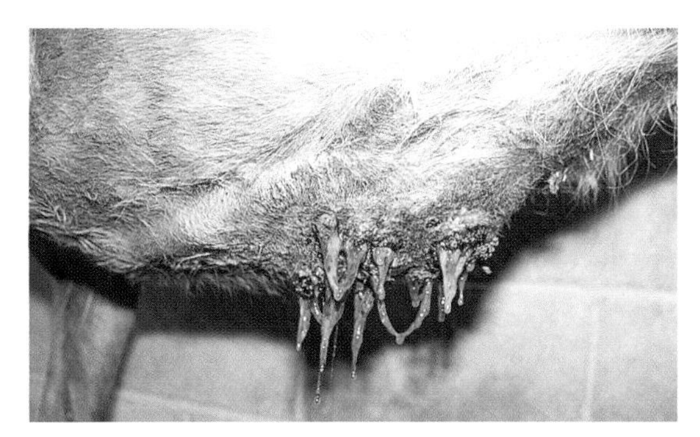

Figure 8.11 'Florida leeches' on the ventral abdomen. The subcutaneous fungal, ulcerative granulomatous lesions were caused by *Pythium insidiosum.*

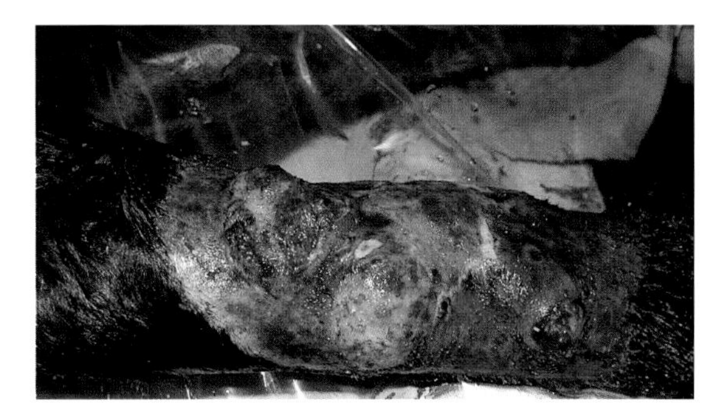

Figure 8.12 Pythiosis. Typical lymphangitis with swelling and oedema of the leg. Lymphadenopathy was present in the inguinal and iliac lymph nodes.

dramatically over a short period, reaching a very large size. Characteristic sticky, stringy serosanguinous discharge which either mats into the hair or hangs from body wall in thick mucopurulent strands (**Fig. 8.11**). Lymphangitis with swelling and oedema develop in chronic cases primarily on legs (**Fig. 8.12**) and ventral abdomen. Joints and tendons may be involved with chronic discharging sinus formation. Lymphadenopathy may occur if the fungal elements gain access to the draining nodes.

Basidiobolomycosis As for pythiosis but growths are more shallow and confined more to the neck and abdomen (**Fig. 8.13**) with no limb lesions.

Differential diagnosis

- Sarcoid (particularly if recurrent interference)
- *Habronema musca* infestation in wounds

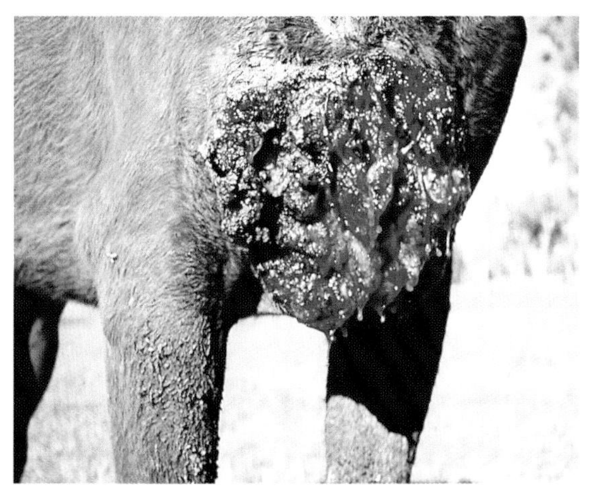

Figure 8.13 Basidiobolomycosis. Severe case with extensive shallow ulceration and exudation confined to brisket and base of the neck. There were no limb lesions.

- Neoplasia (including cutaneous lymphosarcoma)
- Mycetoma
- Botryomycosis (staphylococcal pyogranuloma)
- Exuberant granulation tissue (from any cause)
- Indolent or non-granulating wounds

Diagnostic confirmation

- *Pythiosis* usually has a history of access of horses to water-logged pasture or lagoon creeks; *basidiobolomycosis* occurs more in dry conditions with the organism probably living in the soil.
- Clinical appearance of characteristic mucopurulent strings and 'kunkers' in exudate or in cut surface of lesion.
- Biopsy (collected into 10% formol saline) shows increased collagen and intense eosinophilic infiltration.
- Fungal culture on Sabouraud's agar (using a fresh sample sent on ice) from early lesions identifies organisms responsible.

Treatment

Early treatment is essential as the prognosis is poorer in chronic cases. Surgical excision of the tumour under general anaesthesia is the most common and successful treatment, particularly in chronic cases.[47,62–64] Complete removal of all affected tissue is essential if recurrences are to be avoided. Surgery should be performed again as soon as any new lesions develop (usually manifest as 1–5 mm diameter dark red or black spots). Surgery requires extreme caution on the limbs in particular and iodine-soaked pressure bandages should be applied after excision is complete. Repeat surgery is commonly required when the lesions occur around tendons and joints.

Intravenous sodium iodide[65] is a useful adjunct to surgery. Amphotericin B[66] administered intravenously once daily and topically. For i.v. administration, amphoteracin B is available as vial containing 50 mg lyophilized amphotericin B. The required dose is dissolved in 1 litre of saline and infused intravenously slowly over 1 hour. Intravenous treatment is well tolerated at an average daily dose starting at 0.3 mg/kg rising to 0.6 mg/kg on day 3 and then every other day for the required time (10–80 days). For local treatment of the wound site or fresh lesions: 50 g amphotericin B in 10 ml sterile water + 10 ml dimethyl sulphoxide (DMSO) on a gauze dressing daily for at least 1 week.

Significant benefit may be obtained by surgically removing the bulk of the fungal growth, followed by daily intravenous and topical administration of amphotericin B, with periodic extirpation of small necrotic tracts as necessary. Some strains of *Pythium* have shown resistance to amphotericin B.[67]

Vaccination may provide therapeutic and prophylactic effects[68,69] but vaccines are not manufactured or available commercially and need to be prepared by a suitably qualified laboratory.

Prognosis

Successful treatment depends on the age and physical condition of the horse, previous treatment, age/size/site of the lesion and whether there is bony involvement. Young fresh lesions of 2 weeks' duration respond well to immunotherapy alone. Older lesions respond poorly and all reported cases with bone involvement have died.[70]

chapter 9

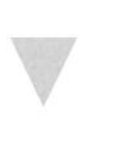

PROTOZOAL DISEASES

Besnoitiosis	121
Dourine (*Trypanosoma equiperdum*)	122

BESNOITIOSIS

Afr; NAm – Cont

Profile

A host-specific protozoal disease due to *Besnoitia besnotii*, or in donkeys *B. benettii*, acquired by ingestion of feed contaminated with cat faeces, or by bites from bloodsucking insects and parenteral injection of blood from acute cases. Horses and donkeys have been reported affected in South Africa and North America.[71,72]

Clinical signs

Exercise intolerance and bilateral nasal discharge.[73] Chronic, pruritic, alopecic dermatitis with generalized thickening and lichenification of the ventral abdominal skin from sternum to scrotum or neck and withers (**Fig. 9.1**) is characteristic of the disease. Multiple papules may be present in subcutis of perineum and abdominal area. The hair is sparse and the skin is inclined to crack and ooze. The worst lesions are usually around the fetlock.

Other signs include an enlarged oedematous prepuce in males. Small nodules may be present on sclera, soft palate, pharynx and larynx.

Differential diagnosis

- Dourine (*Trypanosoma equiperdum*)
- *Culicoides* spp. hypersensitivity (sweet itch) and ventral biting *Culicoides* spp. hypersensitivity
- Equine viral arteritis
- Sarcoidosis
- Lymphosarcoma
- Glanders

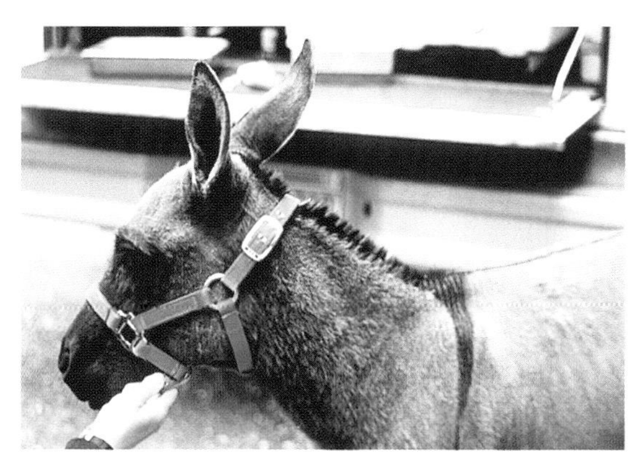

Figure 9.1 *Besnoitia benettii* infection causing extensive dry scaling and thickening of the skin over the withers and neck.

Diagnostic confirmation

- Biopsy reveals spherical *Besnoitia* cysts in dermis with interstitial fibrosis and a chronic plasma cell exudate.[74]

Treatment

Prolonged courses of potentiated sulphonamide (trimethroprim/sulfadiazine) by mouth or injection may help significantly but there are too few reports to provide a definitive treatment.

Prevention

Prevent cat or rodent contact with feedstuffs. If biting insects are present, use insect screens around infected animals.

DOURINE (*Trypanosoma equiperdum*)

Afr; Ind; SAm – Cont

Profile

A venereal protozoal disease with cutaneous manifestations caused by *Trypanosoma equiperdum*. The disease occurs in limited areas of Africa, the Middle East, South America and Asia. Horses have been reported affected in South Africa. The disease has been eradicated from large areas of the world including Europe and North America.

Clinical signs

Insidious onset following prolonged incubation period after infective coitus. Venereal signs are most prominent with swelling of the male and female external genitalia. Characteristic (pathognomonic) 'silver dollar' dermal plaques (2–10 cm diameter) may develop in some cases[74] (**Fig. 9.2**). They develop first in the perineum and then at any site on the skin, with most obvious lesions on the flanks. Plaques are oedematous ('pit' on pressure) and individual lesions may last for hours or weeks. Enlarged oedematous penis and prepuce in male with purulent urethritis.

Weight loss, loss of performance and terminal paralysis after progressive lameness and gluteal muscle atrophy.

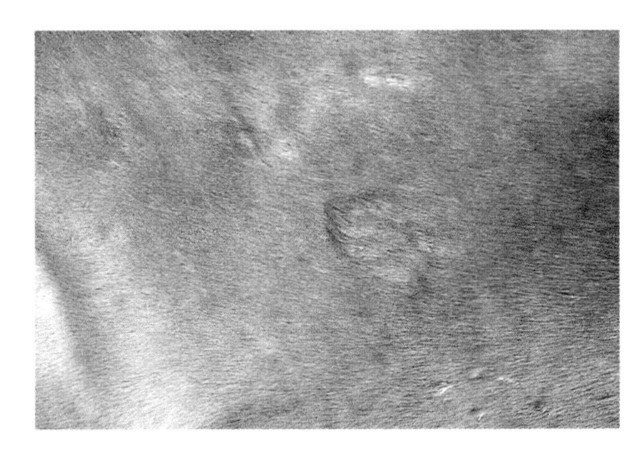

Figure 9.2 Dourine. Characteristic (pathognomonic) 'silver dollar' dermal plaques (2–10 cm diameter) which developed 4 weeks after an infected coitus. Typical systemic and genital signs were obvious. An impression smear taken from the lesion revealed countless trypanosome parasites.

Differential diagnosis

- Urticaria
- Insect bites
- Equine viral arteritis
- Lymphosarcoma
- Rabies (progressive hind-limb and other ascending neurological signs)

Diagnostic confirmation

- History and geographic location.
- Impression smears and sheath washings reveal characteristic *T. equiperdum* organism (characteristic movement can be seen with wet hanging drop preparation under low power).
- Inoculation of blood from infected horse into splenectomized or SCID mice.
- Complement fixation test (CFT).

Treatment

Quinapyramine sulphate or diminazene aceturate can be used but are also very dangerous.

Prevention

Eradication by control of breeding in endemic areas, quarantine and slaughter of infected horses. CFT is used to control importation of the disease into nonendemic areas.

chapter 10

METAZOAN/ PARASITIC DISEASES

Chorioptic mange (leg and tail mange)	123
Psoroptic mange	124
Sarcoptic mange	126
Demodectic mange (demodicosis)	126
Trombiculidiasis (scrub itch/chigger/ harvest mite infestation)	127
Poultry red mite	128
Stickfast or stick-tight fleas	129
Culicoides spp. irritation	130
Ventral midline dermatitis	131
Hypodermiasis (warble fly infestation)	132
Insect bites or stings	133
Myiasis	136
Pediculosis (louse infection)	137
Habronemiasis	139
Parasitic/verminous dermatitis	141
Onchocercal dermatitis (Onchocerciasis/ microfilariasis)	141
Oxyuriasis (pin worm) infestation	143

CHORIOPTIC MANGE (leg and tail mange)

Cont

Profile

A dermatological disease caused by infestation with *Chorioptes equi* which primarily affects the distal limb regions but can extend to abdomen, axilla and groin. It is commonest in winter months in housed heavy breeds with dense feathering on the legs but thin-skinned horses can be affected severely. Carrier horses showing no clinical signs of infestation serve to perpetuate the infection from season to season. The condition is part of the greasy heel syndrome (see p. 202).

Clinical signs

Pruritus, irritation and restlessness with foot stamping and biting at legs are prominent signs (**Fig. 10.1**). Stabled horses are more liable to the infestation, with some remission over grazing periods (although it is likely that these cases remain carriers). The affected horse seeks every opportunity to rub against or kick on posts, fences, concrete steps, walls and rails. Affected groups of horses can often be heard to be stamping their feet all night. Irritation is worse in warmer weather. Rubbing of the leg often causes the horse to bite or chew at the site and affected animals may adopt bizarre positions to achieve this. Patchy alopecia with broken hairs (possibly as result of rubbing and biting) and prominent scaling are common signs (**Fig. 10.2**). Exudation of serum with matting of leg hair, alopecia and scabs may develop over limited or extensive areas. Severe thickening of the skin and secondary bacterial infections arise from

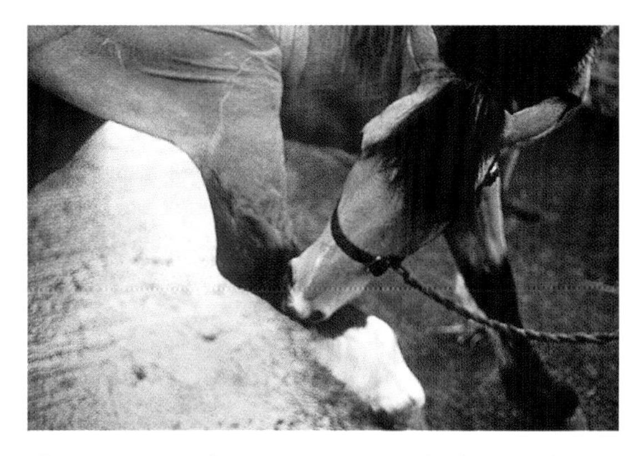

Figure 10.1 Chorioptic mange. The horse is biting at its hind pasterns in response to heavy infestation with *Chorioptes equi*.

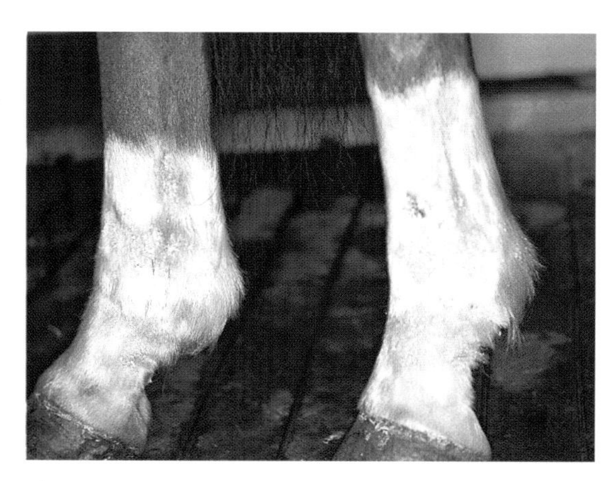

Figure 10.2 Chorioptic mange. Note the extensive scaling and crusting with some areas of acute inflammation which were probably due to self-inflicted trauma.

the long-standing, persistent self-inflicted trauma (see Fig. 16.13).

Whole body (generalized) infestation results in a generally moth-eaten appearance with weight loss, irritability and poor exercise tolerance.

Differential diagnosis

- Dermatophilosis (*Dermatophilus congolensis*)
- Dermatophytosis (*Trichophyton* spp.)
- Trombiculidiasis (*Trombicula autumnalis*)
- Sarcoptic mange (*Sarcops scabei*)
- Lice infestation (*Damalinia* spp. and *Haematopinus* spp.)
- *Culicoides* spp. hypersensitivity (sweet itch)
- *Strongyloides westeri* (parasitic) dermatitis
- Cattle tick (nymphal and larval stages)
- Greasy heel syndrome
- Pastern leukocytoclastic vasculitis
- Pastern folliculitis
- Mercurial and other blister (counterirritants)

Diagnostic confirmation

- Mite is easily recognized in groomings (particularly those obtained from the pastern and palmar cannon regions) and in skin scrapings from fresh lesions (**Fig. 10.3**). They can usually be easily seen with a magnifying lens on a dark tile or under a low-power microscope.

Treatment

Careful clipping of long hair and removal of scabs followed by scrubbing of all affected areas with appropriate insecticidal shampoo or powder may be successful in reducing the numbers of mites and providing some relief of clinical signs. Organophosphates and chlorinated hydrocarbon insecticides are effective but are less available now.

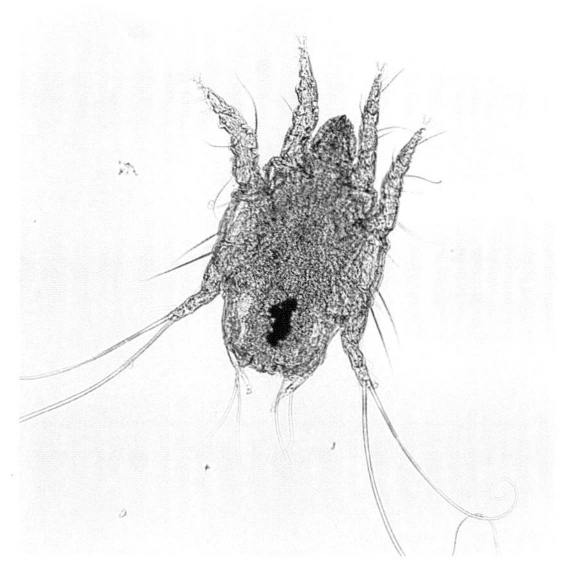

Figure 10.3 *Chorioptes equi.* (× 70)

Oral ivermectin paste (at 0.1 mg/kg daily for 7–10 days or 0.2 mg/kg twice at 2-weekly interval) gives significantly reduced mite numbers but may not cure the problem.[75] Injectable avermectin compounds show some promise as a therapeutic agent but are not yet marketed for this purpose.

Stables where the disease is established show less response to treatments and isolation of infected horses from foals and yearlings should be considered. Mass treatment is useful in controlling large outbreaks or in stables where recurrent infections are common but reservoir hosts (and possible asymptomatic carriers) might make it impossible to eradicate in spite of the short viability of the mite off the host.

PSOROPTIC MANGE

Aus; NAm; Eur – Cont

Profile

A parasitic skin disease (body mange) of young stabled horses caused by the non-burrowing scale and fluid-eating mite *Psoroptes equi* characterized by head-shaking and tail-rubbing. *Psoroptes hippotis* may be a separate species which may cause some cases of ear irritation and headshaking. Older horses may become infected if infected younger horses are introduced into the stable. Mites can also be spread by head collars and rugs.

Clinical signs

Moderate to severe pruritus mostly around the ears, mane, body and tail head (**Fig. 10.4**). Tail-head infestation causes tail rubbing with consequent poor hair density and broken and distorted tail hairs.

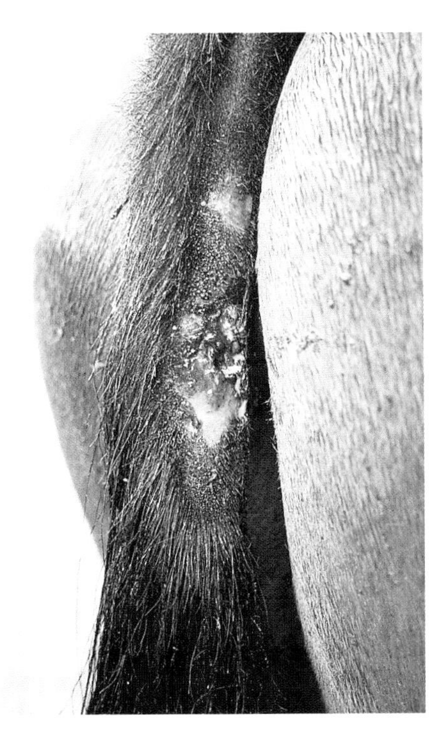

Figure 10.4 Psoroptic mange. *Psoroptes* spp. mites which caused extensive tail-rubbing and severe self-inflicted trauma. This was a severe case.

Irritability, particularly around the head is often reported and some cases of head-shaking have been attributed to this infestation.

Scaling and exudation on the skin is common, particularly along the margins of the ears. Aural discharge, head-rubbing, head-shaking (with a side-to-side shake) and the ears held flat ('droopy' ears) are characteristic of *P. hippotis* (**Fig. 10.5**).

Differential diagnosis

- Culicoides hypersensitivity or allergy (sweet itch)
- Chorioptic mange (*Chorioptes equi*)
- Lice (*Damalinia equi* and *Haematopinus asini*)
- *Oxyuris equi* infestation
- Stickfast flea, *Tyroglyphus* spp. mites
- Spinose ear tick (*Otobius megnini*), cattle tick larvae, other ticks

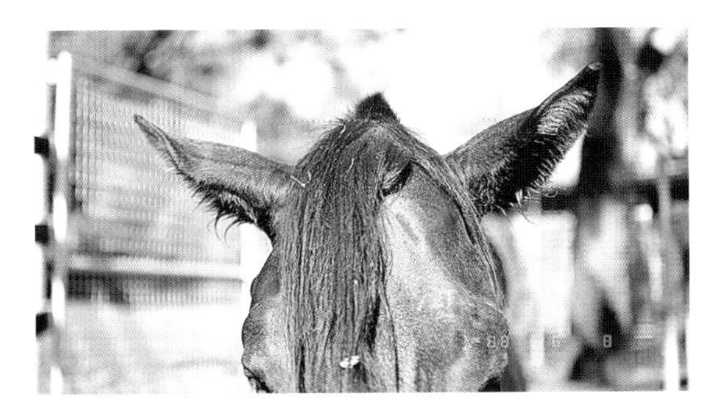

Figure 10.5 *Psoroptes hippotis*. Infestation of the skin of the ears causing a droopy, lop-eared posture. The margins of the ears showed extensive scaling and thickening.

- Atopy (feed or inhaled allergy)
- Conchal cyst
- Idiopathic or photic head-shaking
- Aural haematoma
- Overstrength insecticides

Diagnostic confirmation

- Full samples of ear wax or skin groomings can be examined with a hand lens on a dark tile – small white moving dots will be seen.
- Confirmation by microscopic identification of the mites (**Fig. 10.6**).

Note: Tranquillization may be necessary, as some affected horses resent ear handling but ear resentment is not a pathognomonic symptom.

Figure 10.6 *Psoroptes equi*. (× 70)

Treatment
The general body and tail itch may respond to antiparasitic shampoo containing organophosphate, chlorinated hydrocarbon or synthetic pyrethroid insecticides. The effect of oral ivermectin is uncertain but it may be expected to have at least some effect.

Tranquillization may be required. Clean all accumulated wax and debris from the ears. Proprietary canine antiparasitic ear drops containing gamma benzene hexachloride (Lindane), benzyl benzoate or synthetic pyrethroids can be used with good effect. However, some horses resent the drops more than the condition and can become permanently head-shy after even one or two applications.

Treatment should be repeated in 10 days to ensure that any newly hatched mites are killed.

SARCOPTIC MANGE

Cont; 🚶 – REP

Profile
An uncommon skin disease due to the burrowing mite *Sarcops scabei*. Transmission is by direct contact. It has been eradicated from large areas of the world and is now a rare disease, largely as a result of strict control measures. The removal of effective treatments makes it likely that it will reappear.

Clinical signs
It is characterized by intense pruritus which is associated with a hypersensitivity reaction to the mites and their products in the skin.

Lesions frequently begin on the head, neck and ears and may then spread over the entire body. The earliest lesions are papules and vesicles on skin with intense pruritus. Rubbing and biting leads to excoriation. Alopecia is common with papules and crusts. The skin may become very crusty and thickened (lichenified). Secondary bacterial infections can occur.

Differential diagnosis
- *Culicoides* spp. hypersensitivity (sweet itch) or irritation
- Black fly worry (*Simulium* spp.)
- Chorioptic mange (*Chorioptes equi*)
- Forage/scrub itch/chiggers/harvest mite irritation (*Trombicula* spp.)
- Onchocerciasis (*Onchocerca cervicalis*) (particularly following ivermectin anthelmintic administration)
- Larval cattle tick infestation
- Atopy (feed and inhalant allergy)

Diagnostic confirmation
- *Multiple deep* skin scrapings are required. Microscopic identification of *Sarcoptes scabei* var. *equi* (**Fig. 10.7**). A negative skin scraping may not be significant as the parasite is sometimes very difficult to locate.

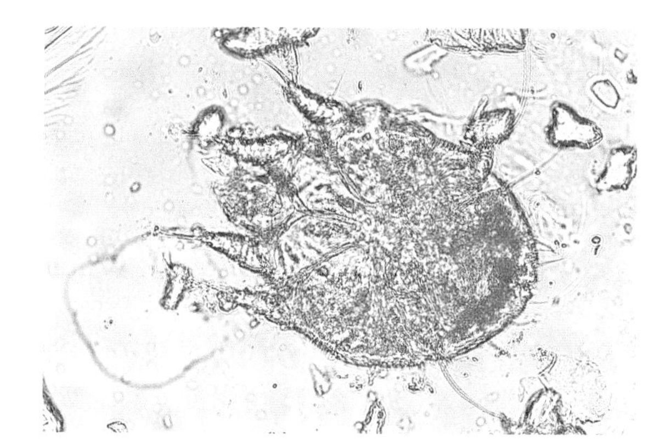

Figure 10.7 *Sarcoptes scabei* var. *equi* (× 70)

Treatment
Topical treatment with chlorinated hydrocarbons or organophosphate insecticides approved for use in horses. Washes containing synthetic pyrethroids are very variable in efficacy. Oral ivermectin at normal dose rates repeated weekly for 3 doses may be effective. Repeated washes and dosing may be needed.

Control
The disease is reportable in some countries. Isolate all infected horses and fumigate all fomites from infected horses; mites can live up to 3 weeks in infested stables and fomites.

DEMODECTIC MANGE (demodicosis)

Profile
Clinically very uncommon disease even though mites can be demonstrated in apparently normal horses. *Demodex caballi* can be found in and around the eyelids and muzzle and *Demodex equi* from the body.

Clinical signs
Asymptomatic, patchy alopecia sometimes with scaling, papules and pustules particularly over the face, neck, shoulders and forelimbs. Some cases of leukotrichia and (possibly) leukoderma around the eyes may be caused by this parasite. Lowering of general body immunity by other conditions (such as debility, concurrent disease, stress or pituitary adenoma) may influence the likelihood of clinical signs developing.

Differential diagnosis
- Other follicular dermatoses
- Onchocercal infestation
- Vitiligo

Diagnostic confirmation
- History
- Skin scrapings (it is best to squeeze the skin firmly during the scraping procedure, which should continue until blood is drawn). The presence of large numbers of mites is suggestive of clinical disease while a single mite may not be significant.
- Skin biopsy of lesions (**Fig. 10.8**).

Note: A positive skin scraping with characteristic clinical features is probably indicative of clinical disease but an alternative diagnosis should be sought unless the animal is immunocompromised.

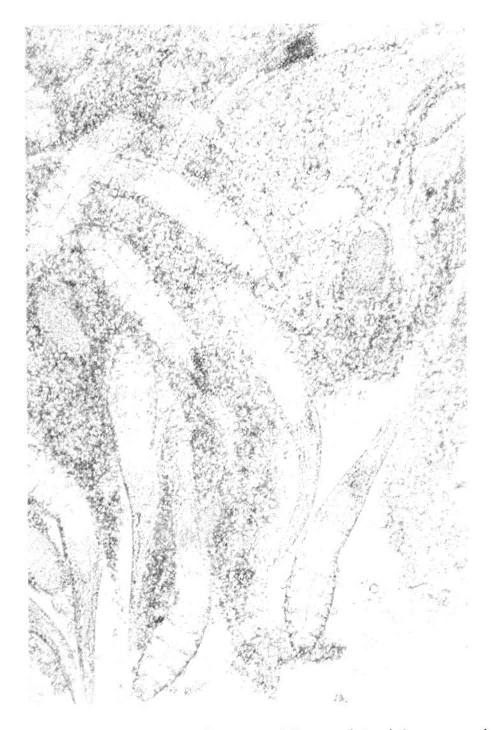

Figure 10.8 *Demodex equi* in a skin biopsy taken from the eyelid of a normal horse.

Treatment
As the condition is usually asymptomatic, it may regress spontaneously. It is in any case largely resistant to therapy. Usually it is not directly treated, though consideration should be given to reasons for impaired immunity and to the treatment of other concurrent disease. Oral ivermectin and washes with organophosphates may be helpful in confirmed cases.

TROMICULIDIASIS (scrub itch/chigger/harvest mite infestation)

Profile
Infestation with *Trombicula* spp. ('harvest', 'chigger', forage or 'srub itch' mites). The mites are capable of living in preserved hay and are commoner on chalky soils in autumn months. The mites are only on the horse for short periods to feed and so even in severe infestations they may be difficult to find. Clinical disease is associated with infestation caused by the nymphal form of the mite.

Note: *Tyroglyphus* spp. mites occur only in grain and can accidentally affect horses.

Clinical signs
The condition usually affects the head (**Fig. 10.9**) and legs of grazing horses in late summer and autumn (especially those grazing on chalky soils). Stabled horses may be infested over the entire body. Irritability, leg-stamping, nose-rubbing and head-shaking reflect the intensely pruritic nature of the infestation. Small papules and wheals on distal limbs, nose, neck and ventral abdomen. Repeated and severe biting at the lower legs results in small or larger hairless areas which may become obviously inflamed and exudative after 2–3 days (**Fig. 10.10**).

Differential diagnosis
- Poultry red mite (*Demanyssus gallinae*) infestation
- *Stomoxys calcitrans* spp. irritation and bites
- Onchocercal dermatitis (*Onchocerca cervicalis*)
- Chorioptic/psoroptic mange (*Chorioptes equi*, *Psoroptes equi/hippotis*)
- Tick larvae infestation

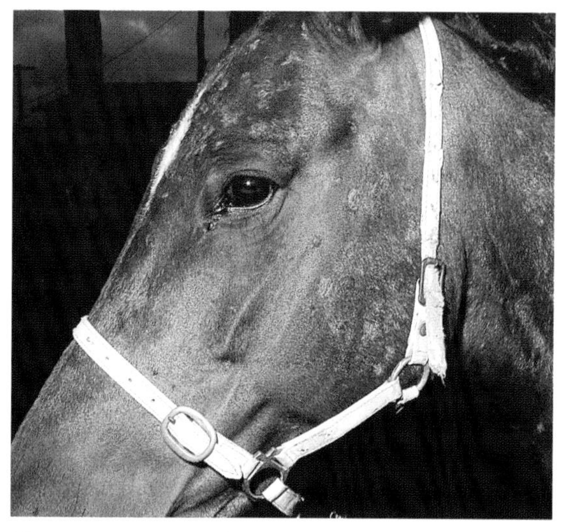

Figure 10.9 Trombiculidiasis. Diffuse dermatitis of the face caused by *Trombicula autumnalis* infestation.

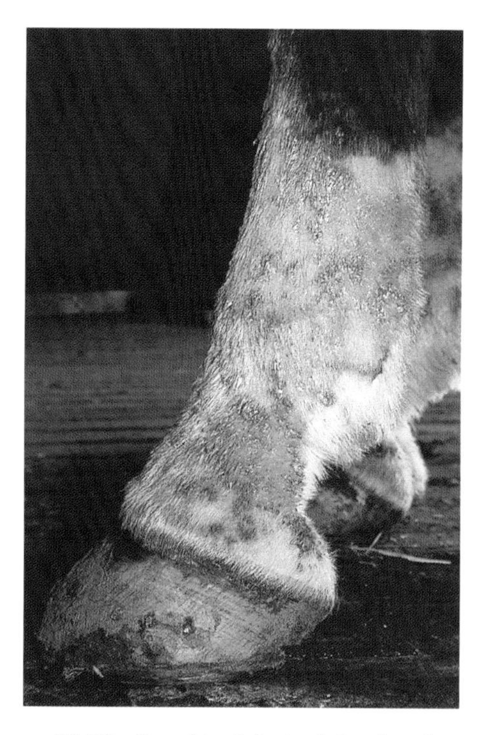

Figure 10.10 Trombiculidiasis. Extensive dermatitis which arose as a result of self-inflicted trauma due to severe and persistent trombiculid mite infestation. Note that the dermatitis was not restricted to the white areas.

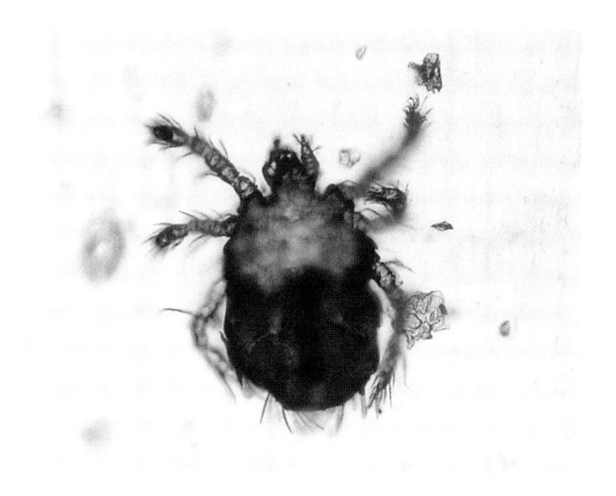

Figure 10.11 *Trombicula autumnalis* (nymphal mite). It is the nymph which causes the most severe problems on horses. (× 40)

- Lice (*Damalinia equi*, *Haematopinus asini*)
- Plant irritation (e.g. thistles)
- Contact sensitivity/allergy

Diagnostic confirmation

- As the mites fall off the host after feeding they are sometimes difficult to find, but aggregations of the red-orange mites feeding at one site make it easier to find on some cases.
- Extensive examination of groomings may be needed at an early stage in the onset of clinical signs. The use of a dark tile is helpful to show up the orange-red nymphs, although some can be colourless (**Fig. 10.11**).

Treatment

Topical applications of insecticidal compounds such as approved organophosphates and chlorinated hydrocarbons are effective in washes or as aerosol sprays. Attention must be paid to the possible source of infection. Horses usually lose infestation quickly and so should only be treated if absolutely necessary. It is better to remove the source of infestation if possible. Mites may live in preserved forage or bedding so infestation can sometimes be 'out-of-season'.

POULTRY RED MITE (*Dermanyssus gallinae*)

Profile

Dermatological disorder due to cutaneous infestation with the poultry (red) mite *Dermanyssus gallinae*. Direct or indirect poultry contact is always present. The mites are blood feeders.

Clinical signs

Severe, often progressive, pruritus over the whole body. Small pruritic skin papules and crusts may be present in areas readily accessible to the mite (legs, face and ventrum). Horses become irritable and stamp and bite at the body and legs (**Fig. 10.12**).

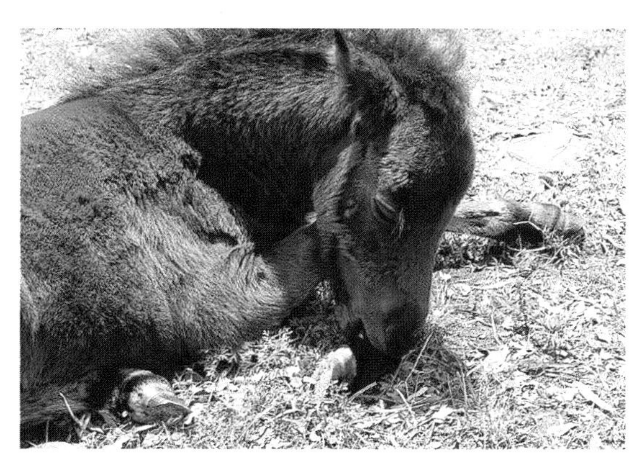

Figure 10.12 Distal limb pruritus due to *Dermanyssus gallinae* infestation. This sign is also characteristic of helminth-related dermatitis in foals due to *Strongyloides westerii* infestation.

Differential diagnosis

- Lice (*Damalinia equi*, *Haematopinus asini*)
- Chorioptic, sarcoptic or psoroptic mange (*Chorioptes equi*, *Sarcoptes scabei*, *Psoroptes equi/hippotis*)
- Culicoides hypersensitivity (sweet itch) and irritation (ventral biting species in particular)
- *Stomoxys calcitrans* fly bites/irritation
- Forage/'scrub itch', harvest (*Trombicula* spp.) mites
- Larval tick infestation
- Larval nematode dermatitis (*Strongyloides westerii*).
- Food allergy/atopy

Diagnostic confirmation

- Poultry contact is always involved. The mites and their eggs can be found in bedding and crevices in walls and wooden poles and poultry perches.
- Groomings show small, mobile, red nymphal mites which are very visible on a black tile. Microscopic identification of mites (**Fig. 10.13**). They are not always present in high numbers and so may be difficult to find.

Treatment

Wash or spray body with approved (licensed) chlorinated hydrocarbon or organophosphate insecticides. Remove horses from proximity to poultry or remove poultry from the stable environment. The effect of such separation may not be obvious for up to 6 months or more as the mites are very robust and can survive well for extended periods away from host chickens.

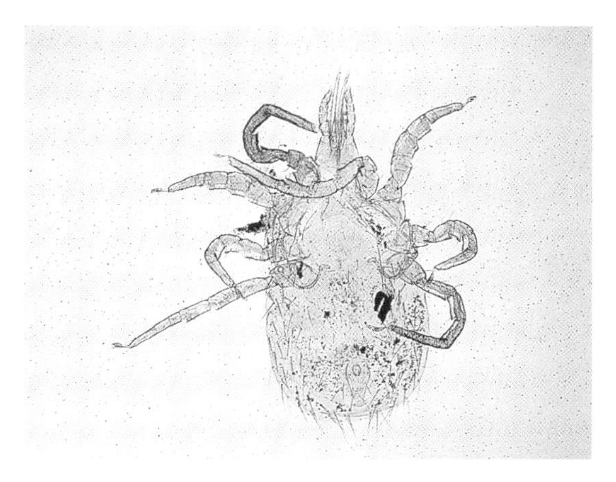

Figure 10.13 *Dermanyssus gallinae* (poultry red mite). (× 40)

Treat building and all equipment with an appropriate insecticide (this may be more difficult than it sounds).

Treat contact poultry accordingly.

Repeat all treatments every 7 days in summer and 10–14 days in winter.

STICKFAST OR STICK-TIGHT FLEAS

Profile

A dermatological condition of horses in close contact with poultry in warm climates caused by the poultry flea *Echidnophaga gallinacea*.

Clinical signs

Prominent pruritus and secondary alopecia and excoriation where fleas attach. Most often affects eyelids, face, ears, chest, shoulders and limbs. Fleas are visible to the naked eye and are firmly attached to the skin.

Differential diagnosis

- *Culicoides* spp. hypersensitivity (sweet itch) or irritation
- Chorioptic, psoroptic and other mange mites
- Lice (*Damalinia equi*, *Haematopinus asini*)
- Other ectoparasites, e.g. spinose ear tick (*Otobius megnini*).

Diagnostic confirmation

- Visible presence of adult fleas with mouth parts buried in horse.

Treatment

Topical wash with insecticidal shampoo, flea powders or aerosols (licensed synthetic pyrethroids, organophosphates and chlorinated hydrocarbons are effective). Remove from poultry contact and/or treat poultry and their housing, otherwise re-infestation will occur.

CULICOIDES SPP. IRRITATION

Profile

Many geographically orientated species of *Culicoides* family which attack horses (also known as 'no-see-ums' or gnats). Individual species tend to attack different areas of the horse. Apart from their nuisance effects they have an important secondary role in the transmission of some important viral (including viral encephalitides) and some other infectious diseases. African horse sickness is probably transmitted primarily by *Culicoides imicola*.

The insects are blood feeders and their life cycle demands warmth, moisture and suitable vegetation conditions for the individual species, so they tend to be very seasonal in most parts of the world. Where this is so, the diseases they transmit and the specific primary effects tend also to be seasonal. Their size and fragility mean that they are most active in calm conditions (with wind speeds less than 6–7 km/h). The various species have preferred feeding times and preferred feeding sites on the host animals. Thus some feed in mornings, others in evenings. Some are ventral feeding, while others prefer to feed on the dorsum of the host.

Note: *All* horses may be attacked by *Culicoides* spp. insects and show signs of irritation which leads to restlessness and even pruritus. This is not the same disorder as affects those horses which have an inordinate allergic response to the bite of relatively few of the midges. Under favourable climatic conditions enormous populations of the flies are present and many horses show severe irritation during these wave attacks. The irritation rapidly abates as the population of flies falls leaving only those horses with hypersensitivity as a serious clinical problem.

Clinical signs

Bites are followed immediately by pain and pruritus which are usually more intense on head, base of mane, tail and over the withers. Ventral biting species bite the ventral abdomen or the limbs and the distribution of the pruritus varies accordingly. Mixed populations of flies are also common so that it is usually impossible without trapping to establish the species involved. Usually most or all of the horses in a group will be affected to some extent (in contrast to the allergic disorder which affects individuals). Self-inflicted trauma can cause moderate to severe superficial skin abrasions and excoriation with serum exudate (**Fig. 10.14**). Individual horses may develop the allergic condition after a single attack, thereafter remaining allergic and become progressively more affected in succeeding seasons. Some breeds are apparently more sensitive and others (such as the Icelandic and Welsh ponies and the Shire horse) are more inclined to develop an allergic reaction.

Differential diagnosis

- Insect irritation, e.g. black-flies (*Simulium* spp.), mosquitoes of many species
- *Culicoides* spp. allergy (sweet itch)

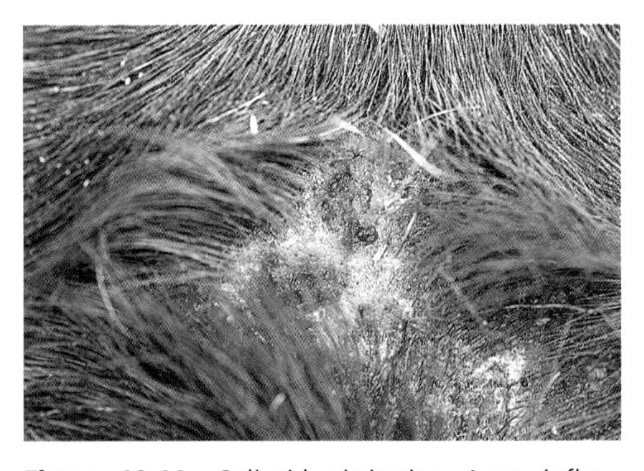

Figure 10.14 *Culicoides* irritation. Acute inflammatory focus due to *Culicoides* spp. bites on the flank. The horse showed no sign of hypersensitivity. Similar intensely pruritic lesions are caused by mosquitoes and a few fly species.

- Dermatophilosis (*Dermatophilus congolensis*)
- Dermatophytosis (*Trichophyton equinum*, *Microsporum gypseum*)
- Lice (*Damalinia equi*, *Haematopinus asini*)
- Onchocerciasis (*Onchocerca cervicalis*)
- Contact hypersensitivity
- Chemical irritation/scald/burn

Diagnostic confirmation

- Seasonal and environmental conditions.
- Presence of large numbers of *Culicoides* spp.: use of a night-light trap will allow identification of the species involved.

Treatment

Use of permethrin and cypermethrin repellents or aromatic oils (such as citronella) and benzyl benzoate can be helpful but are not capable of preventing an attack completely. Suitable stable management and protective rugging, stables with fine mesh filters and overhead fans (to provide an air speed of over 10 km/h) are useful for individual horses. Large groups of paddock horses may be protected by using smoky ('smudge') fires in and around the paddock. Most midges breed in water courses and in shady woodland areas and avoidance of these or controlling the flies within them by drainage and vegetation management, etc. can help.

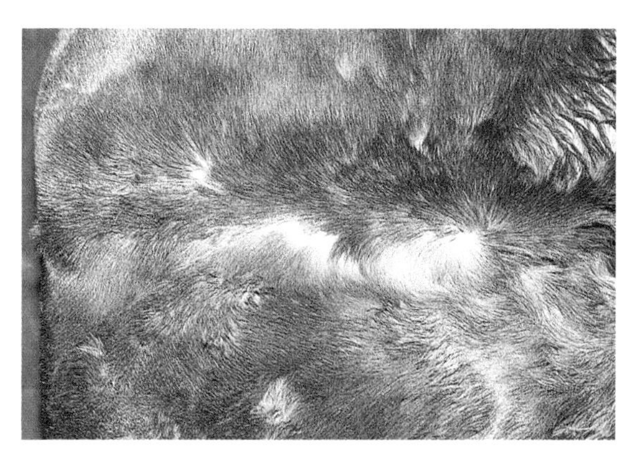

Figure 10.15 *Culicoides* irritation. Ventral midline dermatitis due to ventral biting *Culicoides* spp. midges with self-inflicted trauma caused by rubbing on a water trough.

VENTRAL MIDLINE DERMATITIS

Profile

Specific insect-related dermatitis of grazing horses in summer months in fly-infested areas. The condition is caused by the bites of a variety of insects including *Culicoides* spp., *Haematobia irritans*, *Stomoxys calcitrans* and *Tabanus* spp. Although one species may be prevalent the condition is usually caused by a number of mixed species. The condition is commonest in younger horses (under 3–5 years of age); older horses seem much less prone to it.

Clinical signs

Ventral biting species bite the ventral abdomen along the midline (where the hair is less dense) and particularly around the umbilicus (**Fig. 10.15**). The bites leave sharply demarcated inflamed areas which may be ulcerated, especially as result of self-inflicted trauma. Pruritus varies from mild to extreme, with some horses showing bizarre behaviour and making frantic attempts to rub the ventral abdomen on troughs or fences. Bleeding and crusting with self-inflicted trauma causes skin thickening and alopecia. Localized leukoderma and leukotrichia are common effects of the repeated local trauma. Usually most or all of the horses in a group will be affected to some extent but will vary markedly in their individual responses (by contrast to the allergic disorder, which invariably affects individuals severely).

Differential diagnosis

- Onchocerciasis (*Onchocerca cervicalis*)
- *Culicoides* spp. allergy (sweet itch)
- Dermatophilosis (*Dermatophilus congolensis*)
- Dermatophytosis (*Trichophyton equinum*, *Microsporum gypseum*)
- Lice (*Damalinia equi*, *Haematopinus asini*)
- Poultry or trombiculid mite infestation of bedding
- Contact hypersensitivity
- Chemical irritation/scald/burn

Diagnostic confirmation

- Seasonal and environmental conditions.
- Mixed populations of flies are also common so that it is usually impossible without trapping to establish the species involved.
- Biopsy of the lesions shows prominent eosinophillic infiltration and perivascular inflammation and small areas of superficial epidermal necrosis.

Treatment

Gentle washing and application of soothing creams (usually with corticosteroid) and prevention of further attacks are sensible measures. Parenteral corticosteroids are sometimes required in severe cases. However, in most circumstances it is almost impossible to prevent recurrent attacks. Use of permethrin and cypermethrin repellents or aromatic oils (such as citronella) and benzyl benzoate can be helpful. Thick applications of petroleum jelly or Stockholm tar are used along the ventral midline but make use of the horse unpleasant. Suitable stable management and protective rugging and stables with fine mesh filters are useful for individual horses. Large groups of paddock horses may be protected by using smoky ('smudge') fires in and around the paddock. Fly control measures can be used but are difficult when several species of flies are involved.

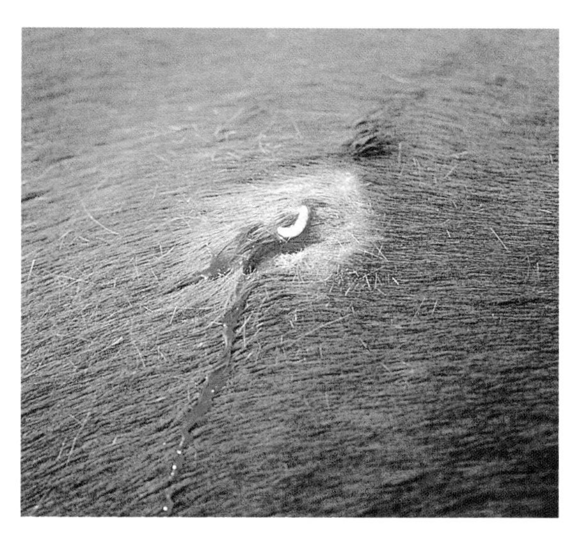

Figure 10.16 *Hypoderma bovis* larva in the skin of a horse.

HYPODERMIASIS (Warble fly infestation)

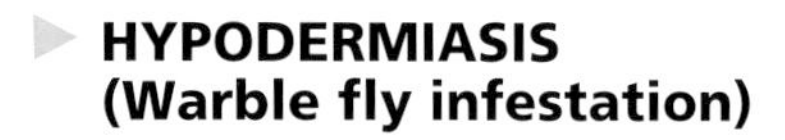

Eur

Profile

Cutaneous nodules caused by migrating *Hypoderma bovis* and *Hypoderma lineatum* larvae. The disease is restricted geographically to the northern hemisphere in areas where control mechanisms for the adult fly are not in operation. Younger horses and those in poor body condition are more likely to be affected. The parasites are bovine adapted and so, while they may cause disease in horses, they seldom mature fully. Aberrant migration can cause significant and unpredictable effects in the central nervous system or elsewhere.

Clinical signs

Early lesions are firm, well-demarcated, warm subcutaneous nodules along the dorsum (particularly in the withers region) in the spring months. Single or a few lesions are usually present but small aggregations may be present. There may be some pain on palpation and saddle resentment. Nodules develop a softer cyst-like structure with a small breathing 'pore' which may be visible and a few will produce a live larva (**Fig. 10.16**). Pruritus may be present during development of larvae. If larva dies or is ruptured *in situ*, the horse may show a severe anaphylactic reaction or gross local inflammation and swelling.

Differential diagnosis

- Infectious granuloma
- Epidermoid and dermoid cyst
- Neoplasia (mast cell, sarcoid or cutaneous lymphosarcoma)
- Foreign body reaction
- Staphylococcal folliculitis/abscess
- (Eosinophilic) Collagen necrosis nodule
- Panniculitis
- Eosinophilic granuloma (insect bite reaction)

Diagnostic confirmation

- Geographical location in winter months
- Contact with affected cattle
- Physical examination of nodular lesion with demonstrable breathing pore in skin or actual larva

Treatment

Medical treatment with ivermectin orally is effective (therefore in a horse where this is used routinely the condition probably will not occur). Topical application of organophosphate insecticides has been successful. There are anecdotal reports of anaphylaxis following drug-induced death of the parasite.

Surgical removal of entire nodule is feasible but may leave a problem area on the saddle region.

INSECT BITES OR STINGS

Profile

Many variations associated with single or multiple stings or bites from individual or swarms of insects. Marked geographical variations reflect the prevalence of the insects. It is not often possible to be certain of the cause unless the episode is observed, but bee stings are identifiable with careful examination of the sites for the remains of the stings.

The role of biting flies in the epidemiology of the equine sarcoid is uncertain, but it seems likely that they have some role in the transmission of the condition.

The common biting and stinging insects include: *Tabanus* spp. (horse fly), *Stomoxys* spp. (stable fly), *Culicoides* spp. (midge, sand fly), *Haematobia* spp. (buffalo fly), *Simulium* spp. (black-flies), *Hippobosca* spp. (louse fly), and various varieties of wasps, mosquitoes, spiders and bees.

Horse flies (*Tabanus* spp.) The life cycle varies from 3–4 months to 2 years. They are mechanical vectors of important viral and other infectious diseases (including equine infectious anaemia). They may also transmit papillomaviruses and fungal infections (dermatophytosis due to *Microsporum gypseum* in particular). The bites produce a marked painful, pruritic skin response showing as wheals, with a central bite mark often with a blood spot.

Stable fly *(Stomoxys calcitrans)* Adult flies resemble the common house fly *(Musca domestica)*, the bush fly *(M. vetustissima)* and the face fly *(M. autumnalis)*. Large biting mouth parts cause considerable skin trauma and leave a relatively large lesion, often in a defined pattern of three or four bites in a chain or group (**Fig. 10.17**). They are capable of mechanical transmission of diseases, including dermatophytosis (ringworm)[55] (see Fig. 8.6, p. 114).

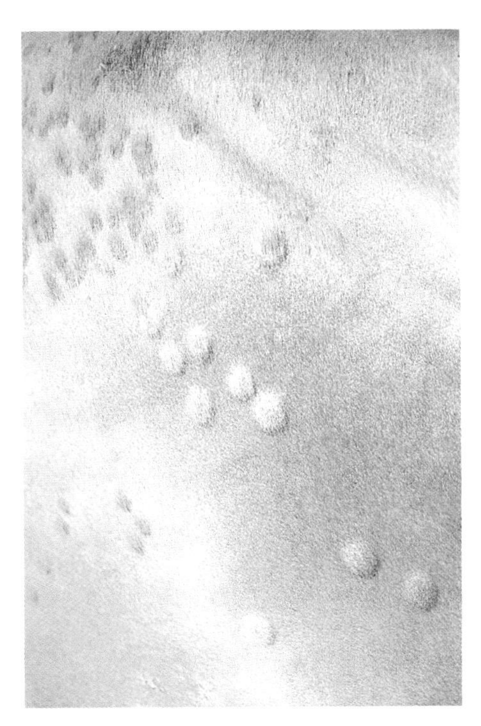

Figure 10.17 Stable fly *(Stomoxys calcitrans)* bites. Notice considerable skin reaction leaving a relatively large lesion, and distinctive patterning of bites.

Buffalo and horn fly (*Haematobia exigua*, *H. irritans)* Subtropical/tropical areas. These flies are small (4 mm in length). Their identification on the horse is recognized by their head-down body position and they tend to feed in small or large groups, aggregating around the shoulders, neck, withers (**Fig. 10.18**), flanks and abdomen of the horse. Both male and female flies are blood feeders, taking up to 20–30 meals daily. After feeding the site often has a small drop of blood.

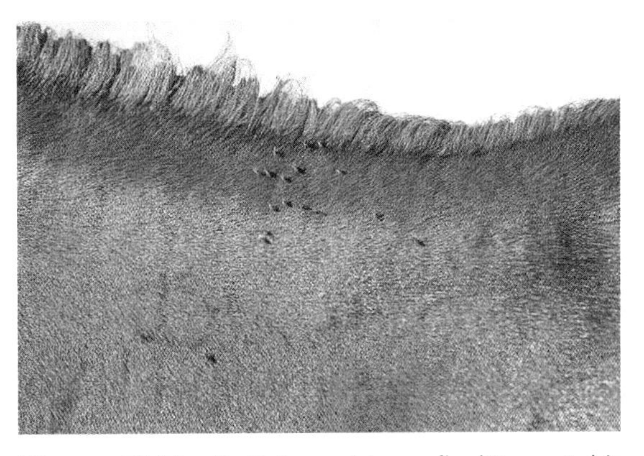

Figure 10.18 Buffalo and horn fly (*Haematobia exigua, H. irritans)* aggregating around the neck and withers. Each bite site often has a small drop of blood.

Black-flies (*Simulium* spp.) Larvae breed in running or still water in spring and summer and they can reach plague proportions following long rainy periods. They cause extreme irritation and inflict painful bites, particularly on the ear flap and head (**Fig. 10.19**) and are most active in the morning and evening. There is a putative association with papillary acanthosis of the pinnae (aural plaques) (see Fig. 6.7, p. 95). Swarm attacks by flies can induce death through release of a toxin capable of causing increased capillary permeability.[76] Hypersensitivity

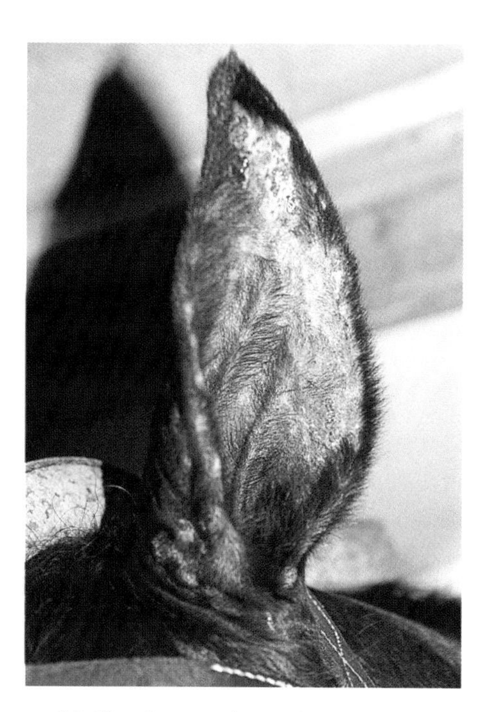

Figure 10.19 Severe dermatitis on the pinnae caused by black-fly (*Simulium* spp.) bites.

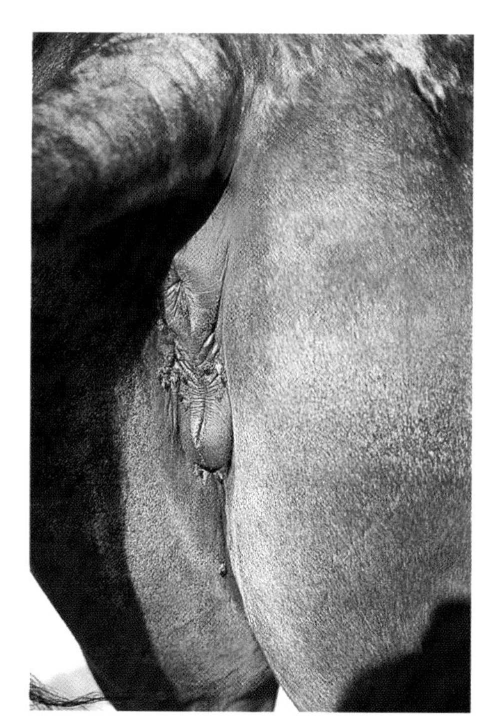

Figure 10.20 Louse flies (*Hippobosca equina, H. maculata, H. rupifes*) in the perineum. The flies are hard to dislodge: note the severe hair loss from the tail as a result of persistent rubbing by the horse in an attempt to dislodge them.

may also occur with a dramatic generalized systemic and dermal response to a single or few bites.

Louse flies (*Hippobosca equina, H. maculata, H. rupifes*). These occur in Europe, Africa and South America. The larvae develop in sheltered dry soil or humus. Adult flies are enthusiastic blood feeders and tend to cluster in the perineum and inguinal regions (**Fig. 10.20**), causing significant lesions with persistent blood loss. They are not easily disturbed and cause local irritation and fly-worry.

Mosquitoes (*Anopheles* spp., *Aedes* spp., etc.) Most attacks are at dusk and early evening but can occur in daylight hours. Multiple bites are common (**Fig. 10.21**). They can transmit viral diseases such as the viral encephalitides, African horse sickness and equine infectious anaemia.

Bees The honey bee *(Apis mellifera)* has been reported to attack horses in the spring and summer, producing oedematous wheals and plaques. Usually single stings are present (**Fig. 10.22**) although swarm attacks have been reported. The potency of bee venom varies between individual bees and also between subspecies in Europe, Africa and North America.[77,78]

Wasps Various species of wasp inhabit and nest in shrubs, trees, brick and stone walls, etc. Accidental knocking of a nest usually precipitates a vicious attack by many wasps. Wasps can each sting several times and so multiple reactions can occur from a single wasp (**Fig. 10.23**); usually such bites are close to each other or at least on one body region. Swarm stings are correspondingly more extensive.

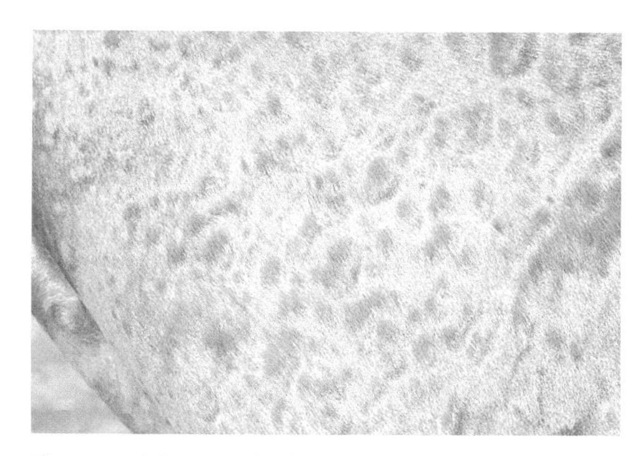

Figure 10.21 Multiple mosquitoes bites showing individual oedematous reactions surrounding a central bite mark.

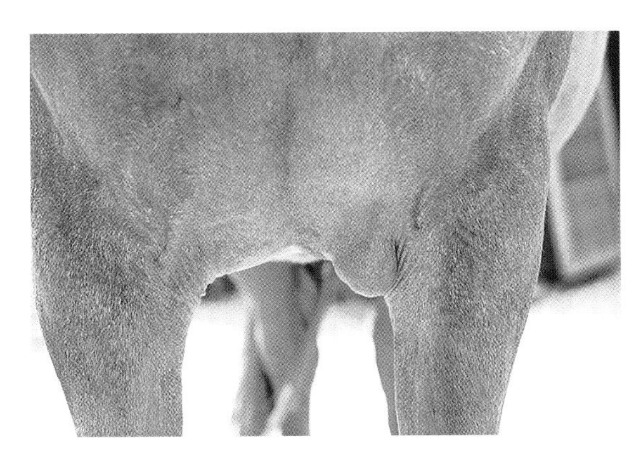

Figure 10.22 Single bee sting in the axilla, with swelling. The sting was identifiable and was removed easily.

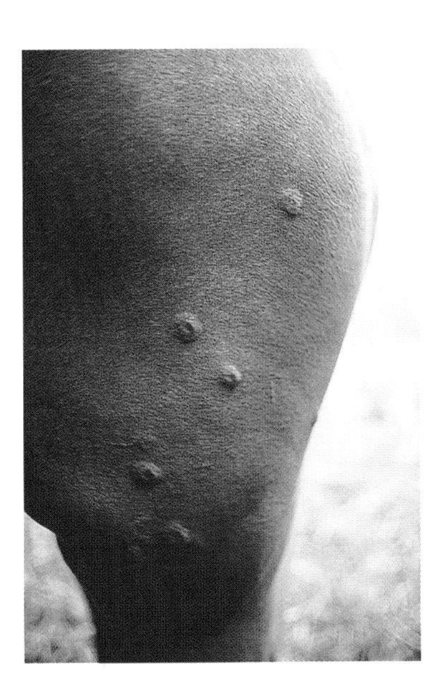

Figure 10.23 Multiple isolated wasp stings. Each sting is very localized and close clipping will reveal a small but distinct central haemorrhagic focus.

Spiders Bites from black widow spider (*Ixeuticus robusta*) and white-tailed spider (*Lampona cylindrata*) and others in various parts of the world cause an acute, hot, extremely painful oedematous swelling. Some induce a prolonged necrotizing effect in the bite area, leading to skin sloughing (Fig. 10.24).

Tick infestation Various ticks are found in many parts of the world. They can cause significant blood loss and debility if present in large numbers.

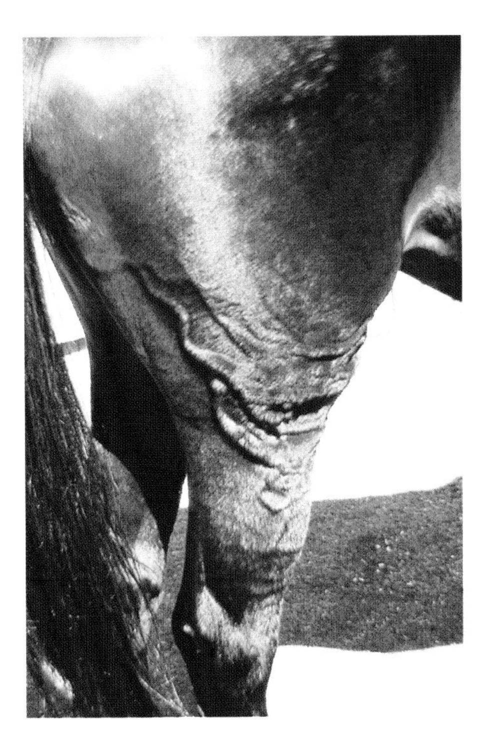

Figure 10.24 Spider bite with extensive local skin necrosis.

Marked local swellings and pain as well as systemic reactions (fever, depression, central nervous signs, etc.) may be encountered. They may also be responsible for transmission of protozoal disease such as babesiosis. The presence of larval ticks (often in enormous numbers) can cause severe pruritus, with stamping and biting at the legs in particular. In spite of the numbers they can be very difficult to find on the horse as they drop off after feeding.

Clinical signs

Biting flies and other insects produce a focal bite and/or some degree of worry or agitation in the horse.

The location and pattern of the bites can be suggestive of the species responsible. Irritability from pain and/or annoyance causes foot-stamping, restlessness, nervous agitation and unpredictable movements. Some horses will actively seek out water, smoke or vegetation to avoid being bitten.

Individual insects such as spiders will cause single episodes of escape behaviour. Both swarm (multiple) bite/stings and some individual bites can be fatal.

Most bites/stings have an obvious central bite mark surrounded by a small circular oedematous plaque. The larger the insect, the larger the puncture and area of oedema, e.g. *Tabanus* spp. are large and may actually draw blood, leaving a visible puncture mark and a small blood spot.

Swarms or individual insects can be involved, with a corresponding number of bites. The nature of the bite and the potency of the venom influences the clinical appearance of the lesion(s). Severe attacks can cause severe systemic effects (cardiac and shock signs) or even death (as in the case of swarm emergence of black-flies in eastern regions of Texas, USA).

Differential diagnosis

- Other causes of transient oedematous nodules with pain.
- Death from swarm attacks may resemble anaphylaxis caused by other factors; skin lesions may not be seen.

Diagnostic confirmation

- History can sometimes be helpful but most stings and bites are similar in appearance.
- Individual severity provides no helpful diagnostic information.
- Bee stings are usually recognized by the sting sac being visibly embedded in the skin but in many cases rubbing of the site causes this to deflate and become invisible.

Treatment

For individual treatment antihistamine injections (tripelennamine and/or acepromazine) can be used. Wasp and spider bites are alkaline while bee stings are acidic and counterirrigation with acetic acid (vinegar) or bicarbonate solutions, respectively, may reduce the immediate painful effects. Analgesic, antibiotic and corticosteroid creams can be applied locally to affected sites. Severe reactions to single or multiple stings/bites may warrant emergency adrenaline medication (3–5 ml subcutaneously of a 1:1000 dilution for a 500 kg horse). Intravenous fluid therapy, flunixin meglumine and corticosteroids may be required.

Control

Manure disposal, slashing of long grass around stable area, removal of rotting vegetation and avoidance of cattle contact will make significant benefits in populations of flies in particular. Spraying stables, walls and yard rails with organophosphates or chlorinated hydrocarbons (where available) is helpful but should be avoided if possible on environmental and safety grounds. Keeping the horses away from the sources of the insects is an effective measure for many of the worst species but is not generally feasible. Protection with meshed windows and a light insect trap inside stables at night may help. Insect repellents (most are synthetic pyrethrins) have a mixed reputation. These are usually effective for up to 7 days, but if a horse is exposed to rain or constant wet periods treatment must be repeated after each wetting or it will be ineffective.

MYIASIS

Profile

Infestation of tissue by fly larvae. Blow-fly strike (*Calliphora* spp.) affects neglected, discharging and infected wounds, rigid limb casts, dirty bandages and necrotic neoplasms. Screw-worm larvae (*Callitroga hominivorax* and *C. macellaria* in North and South America and *Chrysomyia bezziana* in sub-Saharan Africa) cause a more serious disease with infestation of wounds and tumours where they cause extensive tissue destruction.

Clinical signs

Sites of wounds (or plaster casts or dressings) show increasing malodour. The sites are irritating and the horse will often chew and lick at the region, as a result of physical irritation. The larvae are usually obvious on thorough exploration of the wound site but a casual glance may not be enough (**Fig. 10.25**). All wounds should be thoroughly examined during the fly seasons.

The effects of the screw-worm larvae (*Calitroga hominivorax* and *Chrysomyia bezziana*) are particularly severe and may involve extensive tissue destruction and necrosis. The infestation is accompanied by a very unpleasant foetid odour. Self-trauma by biting at and rubbing of the infected site is common and this makes the site more inflamed and more extensive.

Differential diagnosis

- Exuberant granulation tissue (from any cause)
- Botryomycosis (staphylococcal granuloma)
- Habronemiasis (*Habronema musca*)
- Squamous cell carcinoma
- Fibroblastic sarcoid transformation at a wound site

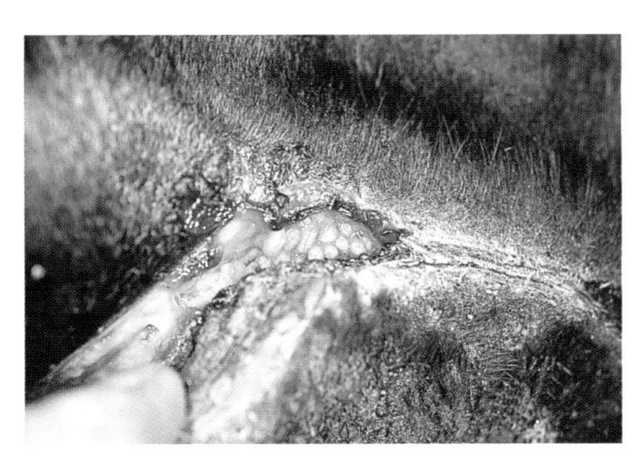

Figure 10.25 Fly strike/myiasis infestation of a wound.

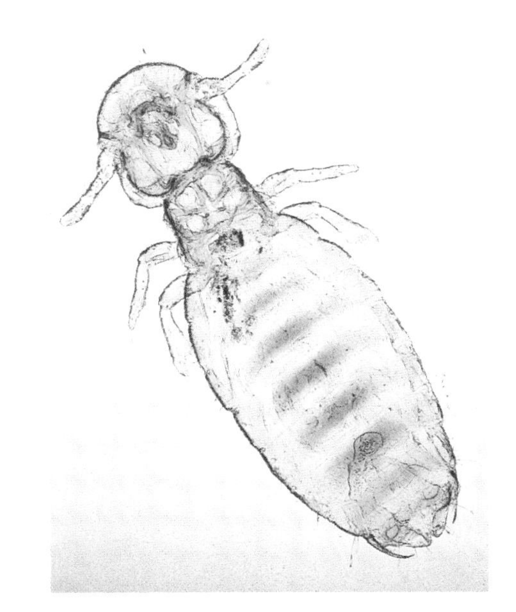

Figure 10.26 *Damalinia equi* louse.

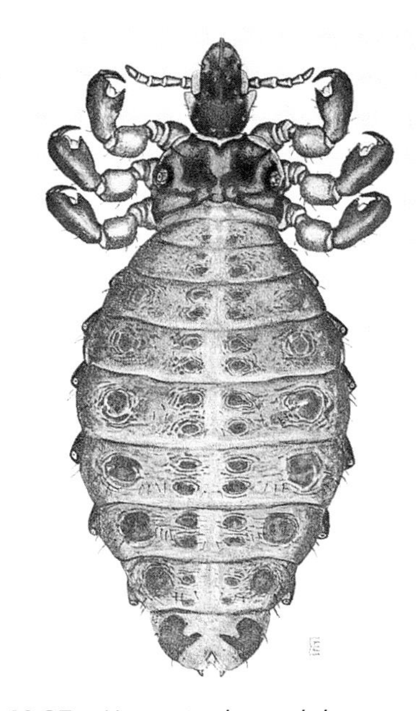

Figure 10.27 *Haematopinus asini.*

Note: All these conditions are possibly subject to fly strike and, although they are not themselves pruritic, the presence of superimposed fly larvae can change this significantly.

Diagnostic confirmation

- Close examination of the wound. The larvae have an obvious breathing pore at one end. They are sometimes very deep within the granulation tissue and may be difficult to find at first.

Treatment

Remove all bandages, cast etc. Clean and irrigate the wound very carefully with saline. Lift out all visible larvae. Insecticidal ointments and lotions (containing gamma benzene hexachloride or organophosphates) are available in some parts of the world and are useful in these cases. Ivermectin (applied topically neat or as a diluted wash in saline) can be effective. It should not be necessary to repeat the procedure unless reinfestation occurs.

PEDICULOSIS (louse infestation)

Cont

Profile

Lice are host-specific obligate parasites and fall into two major groups:

- Biting lice: *Damalinia equi* is a small (<2 mm), not easily visible, pale yellowish scale-chewing louse with a broad flattened head (**Fig. 10.26**).
- Sucking lice: *Haematopinus asini* is about 2 mm long and is a dark coloured, blood-sucking louse with a narrow head (**Fig. 10.27**).

Lice occur worldwide and are particularly severe in winter months when horses are congregated together. Spread is by direct contact or indirectly through grooming brushes, rugs and even via the stable environment, where they can survive for some weeks off the host animal.

Clinical signs

The biting lice (*Damalinia* spp.) prefer the dorsum of the back and the sides of the neck while the blood-sucking lice can be found predominately on the neck, tail and limbs.

Lice of all types cause pruritus which produces irritation, rubbing and biting, dermatitis and unthriftiness with secondary patchy alopecia leading to a 'moth-eaten' appearance of the coat (**Fig. 10.28**). Severe irritation and self-inflicted trauma can produce areas of dermal excoriation and serum exudation. Most obvious sites for the parasites are the side of the neck, the dorsum and the base of the mane and tail, where they can usually be found. These sites are the prime locations for rubbing and biting (**Fig. 10.29**).

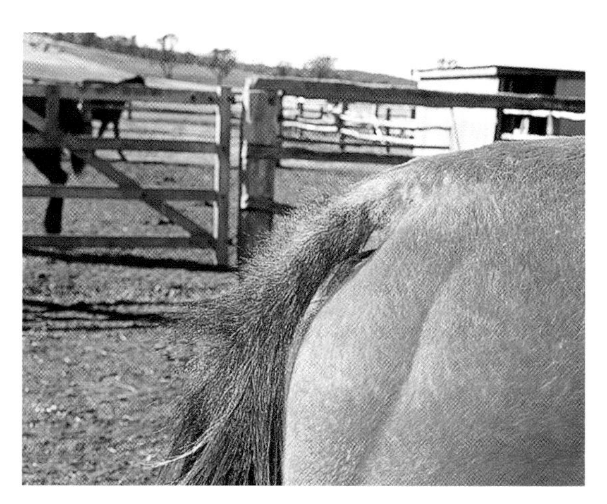

Figure 10.29 Pediculosis. Tail-rubbing caused by lice infestation. Note that the tail itself is less severely affected than the skin of the hind quarters.

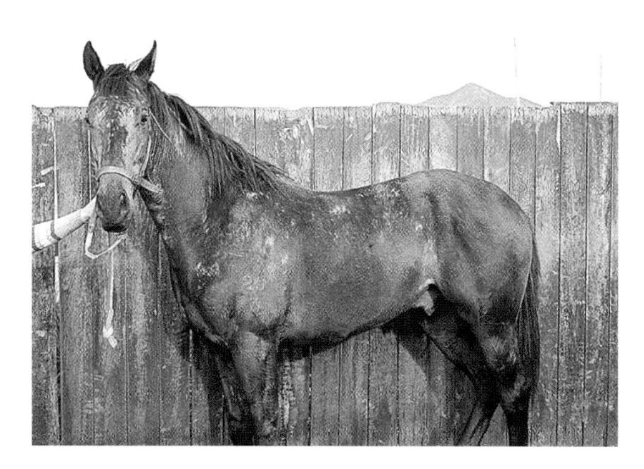

Figure 10.28 Pediculosis. 'Moth-eaten' appearance of the coat of a horse infested with lice.

Loss of condition is common in severely affected horses. Clinically significant anaemia can arise from even marginal burdens of the blood-sucking species. Animals which are stressed, immunocompromised or in poor condition (or combinations of these) seem more liable to developing heavy louse burdens.

Differential diagnosis

- Chorioptic and psoroptic mange
- *Culicoides* spp. irritation and hypersensitivity (sweet itch)
- Dermatophilosis (*Dermatophilus congolensis*)
- Trombiculosis (*Trombicula autumnalis*)
- *Oxyuris equi* infestation (tail rubbing)
- *Dermanyssus gallinae*/*Tyroglyphus* spp. poultry mite infestation
- Trichophytosis and microsporosis (ringworm)
- Stickfast fleas, spinose ear tick (*Otobius megnini*)
- Scalding (diarrhoea/urine/wound fluids, etc.)

Diagnostic confirmation

- *D. equi* is less visible and the eggs are smaller and laid closer to the skin. *Haematopinus asini* adults and the eggs ('nits') can be readily seen with the naked eye (**Fig. 10.30**). Warming of the skin with a hair dryer or lightbulb will usually bring them to the surface and the horse will show a marked irritation with prominent scratch reflexes. Small numbers of lice and the smaller species of biting louse are more difficult to see.
- Groomings can be examined on a black or dark blue tile when the dark brown-red parasites will be seen to move. Microscopic examination will identify the species, which are noticeably different in appearance (*Damalinia* spp. have a relatively broad body with a squarish head (Fig. 10.26) while *Haematopinus* spp. have a longer, narrower body with a sharp conical head (Fig. 10.27).)

Treatment

Whole-body washes or powdering with organophosphate or chlorinated hydrocarbon washes (where available and approved) are very effective. Aerosol insecticides containing organo-

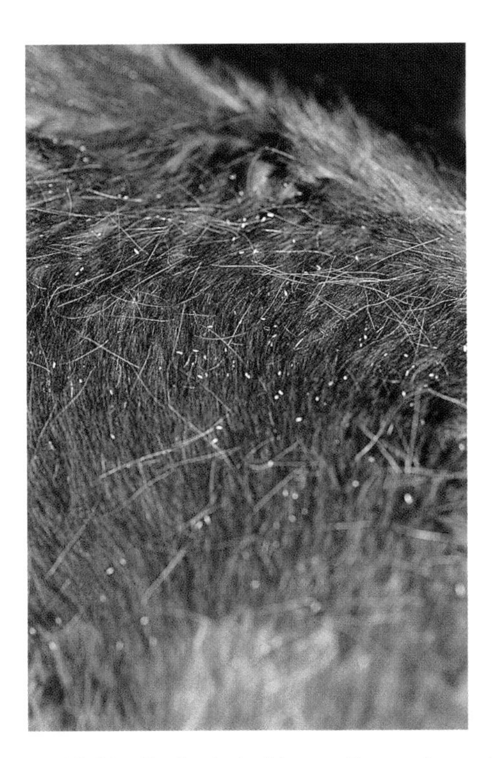

Figure 10.30 Pediculosis. Lice on the coat are visible as small white 'moving' spots. The eggs ('nits') are less visible on the skin. They are attached to hairs, so they may show on magnified hair samples.

phosphates are still widely available for dogs and cats and have been used effectively, but some horses may resent the sound or may show dermal reactions. Pyrethroid louse powders and 'spot' treatments have an unpredictable and often disappointing efficacy. Treatments must be applied to all contact horses simultaneously and must be repeated at 10-day intervals. Oral ivermectin has a limited effect but 'pour-on' ivermectin preparations may be useful. All sprays and pour-on solutions must be applied strictly according to the manufacturer's instructions relating to dosage, concentration, repeat doses and concurrent drug therapy if chemical-induced irritations are to be avoided. Pruritus usually ceases in 24–36 hours following successful treatment. Occasional horses show transient urticaria within 12 hours of pour-on medications.

Coat colour change and loss of hair has been reported after severe louse infestations.[79]

HABRONEMIASIS

Profile

Common cause of ulcerating, cutaneous granulating nodules or wounds in geographical areas where the stomach nematodes *Habronema muscae*, *H. majus* and *Drachia megastoma* occur. It is associated with increased fly population, poor manure collection or disposal and moist patches of long grass. The condition is strongly seasonal, usually with spontaneous remission in autumn/winter. Affected horses are often repeatedly infected in succeeding years, indicating a possible genetic susceptibility. Larval worms are capable of penetrating intact skin.

Clinical signs

The disease occurs in several different forms:

- **Ophthalmic habronemiasis** includes a conjunctival form and a lachrymal form. Conjunctival involvement shows presence of cheesy granules (soft 'kunkers') (**Fig. 10.31**). Involvement of the nasolacrimal duct/sac results in deep circular, granulating ulceration just below the medial canthus of the eye (**Fig. 10.32**). Both forms cause epiphora (tear overflow) and lacrimation (excessive tear production) which may be blood stained.
- **Cutaneous habronemiasis** occurs in two significant forms. Lacrimation and epiphora from any cause wets the facial skin and the resulting excoriated area is colonized by the parasite, causing a rapidly enlarging superficial, granulating skin ulcer (see Fig. 10.32). Facial and ocular irritation results in rubbing and twitching.

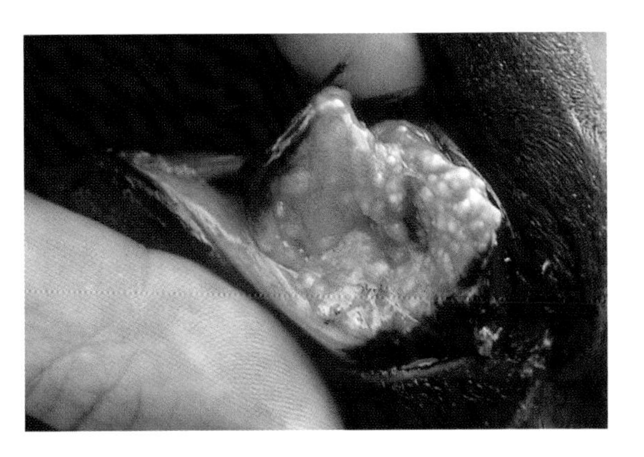

Figure 10.31 Habronemiasis. Conjunctival habronemiasis showing the typical yellow 'granules'.

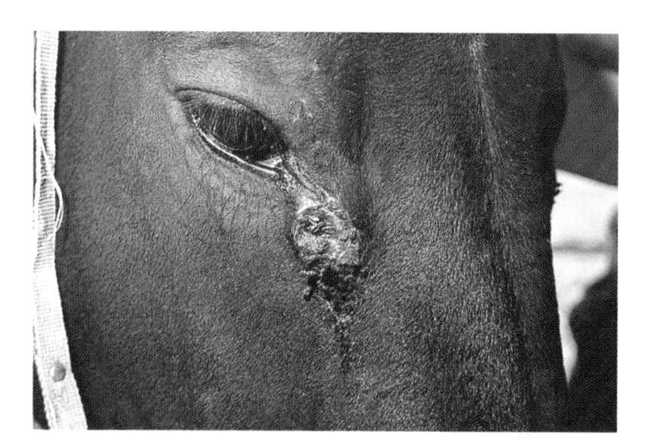

Figure 10.32 Habronemiasis. Habronemiasis of the facial skin below the medial canthus of the eye.

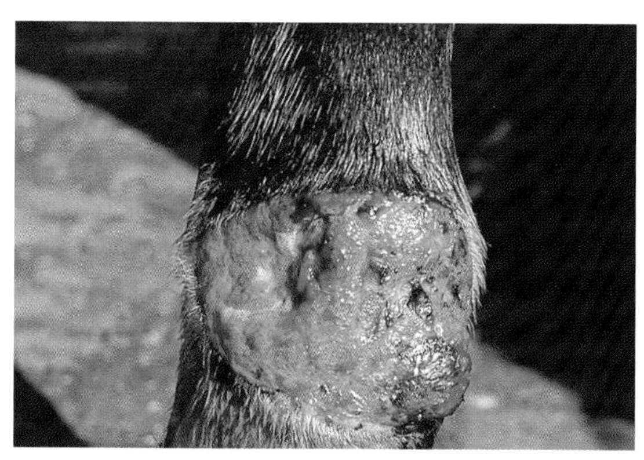

Figure 10.33 Habronemiasis. Habronema infestation of a wound on the cannon resulting in failure of healing. The parasites were visible in washings from the wound surface.

Repeated episodes cause facial scarring and secondary distortion of the eyelids is common.

Wounds which become infested with the parasite fail to heal and may expand with production of unhealthy, exuberant granulation tissue (**Fig. 10.33**), often with an obvious saucer shape. Chewing, biting and rubbing of wounds is very variable; some are severe and others are nonpruritic. A stringy serosanguineous exudate may be seen from some sores. Cheesy, yellow granules may be present on the surface of the wound and in the exudate.

- The urethral process can be affected showing a granulating, ulcerated lesion on the glans penis. Preputial and/or urinary bleeding may be seen or bleeding may occur during service, causing haemospermia which may reduce fertility.

Note: Habronema may be present secondarily to ocular forms of squamous cell carcinoma or to cutaneous pythiosis or other causes of nonhealing wounds and so the combined alternatives should be carefully explored before treatment.

Differential diagnosis

- Exuberant granulation tissue/nonhealing wounds (for any reason)
- Squamous cell carcinoma (facial, penile, palpebral and nictitans forms)
- Sarcoid (fibroblastic and mixed), particularly on the face and at wound sites on the limbs
- Phycomycosis/pythiosis (*Pythium* spp.)
- Botryomycosis (staphylococcal granuloma)
- Foreign body reactions

Diagnostic confirmation

- Characteristic seasonal appearance in geographically endemic area (the parasite will occur in temperate climates under suitable conditions).
- Impression smears and fluid/washes from wounds. False negative smears are common.
- Biopsy may not be very helpful – nonspecific eosinophilia with granulation tissue and intense vascularization.

Treatment

Most lesions resolve spontaneously at the end of the summer months. Surgical removal or curettage is an effective method of treatment on granulating wounds. Oral or topical ivermectin suspended in an aqueous cream base is reportedly effective. Occasionally a second dose is required 3–4 weeks after the initial dose.

Some habronema lesions respond well to cryotherapy, with a single or double freeze–thaw cycle usually being sufficient to kill the larvae, but this may be an over-severe approach.

Ophthalmic forms oral ivermectin and/or corticosteroid eye drops. Lesions on the membrana nictitans (third eyelid) should be curetted and then treated with local application of cortisone drops plus a solution made up with 50% injectable form of ivermectin in artificial tears.

Control

Slashing of long grass in the vicinity of the stable and improved manure disposal will help to control muscid flies and therefore limit the number of cases. Careful attention to horses with a history of the condition is wise as repeated episodes are common and there is some suggestion that there are familial susceptibilities.

PARASITIC/VERMINOUS DERMATITIS

Profile
A diffuse dermatitis involving the distal limbs of young foals after prolonged wet weather where foals are held or handled in old, well-used horse yards, or housed on contaminated bedding or in poor hygienic conditions.[80] Larval forms of the nematodes *Pelodera strongyloides* and *Strongyloides westerii* have been associated with the condition.[80,81]

Clinical signs
Sudden onset of skin irritation and pruritus with stamping, irritability and biting at the legs when mares and foals are congregated in contaminated, wet or boggy yards. Signs of colic such as rolling and biting at legs and flanks can be seen. Interestingly, foals seem to suffer only single or few episodes, seemingly becoming insensitive or resistant to the parasite. Diffuse skin thickening and dermatitis with limb oedema may be present in repeatedly challenged foals. It is reported to cause severe papules, pustules, ulcers, crusts, alopecia and erythema of the limbs, ventral thorax and abdomen, but these represent unusually severe responses.

Differential diagnosis
- Ventral midline dermatitis (biting flies)
- *Culicoides* spp. irritation (ventral biting species)
- *Culicoides* spp. hypersensitivity (sweet itch)
- Chorioptic/psoroptic or sarcoptic mange (usually dorsal pruritus)
- Stable fly (*Stomoxys calcitrans*) bites
- Lice (*Damalinia equina*, *Haematopinus asini*)
- Forage mites (*Trombicula* spp.) or poultry red mite (*Dermanyssus gallinae*) infestation

Diagnostic confirmation
Diagnostic confirmation is difficult.
- History.
- Clinical signs may be suggestive but signs are often not apparently related to skin disease.
- Skin scrapings or washings. Parasite larvae may be seen on or may be recovered from mud washed off the limb into a plastic bag. Positive or negative results may be misleading.
- Skin biopsy shows perifolliculitis, folliculitis and furunculosis. Nematode segments may be present in hair follicles.[82]
- Treatment or removal from the source of infection with subsequent resolution is probably diagnostic.

Treatment
Where severe cases occur, the animals should be washed and removed from the affected yards. Resolution over 3–4 weeks follows improved hygiene and washing of legs in warm soapy water. Topical antibiotic and corticosteroid creams can be used in severe cases if necessary. Control population of *Strongyloides westerii* by regular anthelmintic therapy.

ONCHOCERCAL DERMATITIS (onchocerciasis/microfilariasis)

Profile
Diffuse, seasonal (summer), dermatitis affecting the ventral midline, chest, withers, face and neck due to *Onchocerca cervicalis* microfilaria. The parasite is transmitted by *Culicoides* spp insects and other biting flies. The larvae can be found in the capillaries of the skin of normal horses but type I and type III hypersensitivity reactions appear in some horses affected with microfilaria of *Onchocerca* spp. The clinical disease is rare in horses under 2–3 years old.

Clinical signs
Patchy alopecia with small coalescing papules and thickened, dry scaly skin on the forehead (and less usually the sides of the face; **Fig. 10.34**), pectoral region and ventral midline (**Fig. 10.35**). The condition shows significant pruritus, with severe cases showing marked itching and excoriation, leading to scab formation (the so-called 'bull's eye' lesions on the head). Loss/thinning of mane hair occurs.

The ventral midline shows more consistent alopecia and poor hair regrowth with some leuko- (or melano-)trichia and leuko- (or melano-)derma (see Fig. 10.35).

Tail rubbing is rare.

Severe focal dermatitis with multiple circular inflamed and exudative lesions with moderate to severe pruritus may develop following the death of the microfilaria in the skin after administration of an avermectin anthelmintic (**Fig. 10.36**).

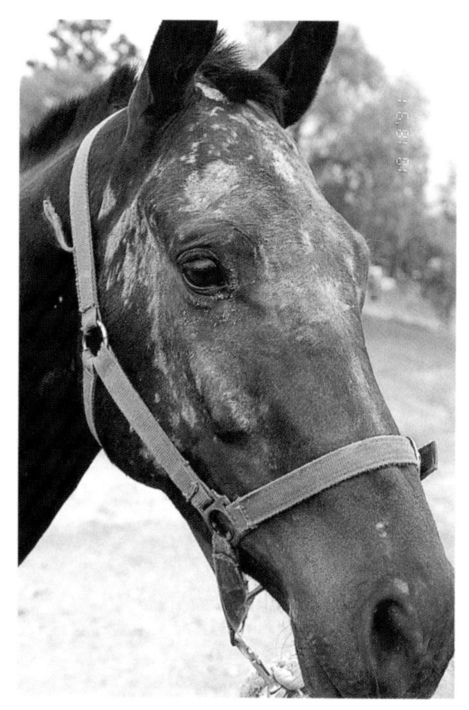

Figure 10.34 Onchocerciasis. Typical alopecic, roughly circular facial lesions of *Onchocerca cervicalis* infection.

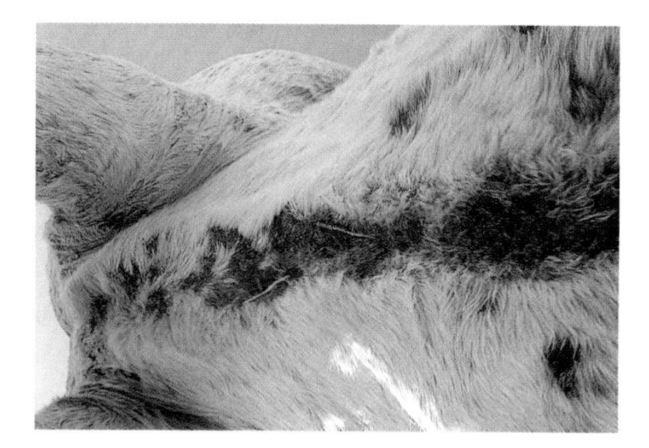

Figure 10.35 Onchocerciasis. Chronic *Onchocerca cervicalis* lesions resulting from irritation and local reaction to the parasites in cutaneous capillaries in the ventral midline.

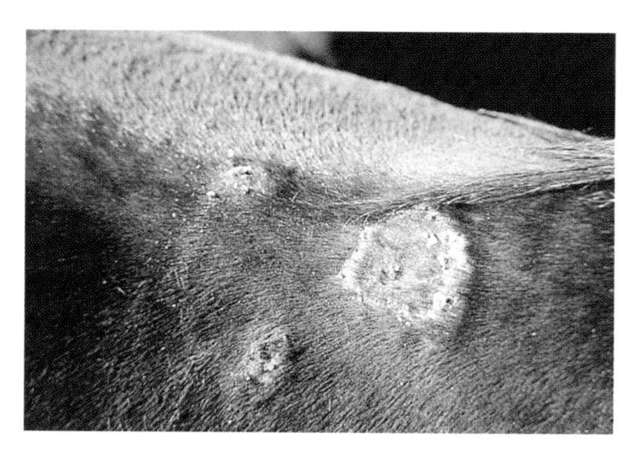

Figure 10.36 Onchocerciasis. Acute focal circular areas of dermatitis resulting from *Onchocerca cervicalis* microfilaria in the skin.

Differential diagnosis

- Ventral midline dermatitis (biting flies)
- Culicoides hypersensitivity (sweet itch)
- Ventral biting *Culicoides* spp. irritation
- Lice (*Damalinia equi*, *Haematopinus asini*)
- Chorioptic/psoroptic/sarcoptic mange
- Trombiculidiasis (*Trombicula* spp.)
- *Boophilus microplus* infestation (cattle tick larvae)
- Nematode dermatitis (*Strongyloides westerii*, *Pelodera strongyloides*)
- *Simulium* spp. (black-fly) irritation
- Unilateral papular dermatosis
- Bacterial folliculitis (*Staphylococcal* spp.)
- Occult sarcoid

Note: As both sweet itch and onchocerciasis are involved with *Culicoides*, both conditions can exist at the same time.

Diagnostic confirmation

- Clinical features.
- History of poor worming regimens (routine use of ivermectin virtually precludes diagnosis).
- Response to ivermectin therapy over several weeks (exacerbation of clinical signs and development of focal suppurative or inflamed areas 24–48 hours after dosing is also supportive of the diagnosis).
- Regresses in winter and returns in summer.
- Biopsy can reveal microfilaria in sections but may be incidental.
- Concentration of larvae using minced biopsy material may also help (but can be misleading also) (see p. 31).

Treatment

Oral ivermectin is extremely effective.[83] Daily dosage for 5 days with fenbendazole or mebendazole at twice the normal dose rate followed by single monthly 'maintenance' treatment is beneficial. Diethylcarbamazine at 1 mg/kg in feed daily for 21 days can be used but is not 100% effective.

Note: Therapy with ivermectin in clinically unaffected and affected horses may cause death of the microfilaria in the capillary beds of the skin. This can cause an acute exudative dermatitis with characteristic circular patterns over the whole body but most severe in the ventral midline and head regions. Severe anaphylactic reactions are also possible.

OXYURIASIS (pin worm) infestation

Profile

Infestation with *Oxyuris equi* which inhabits the terminal regions of the small colon and rectum. Adult worms migrate out of the anus to lay eggs on the perianal skin.

Clinical signs

The adult worms cause anal and perianal irritation. Tail-rubbing causes an acute, excoriated, self-inflicted trauma to the perianal skin and tail-base. Long-term infestation results in excoriation of the base of tail with broken hairs giving a rat-tailed appearance) (**Fig. 10.37**). The horses are often restless and irritable.

Differential diagnosis

- Culicoides hypersensitivity (sweet itch)
- Chorioptic or psoroptic mange
- Lice (*Damalinia equi*, *Haematopinus asini*)
- Dermatophilosis (*Dermatophilus congolensis*)

Diagnostic confirmation

- Poorly wormed, stabled horses
- Examination of perineal area and identification of characteristic triangular operculate eggs from perineal skin using adhesive tape technique (see p. 26).

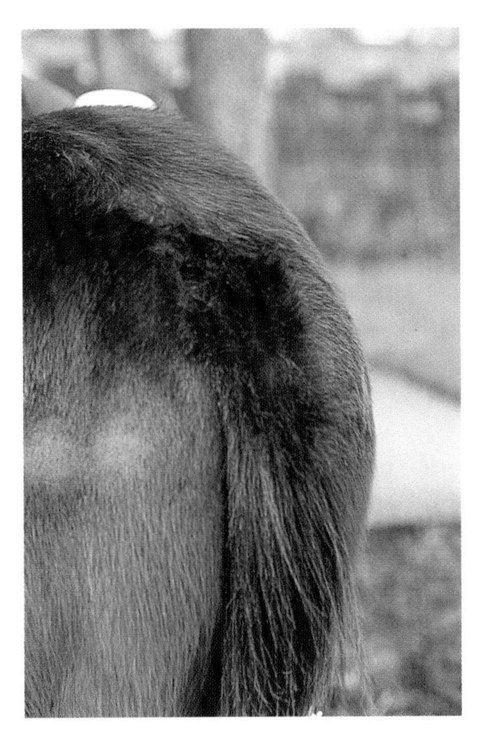

Figure 10.37 Oxyuriasis. Tail-rubbing causing breakage, thinning and distortion of tail hairs due to *Oxyuris equi* infestation.

Treatment

Most modern anthelmintics are effective and any worming programme aimed at ascarids, strongyles and cyathostomes will kill the adult worms. The condition can probably be ignored in horses receiving good anthelmintic regimens involving ivermectin in particular. Improved stable hygiene with clean bedding and regular cleaning of water troughs is important.

Local treatment consists of washing the perineum with soap and warm water to remove the eggs. The itch may be controlled with tranquillizers until anthelmintics have been given.

section B

NON-INFECTIOUS DISEASES

chapter 11

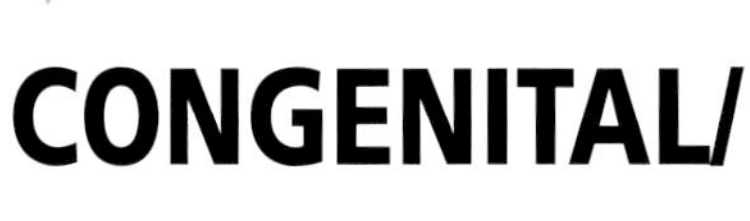

CONGENITAL/ DEVELOPMENTAL DISEASES

Epitheliogenesis imperfecta	145
Epidermolysis bullosa	146
Hyperelastosis cutis (cutaneous aesthenia, Ehlers–Danlos syndrome, dermatosparaxis)	146
Hypotrichosis and mane and tail dystrophy	147
Albinism/lethal-white foal syndrome/ lavender foal syndrome	148
Appaloosa parentage syndrome	149
(Arabian) fading syndrome (pinky syndrome)	150
Conchal cyst	150
Dentigerous cyst	151
Dermoid cyst	151
Epidermoid cysts (atheroma)	152
Calcinosis circumscripta	153

EPITHELIOGENESIS IMPERFECTA

Profile

Rare congenital, inherited cutaneous defect of foals. Possibly a single autosomal recessive gene is responsible.[61,84]

Clinical signs

Clearly demarcated areas with a complete absence of epidermis and skin appendages present at birth. Most obvious defects occur distal to carpus and tarsus but can be over much larger areas (**Fig. 11.1**). Lesions bleed easily and quickly become infected, leading to septicaemia and death. Foals with limited defects have reasonable chance of growing normally, but closure of the fault is difficult.

Differential diagnosis

- Epidermolysis bullosa
- Pemphigus foliaceus

Diagnostic confirmation

- Clinical appearance of complete lack of epidermis and skin appendages over a variable area from birth. There are no other diseases which induce this appearance at birth.
- Negative Nikolsky's sign (transverse finger pressure does not cause the epidermis to 'slip' off the underlying dermis).

Treatment

No treatment is available and even skin grafting of the affected area usually fails to close it. Very small defects can sometimes be closed with repeated surgical reconstructive measures. Cease breeding with mare and stallion.

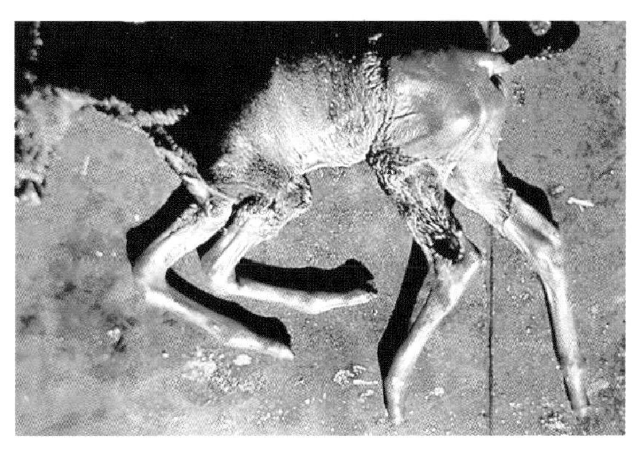

Figure 11.1 Epithelogenesis imperfecta affecting large areas of the skin of a stillborn foal.

EPIDERMOLYSIS BULLOSA

Profile
A group of heritable mechanobullous diseases occurring principally in the Belgian breed of both sexes, characterized by the presence of blister formation following mild trauma.[61,84,85]

Clinical signs
Lesions at mucocutaneous junctions and oral mucosa and elsewhere are present at birth (**Fig. 11.2**). Further lesions develop shortly after birth. Collapsed bullae may be found in the mouth, and separation of hooves at the coronary band is sometimes present. Concurrent dystrophic teeth commonly occur.

Differential diagnosis
- Epitheliogenesis imperfecta
- Bullous pemphigoid
- Pemphigus foliaceus
- Systemic lupus erythematosus-like syndrome
- Scalding and burning injuries

Diagnosis
- Few other conditions are realistically similar.
- Histopathology: cleavage at epidermal–dermal junction.
- Positive Nikolsky's sign (transverse finger pressure *does* cause the epidermis to 'slip' off the underlying dermis)

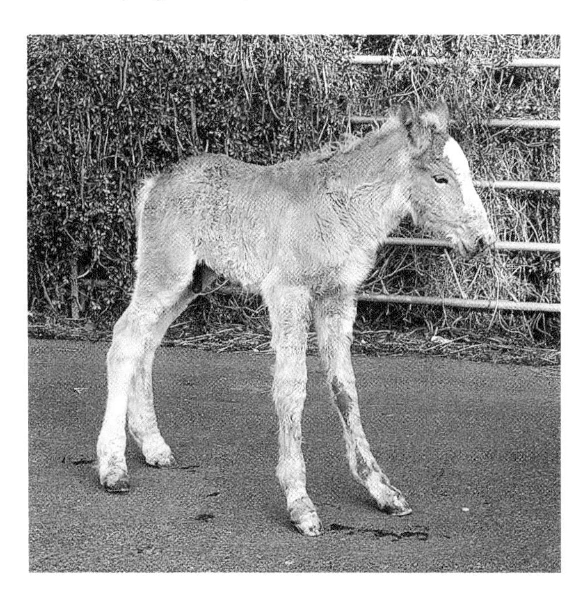

Figure 11.2 Epidermolysis bullosa affecting the medial forelimb region in a Belgian foal.

Treatment
No treatment is possible. Cease breeding from both mare and stallion.

HYPERELASTOSIS CUTIS (cutaneous aesthenia, Ehlers–Danlos syndrome, dermatosparaxis)

Profile
A group of autosomal recessive, inherited, connective-tissue diseases occurring principally in young Quarterhorses which appears at birth or shortly afterwards. At least 9 different subtypes occur in humans and it has been classified on clinical, genetic and biochemical differences. Decreased-collagen as well as fragmentation and disorientation of collagen fibres occur.[84]

Clinical signs
Loose, wrinkled, hyperextensible skin over limited areas of the body or more generalized giving a wrinkle-skin appearance to the whole body (**Fig. 11.3**). There may be sharply demarcated areas of loose hyperfragile skin (**Fig. 11.4**) which tears easily. Damaged or torn skin repairs very slowly with a weak scar formation (and sometimes completely fails to heal) (**Fig. 11.5**). Subcutaneous haematoma and abscesses occur.

Differential diagnosis
- Epitheliogenesis imperfecta/cutaneous agenesis
- Persistent irritation
- Dehydration
- Selenium poisoning

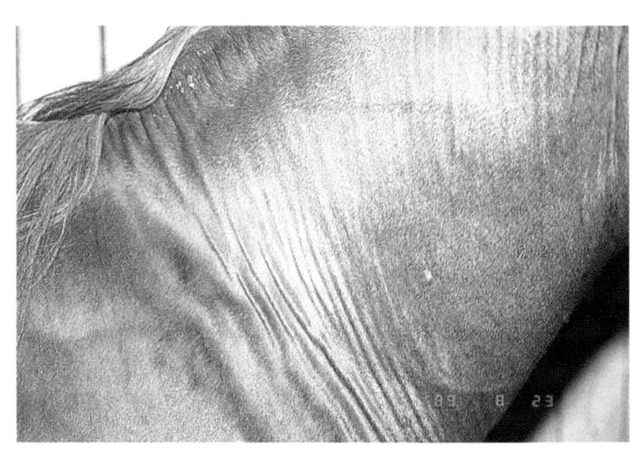

Figure 11.3 Hyperelastosis cutis (cutaneous aesthenia, Ehlers–Danlos syndrome, dermatosparaxis) showing the thin, folded and fragile skin.

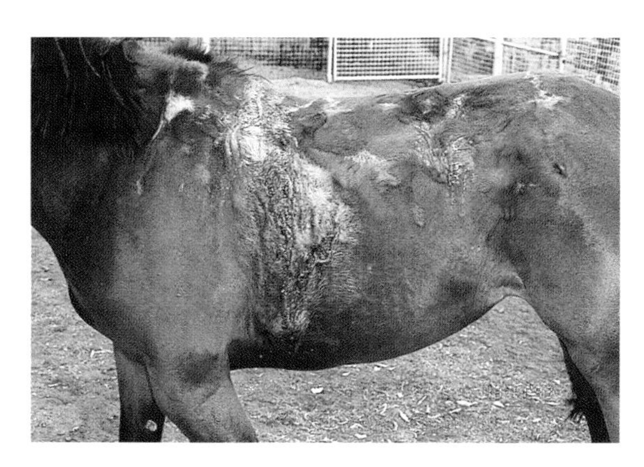

Figure 11.4 Hyperelastosis cutis (cutaneous aesthenia, Ehlers–Danlos syndrome, dermatosparaxis) with extensive skin damage due to minor trauma.

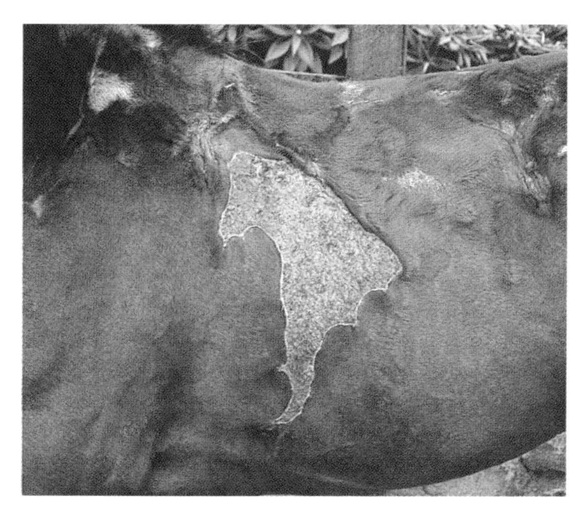

Figure 11.5 Hyperelastosis cutis (cutaneous aesthenia, Ehlers–Danlos syndrome, dermatosparaxis) showing extensive scarring and residual poor skin quality after trauma (same horse as Fig. 11.4, some 3 months later).

Diagnostic confirmation:

- Clinical appearance of loose skin with hyperfragility.
- Biopsy may indicate collagen changes but histopathology has not been well documented in the horse. Thinning of dermis and fragmentation of collagen are the most common reported findings.

Treatment

Affected horses should be removed from breeding programmes. Apart from minimizing trauma and careful, sympathetic wound management, there is no treatment. Wounds in affected areas require collagen-based dressings and a moist wound healing environment. Healing may be delayed for long periods. Skin grafting is theoretically possible but often fails to take over the affected area.

HYPOTRICHOSIS AND MANE AND TAIL DYSTROPHY

Profile

Hypotrichosis is a rare hereditary disease found most often in some lines of Arabian horses in which there is less than the normal amount/density of hair. It does not appear to be linked to hair colour. A commoner manifestation of hair dystrophy/thinning is well recognized in the Appaloosa breed, where the long tail hairs in particular are sparse and brittle. This is regarded as a normal trait in some lines of the Appaloosa horse. Mane and tail dystrophy occurring simultaneously have been recorded in a variety of breeds.

Clinical signs

Hypotrichosis Permanent thinning or almost complete lack of hair particularly around the eyes and extending ventrally towards the muzzle (**Fig. 11.6**). The skin is sometimes slightly scaly and may feel thinner than normal. It seldom affects body hair to any extent.

'Mane and tail dystrophy' shows as a sparse, thin hair density on either the mane or the tail or both with the tail having a rat-tail-like appearance with few, shorter than normal hairs (**Fig. 11.7**).

Differential diagnosis

- Selenium poisoning
- Copper and iodine deficiency
- Chronic/recurrent mild abrasion (e.g. from hoods or other tack)

Diagnostic confirmation

- Clinical appearance and history of sparse hair coat since birth with very little alteration over time.
- Appaloosa or part-bred Appaloosa breeding.
- Biopsy shows reduced numbers of hair follicles but normal skin structure otherwise.

Treatment

None is available. Apart from appearance, there appear to be no detrimental systemic effects associated with this condition. Breeding

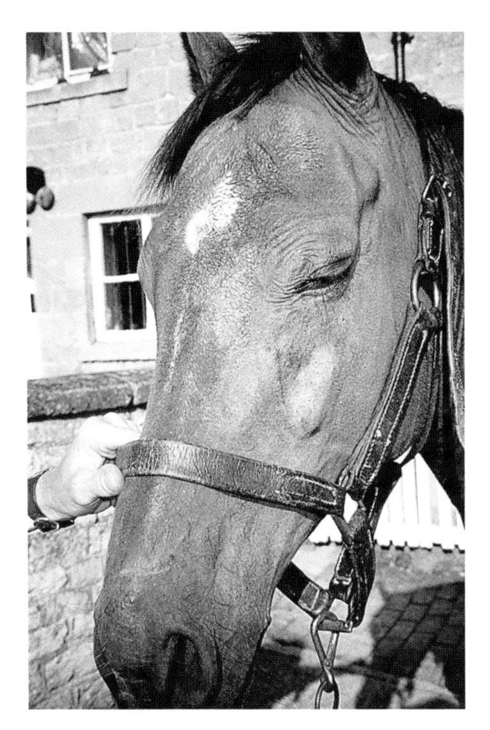

Figure 11.6 Hypotrichosis – poor hair density and quality.

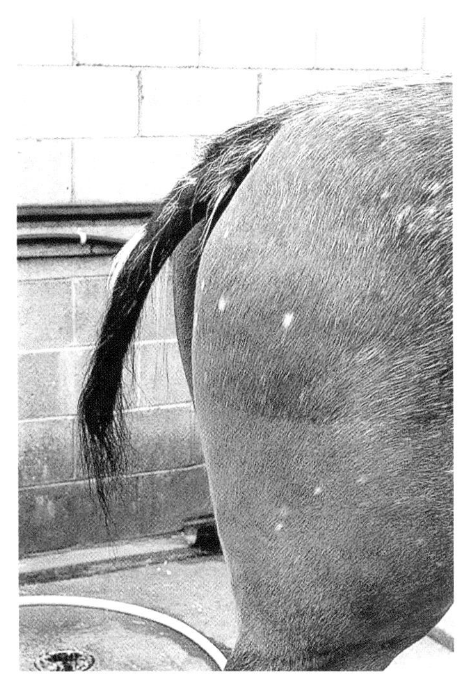

Figure 11.7 Tail-hair dystrophy in an Appaloosa cross gelding.

programmes have failed to identify this trait and it is now accepted in the Appaloosa breed in particular as being normal.

ALBINISM/LETHAL-WHITE FOAL SYNDROME/LAVENDER FOAL SYNDROME

Profile

Albinos have a congenital lack of pigment (melanin) in their skin, hair and iris. This is mostly an inherited condition. Normal melanocytes are present which have a biochemical defect preventing them from synthesizing melanin. Cream-coloured horses lack pigment but are otherwise normal. True albinos have white hair, pink skins and nonpigmented (pink or light blue) irides (and usually have no pigment in the fundus of the eyes). General albinism is an autosomal *dominant* trait and is only viable in the heterozygous state (Ww). While being white-haired, they may have some coloration of the iris (blue or blue/white streaks). When these horses are mated, nonviable embryos (WW) occur in 25% of conceptions and are resorbed or aborted early in gestation. This is best regarded as one form of lethal-white foal syndrome.

Lethal-white foal syndrome occurs with the mating of Overo and Paint horses of the pinto breed and is an autosomal *recessive* trait. These foals are white (albinos) but frequently have concurrent, highly fatal defects of the gastrointestinal tracts such as atresia ani, atresia coli and ileocolonic aganglionosis.[84,86]

Lavender foal syndrome is a rare (supposedly) hereditary disorder of Arabian foals derived from a particular Egyptian line. Most cases have been reported in the United States. It may be coupled with other congenital/genetic defects such as cardiac deformities, wry nose or cleft palate and possible intestinal aganglionosis.

Clinical signs

Partial albino horses are relatively common, showing cream skin and a white hair coat (**Fig. 11.8**). The retina is invariably partially or completely albinotic and the iris may be variously pale blue or white in colour (either completely or partially).

Lethal-white foals are a startlingly white colour at birth. Although they may be apparently normal for the first 1–2 hours after birth, they rapidly develop severe intractable and fatal colic as a result

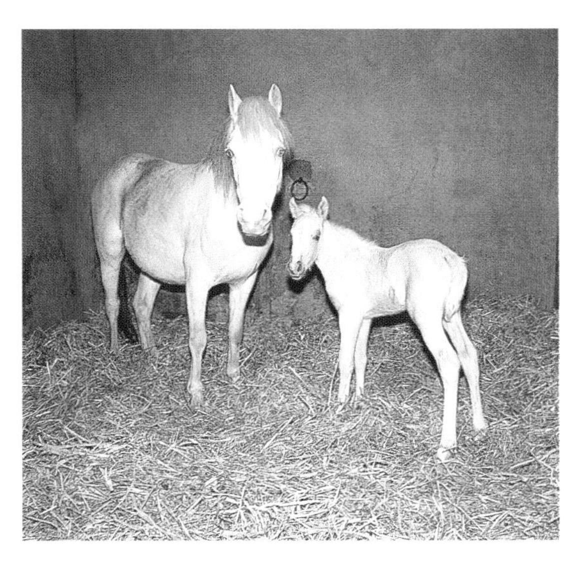

Figure 11.8 Albino foal and albino mare. Both had albinotic retinas and nonpigmented (blue/yellow) irides. Both lived normal lives.

of an incomplete intestinal tract or ileus as a result of intestinal aganglionosis (or both). Concurrent abnormalities of the mouth, pharynx, heart or other structures are also sometimes present.

Lavender foals have a characteristic lavender (bluish/purple) coat colour at birth. They are neurologically abnormal at birth, showing neonatal seizures and convulsions (often even occurring during or immediately after birth). Opisthotonos, paddling, aimless galloping and apparent blindness with a light-hungry and startled expression may be present. No periods of remission or sleep occur. They fail to rise and have no (or reduced/abnormal) suckle reflexes. Death is inevitable.

Differential diagnosis

- Convulsions are similar to neonatal maladjustment/convulsive foal syndrome.
- Idiopathic/benign epilepsy.
- Cerebellar/cerebral hypoplasia syndromes.
- Meningocele/encephalocele.
- Cerebral trauma at or during birth.
- Extensive blood loss at or during birth (visible or invisible) including early cord separation.

Diagnostic confirmation

- Characteristic colour and abrupt onset of associated clinical syndromes of colic and/or intractable seizures.
- Arterial oxygen normal and no evidence of parturient hypoxia.
- Normal haematology/biochemistry.
- Cerebrospinal fluid and electroencephalograms are normal.
- Post mortem examination will identify concurrent developmental abnormalities and intestinal aganglionosis.
- Most cases of lavender foal syndrome show no detectable lesions in any organ, suggesting that it is a functional/physiological disorder.

Treatment

There is no treatment. Albino foals are often normal and survive normally (cream horses are a form of this), although many are mildly photophobic. For lethal-white and lavender foals, attempts to control seizures are fruitless. General anaesthesia gives temporary relief. Attempts to anastomose atretic intestine or enterectomy of affected intestine are a waste of time and effort. Both of these conditions should presently be regarded as 100% fatal within 24–72 hours.

APPALOOSA PARENTAGE SYNDROME

Profile

Appaloosa cross-bred foals often do not have full colour change until 3–4 years of age.

Clinical signs

A previously whole-coloured horse develops white hairs and sometimes overt spots over the rump in particular. Patchy progressive depigmentation of muzzle, eyelids, vulva and prepuce. Hair and skin colour fades progressively with age. Hooves may show banded depigmentation particularly around the hoof wall. Mane and tail hairs may thin out (see mane and tail dystrophy above) but colour changes are not prominent.

Differential diagnosis

- Systemic lupus erythematosus-like syndrome
- Vitiligo/Arabian fading syndrome
- Age-related greying of hair
- Trauma or heat/cold related leukoderma/leukotrichia

Diagnostic confirmation

- Clinical signs coupled with Appaloosa parentage (up to 3 or more generations away).
- Biopsies are unrewarding.

Treatment
It is widely regarded as a normal trait in Appaloosa cross horses.

(ARABIAN) FADING SYNDROME (pinky syndrome)

Profile
Occurs most often in Arabian horses at any age but has also been observed in Welsh mountain ponies.

Clinical signs
Annular or irregular areas of depigmentation of muzzle, lips, periorbital regions (**Fig. 11.9**) and occasionally around perineum, sheath and hooves. Horses occasionally show body patches of depigmentation which may wax and wane in intensity but are usually permanent. The pink skin may be very liable to sunburn.

Differential diagnosis
- Copper deficiency
- Systemic (cutaneous) lupus erythematosus-like syndrome
- Vitiligo

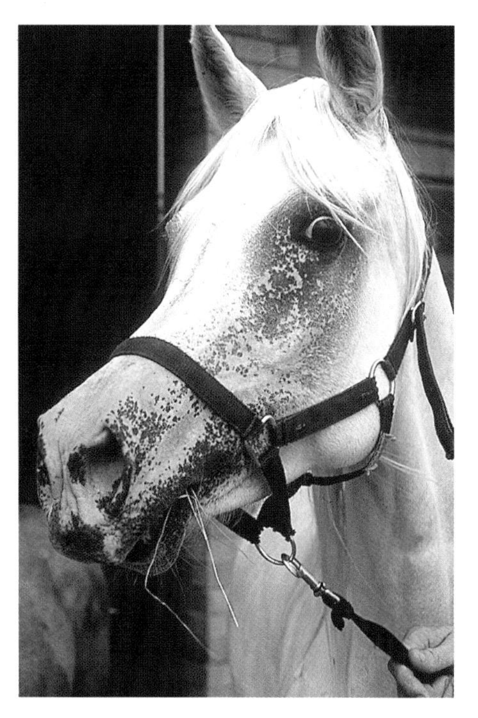

Figure 11.9 (Arabian) fading syndrome (pinky syndrome).

- Appaloosa parentage syndrome
- Trauma, related leukoderma/leukotrichia or freeze/radiation

Diagnostic confirmation
- Clinical appearance in Arabian or Welsh mountain pony breeds.
- Wetting the horse with water allows depigmentation to become more obvious.
- Skin biopsy shows loss of melanin from epidermal basal cells.

Treatment
No effective treatment. Tattoo or hair dyes can be used to mask the true effects but its progressive nature makes it almost impossible to hide permanently. Some horses have shown partial spontaneous recovery.

CONCHAL CYST

Profile
Congenital/developmental abnormality at the base of the ear. May be bilateral.

Clinical signs
Fluctuating, nonpainful swelling at base of the ear or, if fistulated, discharges a glairy, sticky, clear or slightly milky fluid from a tract usually situated on the lower third of the leading edge of the pinna (**Fig. 11.10**).

Differential diagnosis
- Dentigerous cyst
- Foreign body
- Chronic fistula
- Epidermoid cyst
- Psoroptic mange, *Tyroglyphus* spp. nymphs
- Otitis externa/spinose ear tick (*Otobius megnini*)
- Otitis media (suppurative)

Diagnostic confirmation
- Characteristic appearance.
- Histopathology after surgical removal will confirm the diagnosis.

Treatment
Complete surgical removal of the cyst and its duct is the only effective treatment.

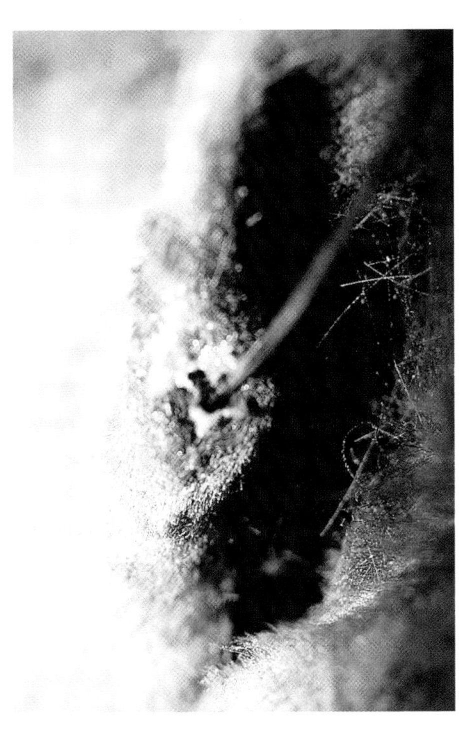

Figure 11.10 Conchal cyst showing the fistula and the character of the discharge. The location is very typical.

DENTIGEROUS CYST

Profile

Congenital or developmental swellings occurring between the base of the ear and eye (temporal region) arising from tooth germ tissue. Occasionally they are also found on the cranial vault or maxillary sinus and contain enamel-forming tissue. They are lined with stratified squamous epithelium and may contain one or more teeth. Drainage may occur near the ear or through the skin adjacent to the cyst.

Clinical signs

Firm, usually fixed nodule between the eye and the ear in the temporal region with an associated fluctuant cyst or a persistent discharging sinus producing a sticky, clear or slightly milky fluid (**Fig. 11.11**). There may be a radiographically obvious dental remnant either associated with the cranium or lying in the adjacent tissues. The former are often fixed firmly while the latter are more mobile.

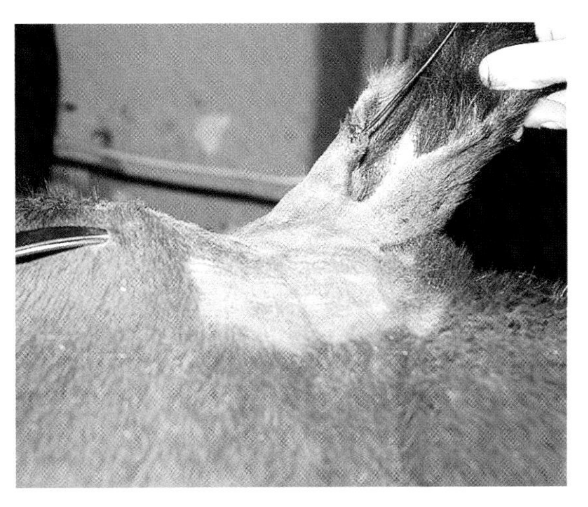

Figure 11.11 Dentigerous cyst with a typical fistula and discharge. The scissors point to an abnormal solid structure which was identified radiographically as an aberrant tooth in a pseudo-alveolus attached to the cranium.

Differential diagnosis

- Conchal cysts
- Other cystic structures
- Neoplasia
- Abscess (usually *Streptococcus equi equi*)

Diagnostic confirmation

- Characteristic appearance.
- Radiography and ultrasonography. May be obvious dental tissue and even an alveolus attached to the cranium.

Treatment

Cautious surgical removal is required (fracture of the cranial vault can occur during attempts to remove the aberrant tooth).

DERMOID CYST

Profile

Congenital or hereditary cutaneous cysts thought to be due to embryonic displacement of ectoderm into the subcutis. Occurs singly and most commonly along dorsal midline. No breed predilection.[87] Usually young horses (< 18 months old) are affected.

Clinical signs

Single or multiple, firm to fluctuant, smooth, dermal nodules (10–15 mm diameter) with normal overlying haired skin. Most are on the dorsal midline between withers and rump (**Fig. 11.12**). Lesions contain a soft cheese-like grey material and sometimes coiled hairs.

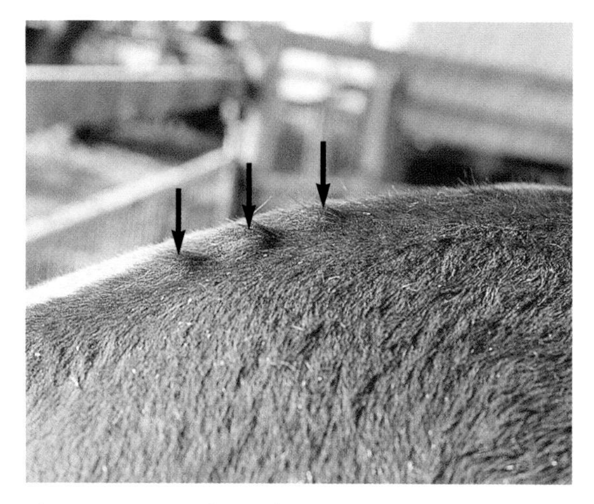

Figure 11.12 Three dermoid cysts in the skin of the croup.

Differential diagnosis

- Epidermoid cysts
- Dentigerous cysts
- Hypodermiasis (*Hypoderma bovis*).

Diagnostic confirmation

- Characteristic location and clinical appearance.
- Excisional biopsy shows cyst wall lined with stratified squamous epithelium containing adnexal structures.

Treatment

Total surgical ablation of cyst wall and contents is effective.

EPIDERMOID CYSTS (atheroma)

Profile

Developmental cystic structure of the epidermis. The commonest site is just above the caudal limit of the false nostril, where it is known as an atheroma. Other sites affected include the limbs and the head.

Clinical signs

Freely movable, well-circumscribed, firm to fluctuant, (usually) solitary nodules (7–30 mm diameter) occurring on head (the area dorsal to the false nostril is by far the commonest site) (**Fig. 11.13**) and legs. They contain a yellow to grey mucoid or porridge-like fluid and no hairs and often remain static for years. A few expand continually but slowly over years. Only very rarely do they reach a size sufficient to cause a problem with air flow in the ipsilateral nostril. It is usually a cosmetic problem only.

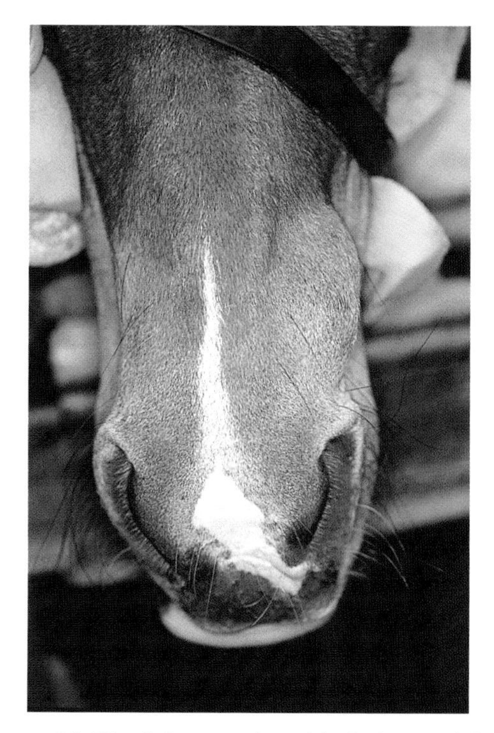

Figure 11.13 Atheroma (nasal inclusion cyst) in a typical location.

Differential diagnosis

- Dentigerous cyst
- Dermoid and conchal cysts
- Foreign body reaction
- Nodular sarcoid

Diagnostic confirmation

- Nonpainful, noninflammatory fluctuant or firm swelling above false nostril is typical.
- Aspiration produces a grey or white sterile creamy liquid.

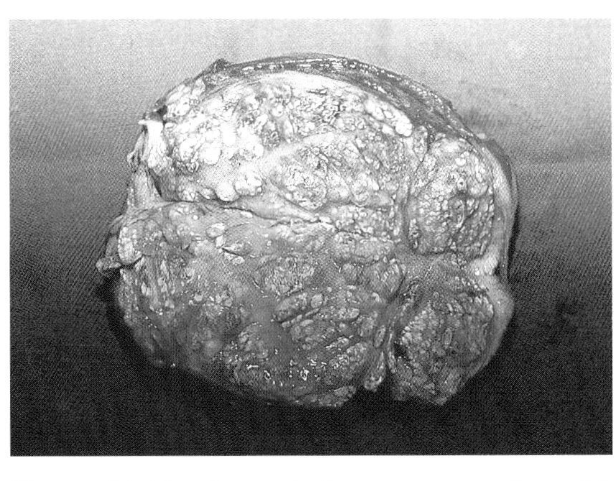

Figure 11.14 The typical appearance of a calcinosis circumscripta nodule surgically removed from the lateral aspect of the stifle.

- Histopathology shows an epithelial lining showing maturation and keratinization typical of epidermis *but* no adnexal structures.

Treatment

Surgical removal is effective.

CALCINOSIS CIRCUMSCRIPTA

Profile

Developmental/congenital condition of young horses (1–4 years) typically occurring over the lateral stifle area and less commonly over other joints such as the carpus and tarsus.

Clinical signs

Firm, nonpainful, nonpruritic, subcutaneous swelling up to 80 mm (or more) in diameter located over the lateral aspect of the stifle or gaskin (or other regions). The circumscribed mass, which comprises an aggregation of calcified granules in a milky-white crumbly base (**Fig. 11.14**), is often clearly attached to the underlying ligament, muscle or joint capsule.

Differential diagnosis

- Acquired bursa
- Foreign body
- Dermoid cyst

Diagnostic confirmation

- Radiographic and ultrasonographic examinations are characteristic.
- Biopsy shows multinodular deposits of minerals within fibrous and granulomatous tissue.

Treatment

Complete surgical removal under general anaesthetic is essential to prevent recurrence but is sometimes not as easy as it might seem initially. There is a high incidence of suture dehiscence.[88]

chapter 12

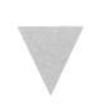

IMMUNE-MEDIATED/ ALLERGIC DISEASES

Urticaria	156
Atopy	160
Food hypersensitivity	161
Pemphigus foliaceus	162
Pemphigus vulgaris (EPV) and bullous pemphigoid (BP)	163
Immune-mediated vasculitis	164
Pastern and cannon leukocytoclastic vasculitis	165
Systemic/cutaneous lupus erythematosus-like syndrome (SLE-like syndrome)	166
Alopecia areata	168
Linear keratosis/linear alopecia	169
Sarcoidosis	169
Erythema multiforme	170
Equine insect hypersensitivity/allergy (sweet itch, Queensland itch)	171
Contact hypersensitivity	173
Drug eruption	174
Lymphoedema	175
(Sterile, nodular) Panniculitis/steatitis	176
Equine cutaneous amyloidosis	176
Axillary nodular necrosis	177
Eosinophilic collagen necrosis/granuloma	177
(Generalized) Granulomatous (enteritis) disease (chronic eosinophilic enteritis)	178
Seborrhoea	179
Purpura haemorrhagica (immune-mediated vasculitis)	180

Inflammatory changes occur in the skin whenever it is injured. These changes are initially related to the specific cause and, secondarily, may relate to autologous changes which develop later. Regardless of the cause, be it heat, cold, infection due to bacterial, fungal, viral or parasitic organisms, radiation, trauma, or allergens, the skin response will be characterized by responses which involve blood vessels, tissue fluids and cells. These changes will be identifiable clinically as the cardinal signs of inflammation, viz. heat, pain, redness, swelling and variable loss of function.

Protection of the host is by means of a structured immune response involving antigens, lymphocytes, antibodies, complement, and other mediators and effector cells. Their normal action is to restore natural body function. Tissues themselves have an immune privilege which severely curtails the extent of self-destruction. Under- or overactivity may lead to serious problems for the host. *Underresponse* leads to failure to control infection and poor elimination of toxic by-products. *Overresponse* causes a loss of, or a reduction in, the immune privilege of tissues (which is responsible for preventing the body destroying itself) and therefore an excessive inflammatory response develops which results in the production of autoimmune disease. Both of these responses are common features of skin disease.

The various ways in which the body can respond have been broadly grouped into four types of hypersensitivity[89] and these have been described in Chapter 1, p. 6). While these are fairly well defined, many reactions are complexes of these and so may show broad variations in clinical features. Types I, II and III all rely on antigen–antibody reactions and are therefore more or less immediate in their clinical effects following introduction of the antigen to a sensitized host animal (usually in less than 4 hours and possibly within minutes). Type IV, however, is cell-mediated and has no immediate antibody–antigen component. Therefore, the responses are delayed for a variable period of time (24–72 hours). The clinical situation, however, is frequently complicated by secondary effects such as self-inflicted trauma and the clinician is only able to examine a single moment in the continuing/continuous process.

Although crusting and scaling (dry dermatoses) are prominent features of many allergic or autoimmune conditions, other signs, including nodules and moist dermatoses, may be present. The diagnosis of allergic or autoimmune disease is not always simple. Indeed, apart from insect hypersensitivity and urticaria, the immune-mediated diseases are not common and are very difficult to diagnose. Their diagnosis may rely on meticulous clinical and historical findings and the elimination of the other more common causes of crusting and scaling in particular.

A very careful examination of the horse's history, a carefully considered series of biopsies of recent lesions, and the assistance of a specialist veterinary dermatopathologist are significant aids to reaching a diagnosis. Knowledge of immune-mediated diseases is being expanded and the similarity to corresponding human disease is evident. However, the horse may present significant or minor variations to the general pattern seen in other species. Similar names are therefore given to some diseases, but it is important to realize that species differences may not entirely justify the name. Extrapolation from the name of the disease to possible diagnostic features and treatment may also therefore not be justified. Further knowledge and research into these diseases may well reclassify them. **Table 12.1** demonstrates the major clinical features of the allergic and autoimmune diseases of the horse.

URTICARIA

Profile

Of all the species of domestic animals, horses show the greatest incidence of urticaria. However, urticaria is a symptom or sign of disease rather than a specific disease entity. It has many different possible causes. In the clinical situation it is usually taken as a single entity even though its clinical manifestations vary from a minor transitory nature to a major, systemic, and possibly even life-threatening problem. Horses between 1 and 10 years of age appear most liable and there is no gender predisposition. Thoroughbred and Arabians are possibly predisposed to urticaria from inhaled allergens.

The aetiopathogenesis is complex, with many suggested or identified causes.[90]

- Degranulation of mast cells and basophils is presumed to be the basic pathogenesis involving the liberation of chemical mediators which cause increased vascular permeability, inflammation and protein leakage with consequent wheal formation.
- Immunological or hypersensitivity reactions in which injected (drugs), ingested (chemical, feeds) or inhaled (pollen, dust, chemicals, moulds) antigens/allergens are delivered to the

Table 12.1 General clinical signs of allergic and autoimmune diseases of the horse

	Scabs and crusts	Erosions and ulceration	Pruritus
Diseases in which hair loss occurs			
Contact hypersensitivity	++	+	+
Drug eruptions	++	+	+++
Systemic lupus erythematosus	+++	+	–
Alopecia areata	–	–	–
Granulomatous enteritis	++	+	++?
Insect hypersensitivity	+++	+++	+++
Linear alopecia	++	–	–
Pemphigus foliaceus	+++	–	+
Pemphigus vulgaris/bullous pemphigoid	bulla	+++	+/–?
Sarcoidosis	+++	+	–
Onchocercal dermatitis	+++	++	++
Vasculitis	++	++	pain
Pastern leukocytoclastic vasculitis	+++	++	pain
Diseases in which hair loss does not initially occur			
Erythema multiforme	+	+	–
Panniculitis (nodular)	–	–	–
Urticaria	–	–	+/–

skin systemically rather than by local contact. Penicillin is the most commonly implicated drug responsible for urticaria.

- Allergic urticaria arises from drugs, food, inhaled allergens (pollens, moulds)[91] or more rarely by direct skin or mucous membrane contact. These should be carefully distinguished from allergic contact dermatitis.
- Physical urticaria arises without any immunological component. Dermatographism arises when a wheal develops from a blunt 'scratch' on skin (**Fig. 12.1**). 'Cold' or temperature-related urticaria can arise from either cold, heat or even light under some conditions. Exercise-induced urticaria may also be encountered following heavy exercise (particularly in hot or very cold conditions).

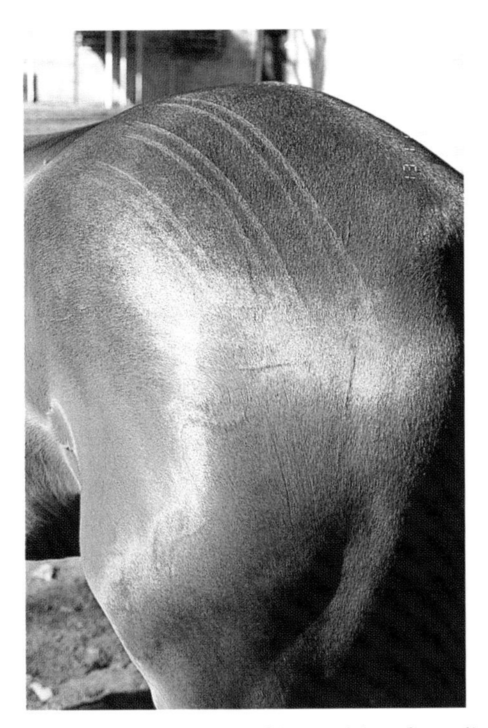

Figure 12.1 Dermatographism arising from light finger scratching over the buttocks.

'Pitting-on-pressure' test

When steady and firm digital pressure is applied to an oedematous swelling or wheal for 10–20 seconds, the imprint/indentation of the finger will remain obvious at the site for several minutes (or longer in some cases) (see Fig. 12.32a,b). Inflammatory or solid/tumour-like swellings do not compress in this way, while fluid-filled swellings are compressible but do not retain the shape of the finger.

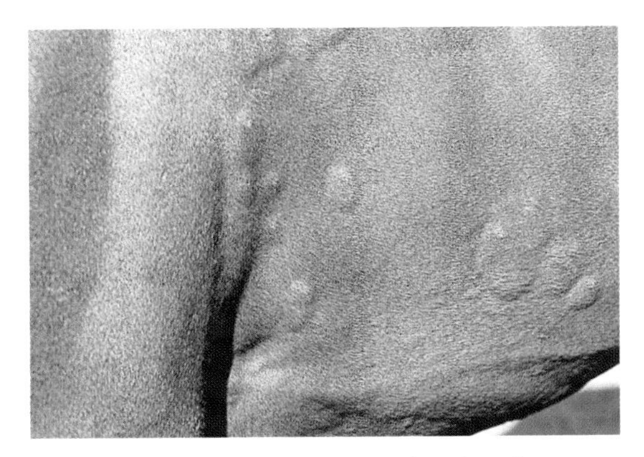

Figure 12.2 Urticaria. Wheals showing the steep-sided, sharply demarcated nature of the typical lesions.

Clinical signs

Onset can be acute or peracute with signs developing within minutes up to a few hours following the instigating factor. Characteristically the signs are oedematous lesions of the skin or mucous membranes called 'wheals' which are flat-topped, papules/nodules with steep-walled sides (**Fig. 12.2**). Typically the lesions themselves will 'pit-on-pressure', but the surrounding skin will usually be normal and will not pit on pressure. This test may be difficult to apply effectively to small urticarial lesions.

Some lesions have slightly depressed centres, but in true urticaria there is no central focus of inflammation (in contrast to insect bites). Pruritus may or may not be present. Some severely affected cases show no pruritus while mild cases with a few lesions sometimes show severe pruritus with extensive self-inflicted trauma suggestive of insect bite hypersensitivity. Hair loss is not usually present unless individual lesions are exudative. Recurrent episodes at random intervals are relatively common (especially when these are due to inhaled or ingested allergens).

Individual urticarial lesions vary in size and shape and quite arbitrarily may be divided into:

Conventional wheals: 2–5 mm in diameter (**Fig. 12.3**).

Papular wheals: multiple, small, uniform 3–6 mm diameter wheals (similar to the appearance of insect bites but without a central focus) (**Fig. 12.4**).

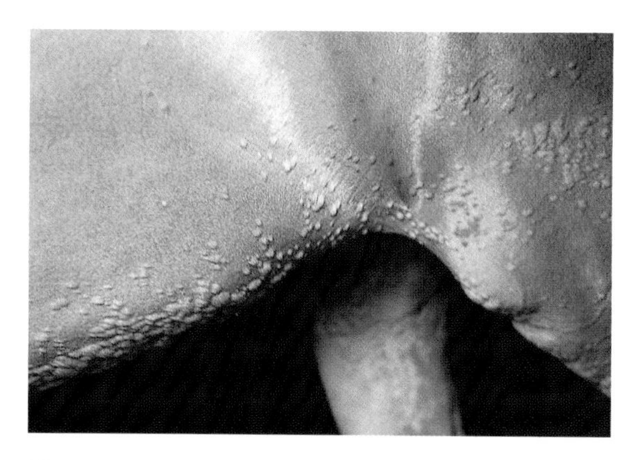

Figure 12.3 Urticaria. Conventional wheals. Lesions are 2–3 mm up to 3–5 mm in diameter.

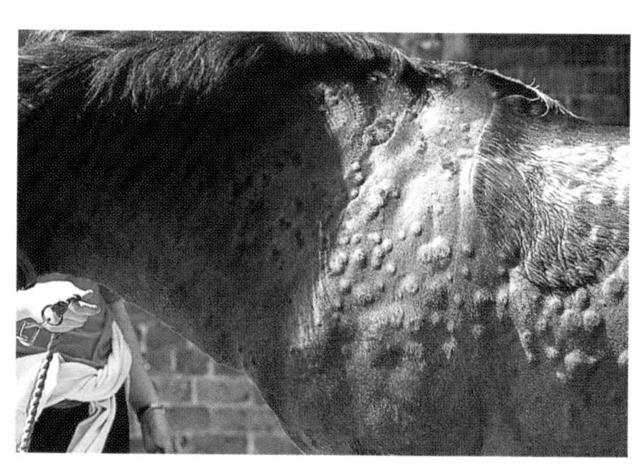

Figure 12.5 Urticaria. Giant wheals. Single and coalesced, multiple wheals up to 20–30 cm diameter.

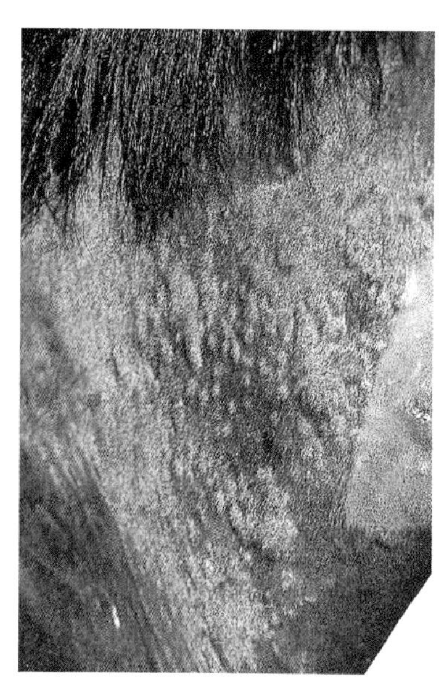

Figure 12.4 Urticaria. Papular wheals: multiple, small uniform 3–6 mm diameter wheals.

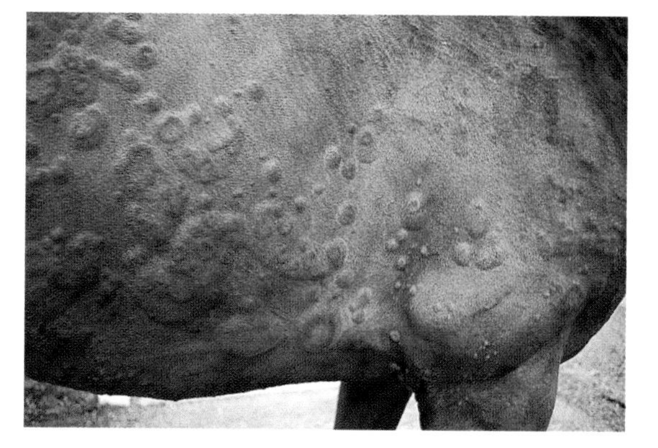

Figure 12.6 Urticaria. Annular wheals. 'Doughnut'-like lesions with a regular or irregular ring of oedema surrounding a depressed, non- (or less) oedematous centre.

Giant wheals: either single or coalesced, multiple wheals up to 20–30 cm diameter (**Fig. 12.5**).

Annular wheals: 'doughnut'-like lesions with a regular or irregular ring of oedema surrounding a depressed, nonoedematory or less oedematous centre (**Fig. 12.6**).

The clinical appearance of the lesions may also present in several different ways depending on the precise location of the response in the skin.

Oozing urticaria Dermal oedema is severe, resulting in oozing of serum from the skin surface and possibly cracking and superficial sloughing of the hair and skin. Care should be taken to distinguish this from an erosive/ulcerative process or a pyoderma or vasculitis. In the early stages the oedematous lesions will still 'pit-on-pressure' in spite of their apparent severity.

Gyrate urticaria The urticarial lesions take on a variety of shapes with some straighter linear, some curvilinear lesions and some serpiginous lesions (**Fig. 12.7**). This has been referred to as the dermal form of 'erythema multiforme' but it should be stressed that this syndrome is not related to 'true' erythema multiforme which is a primary epidermal disease (see Fig. 12.25, p. 171). Drug reactions appear to be the most common cause of this form of urticaria.

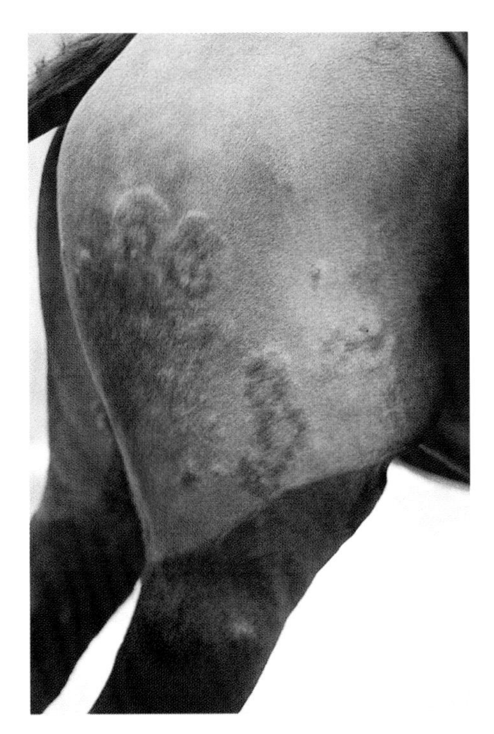

Figure 12.7 Gyrate urticaria.

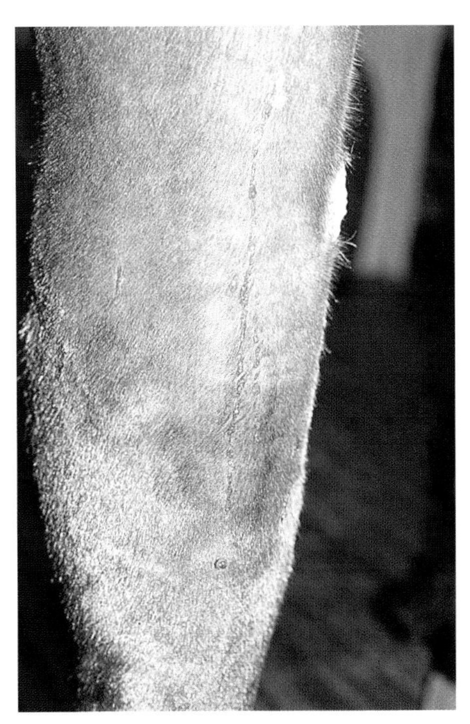

Figure 12.8 Angio-oedema with serum exudation. Note that the oedema is diffuse and ill-defined but it will still pit on pressure.

Angio-oedema (angioneurotic oedema) This is a subcutaneous form of urticaria which tends to be more diffuse owing to lack of restraint of the spread of the fluid through the subcutis (**Fig. 12.8**). It usually involves the head and extremities and is more indicative of systemic and/or serious disease than 'simple' urticaria. Pruritus may or may not be present. It can easily be mistaken for vasculitis and the skin manifestations of the two conditions may in some cases be indistinguishable.

Differential diagnosis

- Insect (mosquitoes/bee/wasp/fly) bites (*Stomoxys* and *Culicoides* are the commonest causes)
- Purpura haemorrhagica
- Erythema multiforme
- Dermatophytosis (*Trichophyton equinum*, *Microsporum* spp.)
- Dermatophilosis (*Dermatophilus congolensis*)
- Haematoma (± haemophilia)
- Lymphangitis
- Abscess/pyoderma
- Cellulitis
- Vasculitis (immune-mediated and photoactivated/actinic)

Diagnostic confirmation

A diagnosis of urticaria is probably unjustified because it is a sign of underlying reactions and it is important to establish the true cause and correct this.

- Clinical signs and history. Recurrence or repeated episodes in response to any possible aetiology (above) is very helpful.
- Biopsy is often unrewarding and can even be misleading. The extent of self-inflicted or secondary trauma can further complicate the problem of diagnosis if reliance is made on biopsy. Biopsy specimens are often of lesser diagnostic value because oedema fluid leaks out into the fixative. However, the section may show non-specific lymphocyte and eosinophil infiltration.
- A dermatographism check can be made by scratching the skin with the blunt end of a ballpoint pen and observing for a reaction within 10–15 minutes (a positive reaction is reflected by a marked oedematous wheal which follows the path of the scratch).
- 'Cold' urticaria can be induced by applying an ice cube to the skin for a few minutes, and an urticarial wheal developing in < 15 minutes is a positive reaction.

- Other allergens can be detected by enzyme-linked immunosorbent assay (ELISA) or radioallergosorbent test (RAST) on a blood (serum) sample. Tests are designed to detect specific IgE proteins which reflect allergic responses. The tests are not widely standardized and in many ways are too sensitive for practical use. They commonly identify groups of proteins, etc., to which the horse is variously 'allergic' (see p. 32, Chapter 3).
- Suspected food allergy can only be traced by using a hypoallergenic diet (such as alfalfa hay only with distilled or boiled water) for 3 weeks and then challenging the horse with specific single components of the diet for 3 weeks until a positive is identified. Confirmation of this will require a second challenge after withdrawal for 3 weeks. Positive reactions can develop quickly but can also take 2–3 weeks to appear, so it can be a very time consuming process.
- 'Contact' causes are rare in horses but during diagnostic tests the horse should be kept in a clean stable on paper bedding and all contact with possible sources of insects or other allergens should be avoided.

Treatment

Treatment is often frustrating, with recurrences occurring at regular or irregular intervals.

1. Initial attack. A short course of systemic corticosteroids administered intravenously often has a dramatic benefit. It can be repeated 2–3 times over several days if necessary.
2. After each recurrence a full further investigation *must* be undertaken. The early episodes are often the clearest and least complicated. Every effort must be made to establish the likely cause by dietary and management manipulation. All extraneous drugs and supplements should be withdrawn.
3. If the condition persists after 4–6 weeks, reassess again and possibly evaluate by skin testing (Chapter 3, p. 33) for atopic disease (IgE) or specific ELISA or RAST tests for IgE. Identify possible/probable causes from the panel of positive results and attempt to avoid them.
4. Hyposensitization and neutralization may be attempted but this is not generally available and carries risks. It may hold some promise for inhaled allergic urticaria. The specific dose of the allergen used and the required frequency of challenge are variable according to the individual response but usually have to be maintained throughout life.

Long-term treatment

Twice-daily doses of oral corticosteroids (preferably prednisolone or methylprednisolone) should be manipulated so as to obtain an acceptable effect. The dose should then be reduced to reach a minimal effective therapeutic dose. Double this daily dose should then be administered on alternate mornings only (see Chapter 4, p. 48). Antihistamines including oral hydroxyzine hydrochloride or parenteral tripelennamine are very disappointing in the horse. If effective, a remission in 3–4 days will be achieved and the drug can then be reduced to a minimum effective daily dose. Major side effects include sedation and/or hyperactivity. The drugs should not be used in pregnant mares as there is a suggestion of teratogenicity.

ATOPY

Profile

A genetically mediated (inherited) pruritus associated with a type I hypersensitivity reaction to pollens, grasses, weeds and trees, moulds, dust, feathers, cotton, wool and other fibres. Arabians and Thoroughbreds in early adulthood appear to be predisposed to the condition.[92] There is debate whether the classical disease exists in the horse. Although it is considered to be a rare disease, it may in fact be underdiagnosed.

Clinical signs

Recurrent pruritus unrelated to season without obvious or histological primary lesions other than self-mutilation. Horses often bite unrelated regions in subsequent attacks (**Fig. 12.9**).

Secondary lesions are invariably related to self-inflicted damage and include excoriation, alopecia, lichenification and hyperpigmentation (melanoderma) or scarring.

Differential diagnosis

- Ectoparasites (pathogens and incidentals)
- Food or other (insect) hypersensitivity

Diagnostic confirmation

- Absolute elimination of all other causes of pruritus. The last resort for diagnosis. Early elimination of insect and food hypersensitivity by exclusion.
- Intradermal testing (limited use, related to availability of antigens) using locally important antigen possibilities (moulds, pollen and dusts). This

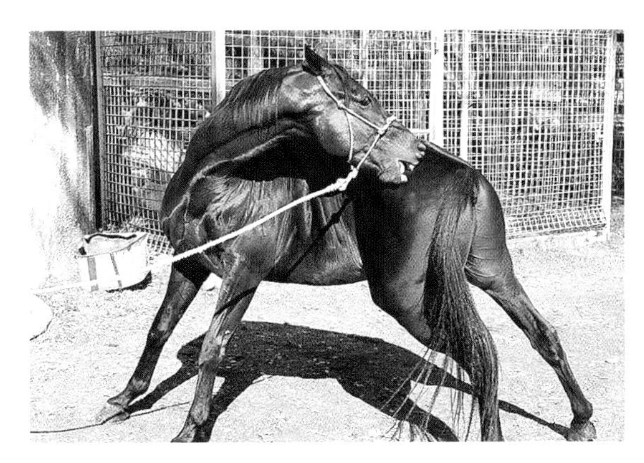

Figure 12.9 Atopy. A young horse with recurrent self-mutilation for which no other cause could be established.

will identify the specific reactivity of the animal to the allergens.
- Serum testing (RAST) gives particularly poor reliability, with false positives and false negatives and poor repeatability.
- Skin biopsy shows only nonspecific superficial to deep perivascular dermatitis with eosinophilia.

Treatment

If the allergen can be determined, it may be possible to avoid contact. Hyposensitization is possible in some cases using injections of increasing strength but these are not without hazard and need to be maintained for years.

Systemic glucocorticoids are useful (prednisolone is probably the best) (see Chapter 4, p. 48).

FOOD HYPERSENSITIVITY

Profile

This is suggested to be a complex type I, II and III hypersensitivity reaction in response to individual and groups of foodstuffs. It is suspected that protein components are more liable to induce the response, but grains and cereals are possible causes. There is no sex, breed or age predilection.

Clinical signs

Recurrent generalized pruritus, perineal pruritus and/or urticaria related to ingestion of the allergen (feed type). Urticarial responses to specific feed components are probably the commonest manifestations of food allergies (see Figs 12.3 to 12.6). Barley and oats are particularly reported as being a cause but this may reflect the higher number of horses receiving these.

Secondary lesions such as papules and plaques with crusting and exudative excoriation are invariably related to self-inflicted damage. Skin thickening and extensive flaking can arise with long-standing cases. Repeated episodes can result in skin scarring and altered pigment of both skin and hair.

Differential diagnosis

- Ectoparasites (pathogens and incidentals) – lice and mites in particular
- Cutaneous onchocerciasis (*Onchocerca cervicalis*)
- Oxyuriasis (*Oxyuris equi*)
- Atopy
- Insect hypersensitivity

Diagnostic confirmation

- Early clinical elimination of insect/parasite infestation.
- Food exclusion trials.
- Intradermal testing (limited use, related to availability of antigens) using locally important antigen possibilities (moulds, pollen and dusts). This will identify the specific reactivity of the animal to the allergens (Chapter 3, p. 33).
- Serum testing (RAST) gives particularly poor reliability with false positives and false negatives and poor repeatability.
- Skin biopsy shows only nonspecific superficial to deep perivascular dermatitis with eosinophilia.

Treatment

Feed exclusion trials should start with the feeding of good quality hay to which the horse has had no previous exposure. This is fed alone for 3 weeks. If an improvement is produced by this, a tentative diagnosis can be made. Re-introduction of the original diet can then be made and a diagnosis confirmed if the condition returns. Not many owners are willing to undergo this, however, preferring to maintain a diet on which there is no problem. If the allergen can be determined, it may be possible to avoid it completely. Systemic corticosteroids can be administered to control the condition but response is typically poor. Elimination of contact with the specific allergen must be the prime objective. Hyposensitization is possible in some cases using injections of increasing strength but these are not without hazard and need to be maintained for years.

PEMPHIGUS FOLIACEUS

Profile
An autoimmune disease characterized by an exfoliative dermatitis due to a type II hypersensitivity due to autoantibodies directed against the cell membrane of the epidermal cells. Commonest in Appaloosas but not restricted to them.

Clinical signs
Early cases Transient vesicles and pustules with superficial erosions forming epidermal collarettes (**Fig. 12.10**). Variable erythematous scaling and crusting commonly begins around the face and/or limbs. Inflammation is particularly severe on the skin of the limbs (**Fig. 12.11**). Acute inflammation of the coronary band, chestnut and ergot is a common but not consistent finding resulting in variable lameness. Gradual extension to the whole body over some days or weeks is common with marked alopecia but only mild pruritus. The acute skin lesions may be painful or pruritic (as manifest by persistent rubbing) and secondary excoriations may then be misleading.

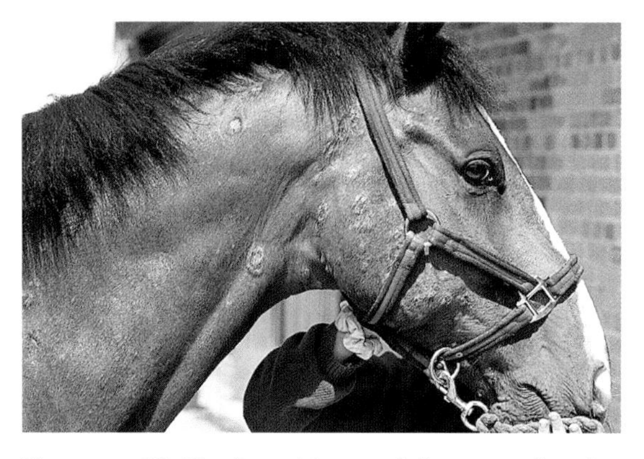

Figure 12.10 Pemphigus foliaceus showing circular erythematous and exudative lesions which developed into epidermal collarettes.

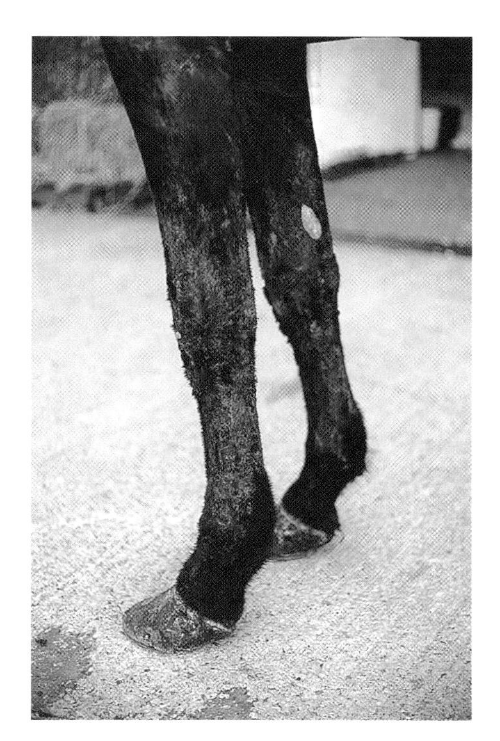

Figure 12.11 Pemphigus foliaceus. Severe and extensive lesions on the skin of the limbs.

Advanced/chronic cases Severe, diffuse crusting and scaling with extensive alopecia (**Fig. 12.12**).

Systemic signs include lethargy, anorexia, ventral/limb oedema, fever, depression and chronic weight loss.

Differential diagnosis
- Dermatophilosis (*Dermatophilus congolensis*)
- Dermatophytosis (*Trichophyton* spp., *Microsporum* spp.)
- Staphylococcal folliculitis
- Onchocerciasis (*Onchocerca cervicalis*)
- *Culicoides* spp. dermatitis (nonallergic and allergic forms (sweet itch))
- (Generalized) Granulomatous enteritis syndrome
- Systemic lupus erythematosus-like syndrome
- Bullous pemphigoid/pemphigus vulgaris
- Exfoliative eosinophilic dermatitis
- Papular dermatitis
- Sarcoidosis
- Epitheliogenesis imperfecta
- Epidermolysis bullosa
- Coronary band dystrophy
- Drug eruptions
- Chemical dermatoses
- Seborrhea

Diagnostic confirmation
- History and clinical appearance are characteristic.
- Haematology and biochemistry are usually normal or at least nonspecific.

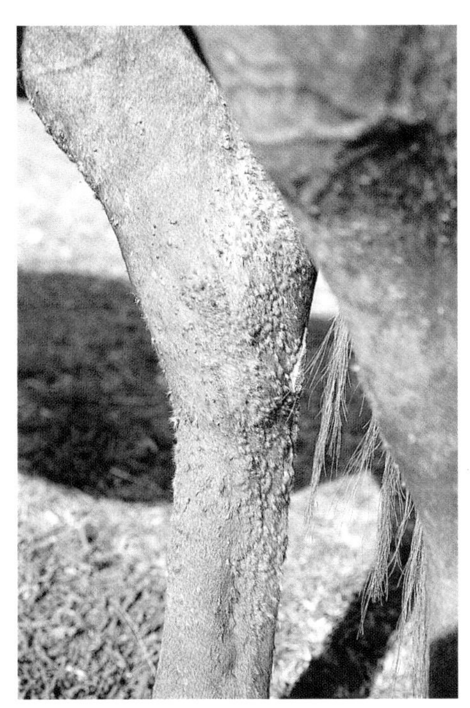

Figure 12.12 Pemphigus foliaceus. Advanced, chronic form showing extensive scaling, alopecia and thickening of the skin.

- Direct impression smears from fresh lesions show only acanthocytes and neutrophils.
- Biopsy is characteristic.[93]
- Direct immunofluorescence testing shows intracellular deposits of immunoglobulin in epidermis. Lesion selection for histopathology is very important. Intact vesicles or pustules are preferred. Sample perilesional skin if vesicles or pustules are not obviously present.[61] Michel's fixative (buffered ammonium sulphate solution) provides good preservation of immunoglobulins and complement.[94] In some cases acanthotic epidermal cells can be identified in fluid from intact blisters.

Note: To protect intact vesicles or surface scabs do not wipe or shave the skin prior to biopsy as it might damage an intact vesicle or pustule. Multiple sites should be sampled, with the surface scabs being included as far as possible.

Treatment

Prognosis is very poor with recovery very rare, but younger horses may respond better and carry a marginally better prognosis.[95] Treatment includes high-dose (immunosuppressive dose) corticosteroid therapy (prednisolone at 2.2–4.4 mg/kg daily) for weeks (see principles of therapeutics, Chapter 4, p. 48). Dose reductions are usually unrewarding with rapid relapse. Attempts should be made to change to alternate-day therapy. It is likely that treatment will be required for the rest of the animal's life. If the horse fails to respond to corticosteroids, consideration should be given to using gold injections.[23]

PEMPHIGUS VULGARIS (EPV) AND BULLOUS PEMPHIGOID (BP)

Profile

Rare vesicobullous, ulcerative diseases which may affect the oral cavity, mucocutaneous junctions and skin (or combinations of these). It is a type II hypersensitivity reaction. The two clinical diseases have many similarities[96] and are often described together.

Clinical signs

Initial signs are transient, fragile vesicles and bullae in skin and mucocutaneous junctions. These rapidly burst and leave crusts and ulcers with epidermal collarettes. Most prominent lesions occur around the oral and vulval mucous membrane–skin junctions (**Fig. 12.13**). Lesions may also occur at junctions between skin and keratinized areas such as the coronet and around the ergots and chestnuts. Diffuse lesions may be present in groin and axillae. The lesions may be very extensive with serum exudation and gross oedema (particularly of the limbs) but are seldom either painful or pruritic.

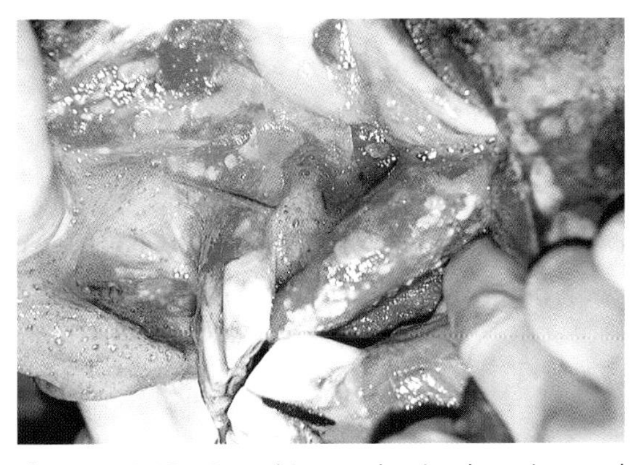

Figure 12.13 Pemphigus vulgaris ulceration and bulla formation in the oral mucosa. Note the lesions also at the mucocutaneous junction of the commissure of the mouth.

Systemic signs are present in severely affected horses including anorexia, depression and intermittent or persistent pyrexia.

Differential diagnosis

- (Generalized) Granulomatous enteritis syndrome
- Pemphigus foliaceus
- Vesicular stomatitis
- Chronic dermatophilosis (*Dermatophilus congolensis*)
- Chronic chorioptic mange (*Chorioptes equi*)
- Oral irritations and toxic burns
- Renal failure (oral ulceration)

Diagnostic confirmation

- History and clinical examination are suggestive but diagnosis is usually made after exclusion of all other possible disorders.
- Skin biopsy is very useful. Shave biopsy is probably the best sample. If possible a whole, intact vesicle or bulla should be obtained. Tissue can be examined directly or by immunohistochemistry (with immunofluorescence).
  - In **bullous pemphigoid** multiple biopsies of fresh lesions must be taken. They will show characteristic subepidermal vacuolar alteration and subepidermal clefting with vesicle formation.
  - Direct immunoglobulin testing of biopsy sections show linear deposition of immunoglobulins and complement at the basement membrane of skin or mucosa.
- Serum samples can be tested for anti-horse globulins (Coombs' test) but results are variable.

Treatment: High doses of systemic corticosteroids such as prednisolone may have to be maintained for life. Once an improvement has been obtained using high doses, progressive reduction may establish a minimal therapeutic dose.

The prognosis is very poor and most cases are euthanased.

IMMUNE-MEDIATED VASCULITIS

Profile

Uncommon disorder characterized by purpura, oedema, necrosis and ulceration of lower limbs and oral mucosa due to combined type I and type III hypersensitivity reactions.

Clinical signs

Signs occur characteristically (but not exclusively) 2–4 weeks after respiratory infection due to *Streptococcus equi*. Most prominent signs occur on coronet, pastern and fetlock (**Fig. 12.14**). The lips and periorbital tissues are also affected in many cases. Focal and diffuse areas of oedema, erythema, necrosis and ulceration develop. There is no pruritus and while pain is shown only in the earliest stages in some horses it remains a problem for many weeks.

Systemic signs of pyrexia, weight loss, depression and anorexia are often present.

It may become chronic or recurrent and some cases completely fail to resolve.

Differential diagnosis

- Dermatophilosis (*Dermatophilus congolensis*)
- Dermatophytosis (*Trichophyton* spp.)
- Staphylococcal or streptococcal pastern folliculitis
- Purpura haemorrhagica
- Pemphigus foliaceus
- Bullous pemphigoid/pemphigus vulgaris
- Drug eruption
- (Generalized) granulomatous enteritis syndrome
- Leukocytoclastic vasculitis
- 'Greasy heel' syndrome

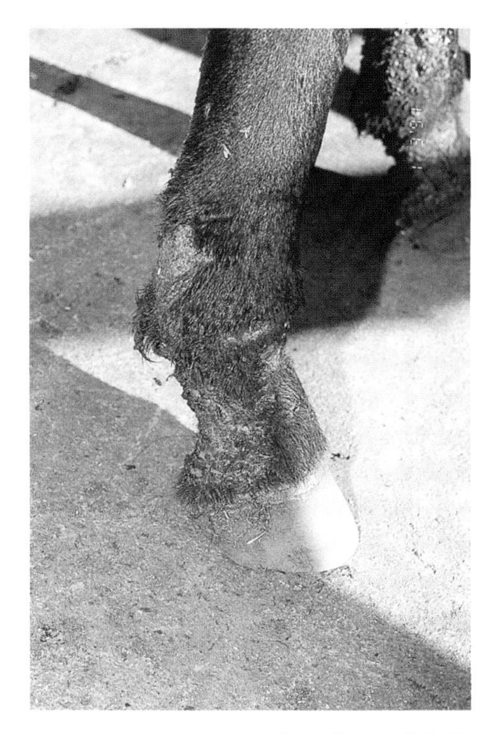

Figure 12.14 Immune-mediated vasculitis lesions on the distal limb (note that the lesions are not restricted to nonpigmented skin).

Diagnostic confirmation

- Clinical appearance.
- Clinical pathology (haematology and biochemistry) shows normal platelet counts, with mild anaemia and panleukopenia. Serum proteins are often abnormal.
- Biopsy shows neutrophilic, eosinophilic, lymphocytic infiltration and mixed vasculitis. Diagnostic biopsies are best taken within 24 hours of a fresh lesion occurring.

Treatment

If possible treat the underlying disease. Provided diagnosis is very rapid, oral prednisolone (with a long course of antibiotics) should be given twice daily until regression occurs and then reduced to the lowest possible alternate day dose. After full remission the dose can be gradually reduced. Recurrences are common and some cases fail to respond and succumb.

PASTERN AND CANNON LEUKOCYTOCLASTIC VASCULITIS

Profile

Specific sporadic disease of equine skin which is probably more common than realized. Mature horses are usually affected without sex predilection. The nonpigmented extremities are most frequently affected and the disease usually occurs in summer in regions with plentiful sunlight.[97]

Aetiology and pathogenesis are uncertain, but IgG deposition and/or C3 portion of complement have been detected in the earliest stages by direct immunofluorescence of affected vessel walls. Percutaneous absorption has not been ruled out, but unpigmented skin involvement suggests a role of ultraviolet light. However, the disease is not a true photosensitization. Records of affected horses also indicate no known contact with photosensitizing compounds and liver function is usually normal.

Clinical signs

Acute onset of erythema, oozing and crusting which is clearly demarcated and restricted to the white areas of the distal limb (and particularly the lateral aspect of the hind pasterns) (**Fig. 12.15**). Pigmented limbs are seldom, if ever, affected. The outward appearance of the disorder may belie the severity and extent of the inflamed skin, which can only be truly appreciated by close clipping of the hair.

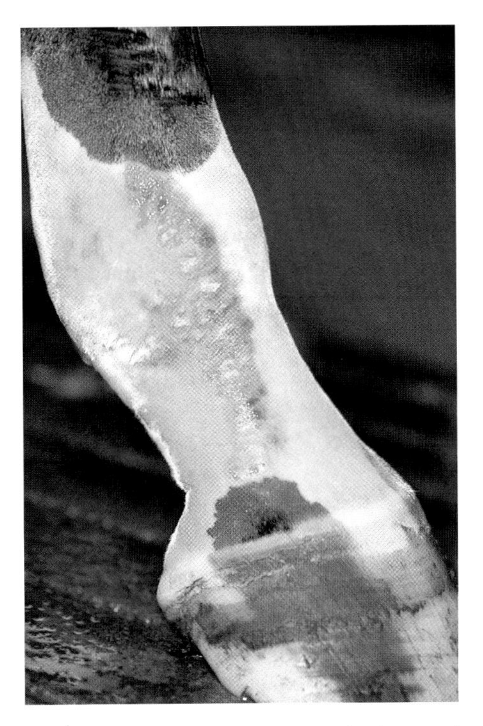

Figure 12.15 Pastern and cannon leukocytoclastic vasculitis characteristically affecting only the lateral aspect of the pigmented hind limb. The left leg is obviously unaffected and there is no abnormality on the medial aspect of the white leg. The full extent of the disorder can be appreciated after close clipping.

The condition is more painful than pruritic. Erosions, ulceration and oedema of affected limbs is more extensive than might be expected for the size and extent of the lesion. The exudate takes on a warty appearance and character and removal of the scabs and crusts is quite difficult.

Differential diagnosis

- Pastern folliculitis (mixed *Staphylococcus* spp.)
- Dermatophilosis (*Dermatophilus congolensis*)
- Photosensitization – especially due to plants. Careful history to eliminate plant aetiology
- Actinic dermatitis – liver function tests
- Pemphigus foliaceus

All horses showing dermatitic lesions restricted to nonpigmented skin *must* be tested for liver function.

Diagnostic confirmation

- Clinical appearance on the lateral aspect of a nonpigmented pastern is typical
- Biopsy is usually nonspecific unless the earliest

lesions can be identified. Acute changes show leukocytoclastic vasculitis with vessel wall necrosis and thrombosis. Epidermal changes include hyperplastic and degenerative changes and, in chronic cases, papillomatosis has been reported.

Treatment

High (immunosuppressive) doses of corticosteroids (see Chapter 4, p. 48) daily for up to 2 weeks with a gradual withdrawal over 4 weeks and repeated use of emollient cream and keratolytics such as salicylic acid can be helpful. There are occasional recurrences during or soon after treatment, requiring further courses of corticosteroids. Protect affected areas from direct or reflected ultraviolet light by stabling in daylight and using leg wraps. Soothing creams containing antiseptics, antibiotics and steroids and factor 20+ sun-block lotions can be helpful.

SYSTEMIC/CUTANEOUS LUPUS ERYTHEMATOSUS-LIKE SYNDROME (SLE-like syndrome)

Profile

A rare, incompletely defined disease in horses which differs in several ways from classical forms encountered in humans and dogs. The syndrome has some features of both discoid lupus erythematosus (DLE) and systemic lupus erythematosus (SLE). Multiple organ involvement including the skin is characteristic. A variable number of cases have significant anti-nuclear antibody (ANA).[98] True lupus cells have not been detected in horses. In some equine cases the disease appears as a more benign form.

The pathogenesis is probably multifactorial. 'Autoimmune disease' results from the interaction of genetic, immunological, environmental and possible infective relationships as well as iatrogenic causes involving drug administrations. These would seem to be a reasonable basis for induction of the disease. The aetiopathogenesis might include the following:

- Immunological aspects involving antibodies (IgG and IgM) and complement C3 portion have been observed at the epidermal–dermal skin junction and have also been seen in small superficial blood vessels. Circulating anti-nuclear antibody (ANA) may be present (but may be positive in horses not showing the clinical signs also).
- Trigger factors including infections, changes in environment, extremes of temperature, drugs, stressful events such as pregnancy, heavy work, etc. are usually reported.
- Underlying systemic disease such as lymphosarcoma (or other internal neoplasm) or other chronic inflammatory processes may also be active trigger factors.
- Virus-like particles have been seen in electron-microscopic studies of both SLE and DLE in other species but are not described in the horse.

Clinical signs

Erythema, scaling and exudation occur early (**Fig. 12.16**) and the skin of long-standing cases has a wrinkled, leathery appearance with extensive scaling (**Fig. 12.17**). Haired areas may show various degrees of alopecia. There is often a sharp demarcation between pigmented and depigmented areas. Apparent photosensitization can be present involving the depigmented areas and this makes the diagnosis difficult. Rapid or insidious depigmentation occurs around the eyes, lips, nostrils (**Fig. 12.18**), vulva, anal ring and prepuce. Pruritus is not a common sign but can be present.

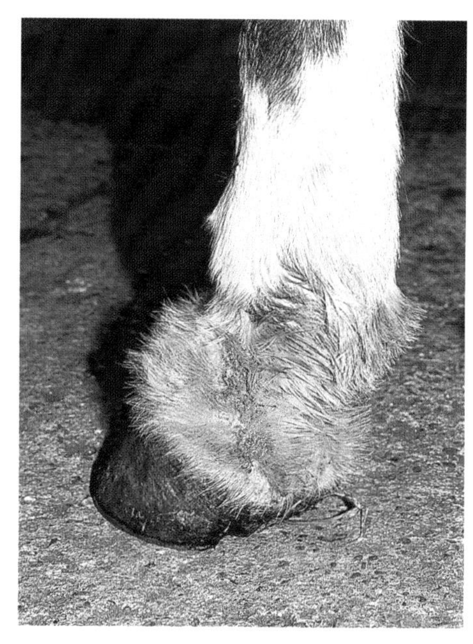

Figure 12.16 Systemic lupus erythematosus-like syndrome showing diffuse, severe, exudative, dermatitis affecting the distal limb region. All four legs showed similar signs (including two which were pigmented).

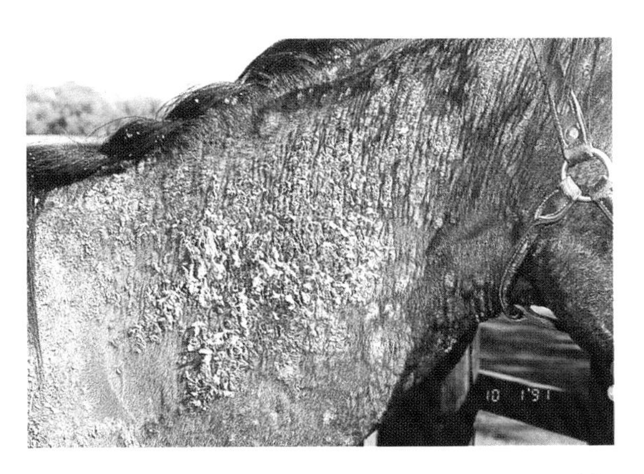

Figure 12.17 Systemic lupus erythematosus-like syndrome showing chronic skin involvement with roughening and thickening of the skin and a leathery appearance

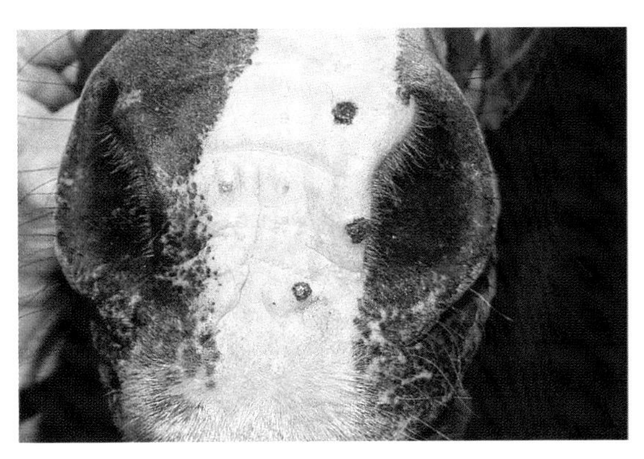

Figure 12.19 Systemic lupus erythematosus-like syndrome. Typical focal areas of haemorrhage and necrosis in the skin of the muzzle.

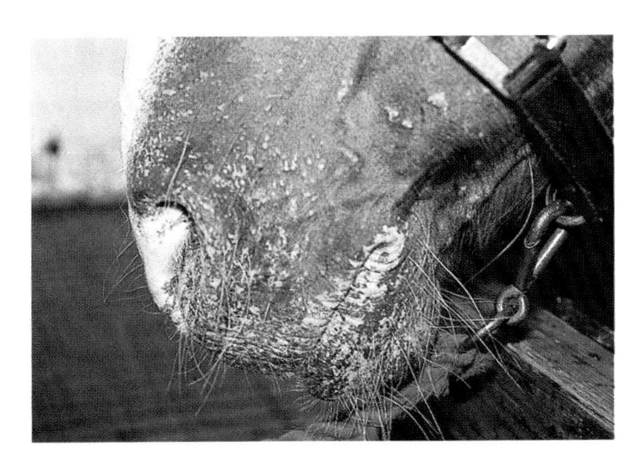

Figure 12.18 Systemic lupus erythematosus-like syndrome. Insidious depigmentation of the mouth and muzzle accompanied by miliary ulcerative foci in the skin.

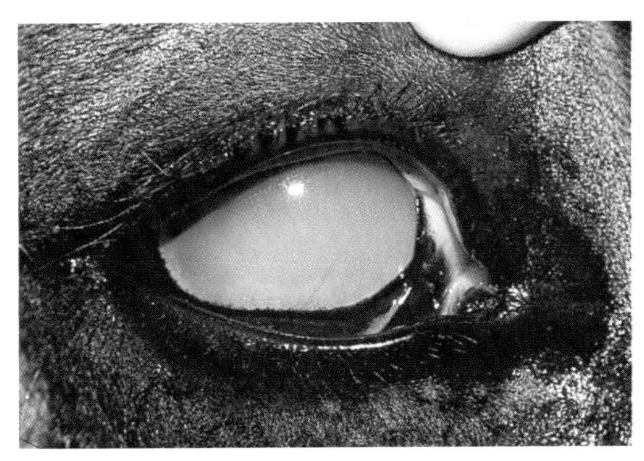

Figure 12.20 Systemic lupus erythematosus-like syndrome showing severe hypopyon (accumulation of inflammatory debris in the anterior chamber of the eye). This showed a remarkable improvement over 3–4 days when it was only just visible but it returned overnight some 3 days later.

The more severe SLE-like cases show various multiple organ involvement including prominent lameness (polyarthritis), uveitis and pyrexia and weight loss is common. Petechiation of mucous membranes, skin (**Fig. 12.19**), hypopyon (inflammatory debris in the anterior chamber of the eye) (**Fig. 12.20**) and hyphaema (blood in the anterior chamber of the eye) can be present in severe cases. Significantly, the intraocular changes can fluctuate over a relatively short time.

Involvement of several organ systems simultaneously is a strongly suggestive feature of the disorder, but some cases have limited overt signs.

Differential diagnosis

- Drug eruptions
- Occult polysystemic infections (including borreliosis or Lyme disease) or neoplasia (including internal forms of lymphosarcoma)
- Chronic *Culicoides* spp. hypersensitivity (sweet itch)
- Chronic/recurrent dermatophilosis (*Dermatophilus congolensis*)
- Other depigmentation diseases
    - vitiligo
    - Arabian fading syndrome
    - Appaloosa parentage

- (Generalized) granulomatous enteritis syndrome
- Sarcoidosis
- Leukoderma, scarring or chronic irritation
- Scalding (urine/faeces/wound fluids)

Diagnostic confirmation

- No single test or sign should be taken as pathognomonic. A full range of diagnostic aids should be employed as some may show false positive or false negative results.
- Multiple organ involvement is typical.
- Biopsy of skin (taken into formalin for conventional histopathology and possibly Michel's medium for immunofluorescent studies) is characteristic.
- Serum can be tested for antinuclear antibody (ANA) with variable results. Coombs' test may be positive in some cases.
- Blood analysis is usually nonspecific. High plasma fibrinogen, hypergammaglobulinaemia and hypoalbuminaemia with elevated white cell counts with a left-shifted neutrophilia are possible.

Treatment

Attempts should be made to diagnose and then treat or remove any possible trigger factors or underlying disease. Treatment with antibiotics should always precede and run concurrently with corticosteroid treatment. Prolonged treatment courses are needed. False cases may recover, while confirmed positive cases seldom undergo remission for anything other than short periods. Acute and severe remissions and deterioration are common. The systemic signs may be more serious than the cutaneous signs.

ALOPECIA AREATA

Profile

A rare, cell-mediated, autoimmune skin disease. Increased awareness of the disease has resulted in more identified cases.[99] The aetiopathogenesis seems to involve the presence of T lymphocytes directed against the hair matrix and root sheath and the epithelium of hair follicles. There is some suggestion of an hereditary factor as some 20% of cases are genetically related.

Clinical signs

Insidious or rapid onset of a nonpruritic, diffuse thinning of the mane and tail and development of one or more reasonably circumscribed areas of partial or complete alopecia (**Fig. 12.21**). Affected areas may coalesce to produce extensive alopecia without any overt signs of inflammation. Defective hoof growth may occur. Spotted leukotrichia or melanotrichia may be associated with hair loss in affected areas.

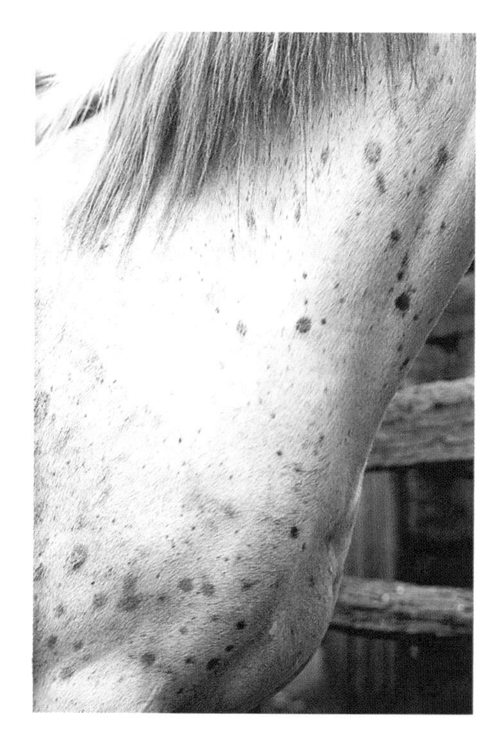

Figure 12.21 Alopecia areata. Notice the focal generally circular areas of alopecia (this revealing the normal black skin of this grey horse).

Differential diagnosis

- Dermatophytosis (*Trichophyton* spp., *Microsporum* spp.)
- Dermatophilosis (*Dermatophilus congolensis*)
- Occult sarcoid

Diagnostic confirmation

- Nonspecific alopecia with mane and tail dystrophy.
- Biopsy shows lymphocytic bulbitis with T cell accumulations at hair bulbs and 'miniature' hair follicles. In early cases it occurs in anagen phase, whereas in chronic cases it is in telogen phase.
- May show defective keratinization in old lesions. Inflammation may be minimal and

section may reveal only small telogen follicles lacking hair.

Treatment

Spontaneous remission has been recorded but the chance of complete and permanent remission is poor. There is no effective treatment.

LINEAR KERATOSIS/LINEAR ALOPECIA

Profile

Idiopathic, possibly inherited dermatosis characterized by unilateral, linear, vertical bands of hyperkeratosis on neck, thorax and upper hind leg. The disorder is rare and its pathogenesis is unclear. Most cases occur in Quarterhorses between 1 and 5 years of age.

Clinical signs

One or more vertically arranged bands of alopecia and hyperkeratotic papules and plaques associated with scaling/crusting most often occurring on the neck (**Fig. 12.22**) or the buttock (**Fig. 12.23**). The lesions are asymptomatic with no pruritus or pain.

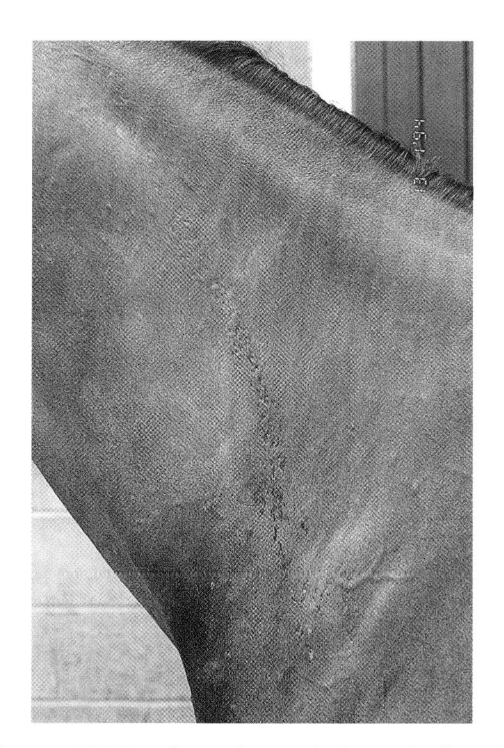

Figure 12.22 Linear keratosis in a single well-defined line down the side of the neck.

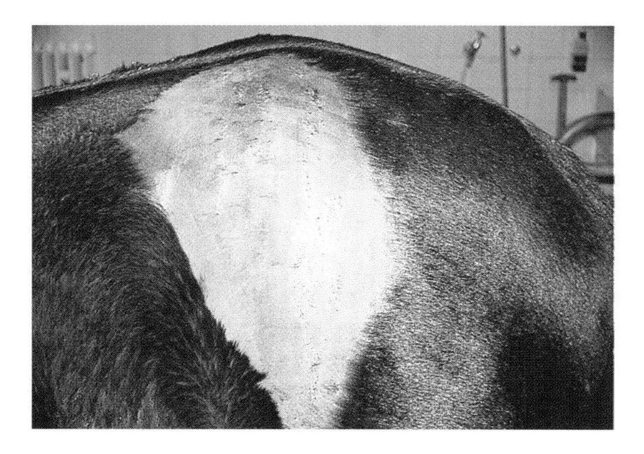

Figure 12.23 Linear keratosis showing multiple linear areas on the buttock (note that this was only obvious after the hair-coat had been clipped away).

Many cases are only detected incidentally after clipping out and may give the impression of a healed traumatic lesion/scratch etc.

Differential diagnosis

- Chronic hyperkeratosis from irritant drugs, e.g. mercurial blister or repeated trauma
- Dermatophilosis (*Dermatophilus congolensis*)
- Clipper rash/recent trauma (e.g. scratch)

Diagnostic confirmation

- Clinical appearance is very typical.
- Biopsy shows variably regular papillated epidermal hyperplasia with marked compact orthokeratotic hyperkeratosis. Primary change is a lymphocytic mural folliculitis.[100]

Treatment

No treatment has any noticeable effect. Keratolytic agents such as salicylic acid creams may temporarily reduce the amount of hyperkeratosis.

SARCOIDOSIS

Profile

A rare systemic granulomatous disease showing exfoliative dermatitis, (severe) wasting and sarcoidal granulomatous involvement of multiple organ systems. No age, breed or sex predilections are known. The cause and the pathogenesis are unknown[101] and no infectious agent has been identified. All described cases have so far (initially at least) been presented for investigation of skin disease. The condition is not related to the equine sarcoid but may be a part of the generalized granulomatous enteritis/dermatitis syndrome (see p. 178).[102]

Clinical signs

The commoner skin lesions include generalized, extensive scaling and crusting of skin (**Fig. 12.24**) with variable alopecia of the face and limbs (in particular). These signs may more rarely be focal (limited areas) or multifocal (many areas but discretely demarcated). A second rarer form has skin lesions consisting of nodules or large tumour-like masses. Both skin forms may be present at the same time. Generalized wasting disease and ill thrift are common concurrent signs. Poor appetite and persistent or undulant low-grade fever are reported. Peripheral lymphadenopathy and variable organic signs (including mediastinal and pulmonary granulomatous masses) may be detected. The presence of these may account for the poor exercise tolerance and various degrees of dyspnoea. Liver and intestinal involvement are relatively common, giving rise to icterus and diarrhoea respectively. Other organs are only rarely involved and so far no ocular, cardiac, splenic or central nervous lesions have been described.

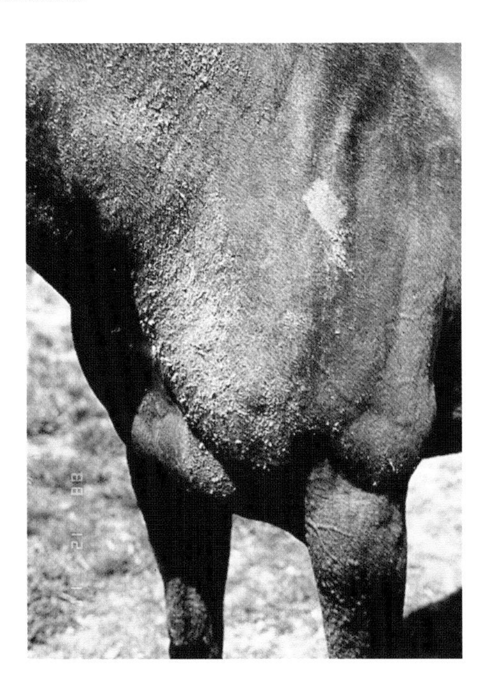

Figure 12.24 Sarcoidosis showing the typically extensive scaling and crusting of large areas of the skin surface.

Differential diagnosis

- Dermatophilosis (*Dermatophilus congolensis*)
- Dermatophytosis (*Trichophyton* spp.)
- Pemphigus foliaceus
- Seborrhoea
- Exfoliative eosinophilic dermatitis
- Immune-mediated diseases including systemic lupus erythematosus-like syndrome
- Erythema multiforme
- Food sensitivity/allergy
- 'Hairy vetch' disease in USA
- Verrucose sarcoid

Diagnostic confirmation

- History and clinical examination. The diagnosis is most often made by exclusion of all other options.
- Haematology: Leukocytosis, increased fibrinogen and hyperglobulinaemia. Mild or more severe anaemia. Abnormal kidney and liver function tests.
- Skin biopsy shows dermatitis with frequent multi-nucleated histiocytic giant cells. Perifollicular and mid- or superficial dermal sarcoidal granulomata are characteristic.
- Organ biopsy: Mesenteric and thoracic lymph nodes, lungs, gastrointestinal tract and liver may be affected with sarcoidal granuloma. These are very characteristic nonsuppurative, noncaseating granulomata which may be microscopic. They consist of aggregations of multinucleated giant cells, neutrophils (in low numbers), lymphocytes and plasma cells.

Treatment

Change feed first – a similar or identical syndrome has been caused by hairy vetch in field cases and in some cases of feed allergy. The former has not, however, been reproduced experimentally. No effective treatment is described, but a few horses have experienced spontaneous remission for no apparent reason. Prolonged oral prednisolone may be helpful and immune-stimulating drugs such as levamisole have been used with variable (largely unsubstantiated) results.

ERYTHEMA MULTIFORME

Profile

Rare, acute, self-limiting, urticarial, maculopapular or vesicobullous dermatosis. The complex arises secondarily to other triggering influences such as drugs, infections (especially herpesvirus) and tumours (particularly reticular neoplasms). Some cases are mistakenly identified as gyrate urticaria (and vice versa). It should be considered to be a type of allergic response, being very similar to graft-versus-host reaction, but many cases are classified as idiopathic when no underlying cause can be found. Most cases in horses are attributed to drug reactions (trimethoprim sulphur combinations and ceftiofur in particular)[103] but in many cases no explanation can be found.[104]

Clinical signs

Asymptomatic, cutaneous, more or less symmetrically distributed skin eruptions with a characteristic 'wheal-like' lesion similar to an urticarial plaque develop rapidly from an initial, more typical urticarial lesion. Lesions show a variable appearance with serpiginous or circular doughnut-like rings (**Fig. 12.25**). Mucous membranes of mouth and nasal cavity, vulva and conjunctiva may be involved.[106] The lesions frequently persist for weeks without showing any scaling, crusting or alopecia in many horses. Some cases appear to undergo some remission of signs over some months or years, while others become progressively worse. No case can be considered to be in full remission or cured as recurrences are likely.

Differential diagnosis

- Urticaria (particularly the gyrate form)
- Amyloidosis
- Mastocytoma
- Lymphosarcoma
- Drug eruptions/reaction

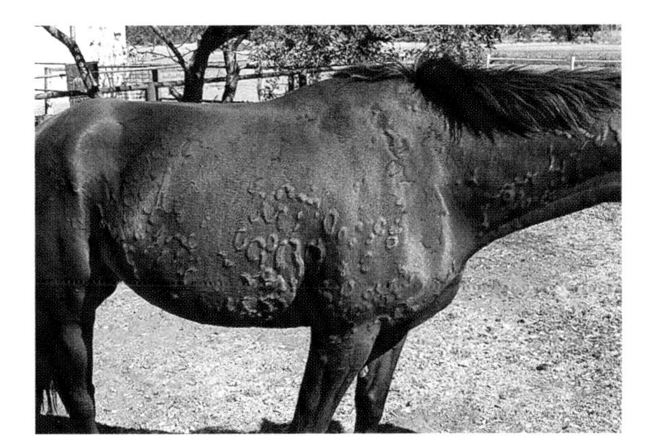

Figure 12.25 Erythema multiforme. Note the serpiginous (expanding) lesions over the chest wall in particular.

Diagnostic confirmation

- Characteristic lesions over the whole body.
- Skin biopsy: Hydropic interface dermatitis with migration of lymphocytes into epidermis leading to necrosis of keratinocytes. The major dermal changes include oedema of superficial dermis and presence of leaked red cells in superficial dermis with necrosis of keratinocytes.

Treatment

Treatment is not usually warranted. Systemic corticosteroids have little benefit unless in high doses. The condition may run a benign natural course over 2–3 months or more. While some cases recover spontaneously others have persistent lesions. Recurrence is reported.

EQUINE INSECT HYPERSENSITIVITY/ ALLERGY (sweet itch, Queensland itch)

Profile

By far the most common skin allergy in horses. Due to hypersensitivity to bites of *Culicoides* spp. midges. No sex or hair/skin colour predilection. Cases in foals and young horses are rare. Most horses become affected after 4–5 years of age and the condition worsens with advancing age. Certain breeds seem particularly sensitive (e.g. Shire, Icelandic and Welsh ponies), suggesting a genetic basis to the hypersensitivity.

The neck/tail form is probably the consequence of neck-and-tail-biting *Culicoides* spp. midges. The ventral abdomen form is due to ventral-biting *Culicoides* spp. midges but can be due to other insects. Hypersensitivity is commoner due to the dorsal biting insect.

Note: *Culicoides* spp. insects also cause a primary bite irritation in all horses but not all horses develop an allergy/hypersensitivity (see p. 130).

Clinical signs

Clinical signs are characteristically seasonal and gradually become worse over succeeding years. The first signs may develop at any age.

General signs Pruritus is always present and is worse in the early evening (dusk) and early morning. Tail switching, rubbing and restlessness are always shown. Loss of weight due to constant irritation.

Acute form Pruritus with aggressive rubbing of

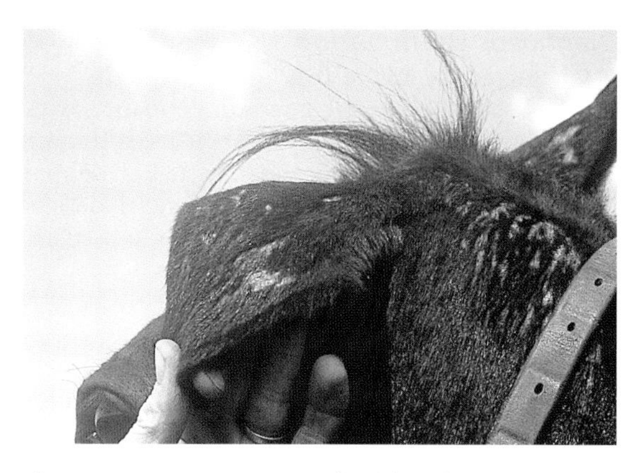

Figure 12.26 Acute culicoides hypersensitivity (sweet itch/Queensland itch) showing papules on the ears and crest under the mane.

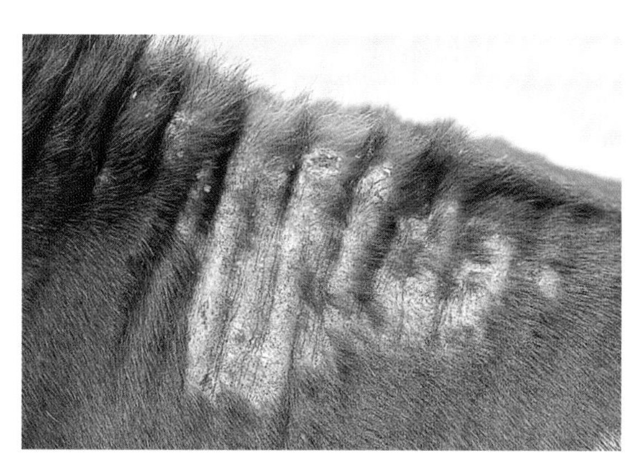

Figure 12.28 Chronic culicoides hypersensitivity (sweet itch/Queensland itch) showing severe rugae formation with thickened skin and profound hair loss in the withers region. Note the fresh lesions resulting from recent self-inflicted trauma.

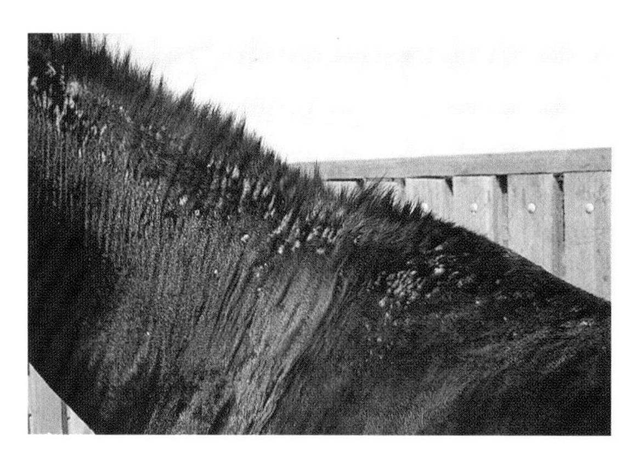

Figure 12.27 Acute culicoides hypersensitivity (sweet itch/Queensland itch) showing papules along the upper part of the neck and sparse, broken and damaged mane hairs.

the tail-base, neck (mane-base), head and back. Papules occur along the back of the horse from ears (**Figs. 12.26** and **12.27**) to tail. Self-inflicted trauma causes exfoliation, exudation of serum and patchy alopecia. Crusting and melanotrichia are common effects. The species of midge largely dictates the location of the clinical features but most show a sparse, severely thinned tail and mane hairs which are often broken and distorted (**Fig. 12.27**). Ventral-biting midges may cause a similar response on the ventral abdomen.

Chronic form Variously thickened (lichenified) skin with rugae on withers (**Fig. 12.28**), neck and tail-head (**Fig. 12.29**). Chronic hair loss and coarsening of hair coat quality in affected areas. The tail may develop a rat-tailed appearance. Acute episodes superimposed on the chronic effects are commonly encountered.

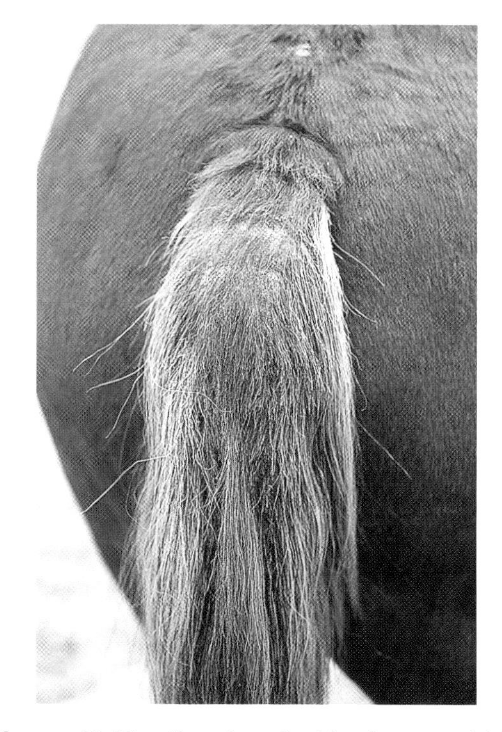

Figure 12.29 Chronic culicoides hypersensitivity (sweet itch/Queensland itch) showing the result of chronic repeated tail rubbing resulting in hair loss and skin thickening over the tail-base. This photograph shows the early recovery stage occurring in the winter months.

Differential diagnosis

- Lice infestation (*Damalinia equi*, *Haematopinus asini*)
- Chorioptic and/or psoroptic mange (tail forms)
- *Oxyuris equi* infestation
- Fly bites. *Stomoxys* spp., *Simulium* spp., *Haematobia exigua*
- Dermatophilosis (*Dermatophilus congolensis)*
- Dermatophytosis (*Microsporum gypseum)*
- Onchocercal dermatitis (*Onchocerca cervicalis*)
- Unilateral papular dermatosis,
- 'Stickfast' flea, spinose ear tick, cattle tick larvae, bee stings
- Chemical irritation
- Besnoitiosis
- Mane and tail dystrophy
- Anhidrosis

Diagnostic confirmation

- Characteristic clinical signs.
- Seasonality (summer months and improving in winter or colder periods).
- Elimination of all other ectoparasitic possibilities.
- Biopsy shows mild to severe eosinophilic folliculitis and dermatitis.
- Intradermal skin testing using aqueous whole-insect antigen is reported to give reliable positive results but is not available for general use.
- Identification of biting insects is important as not all *Culicoides* bite dorsal areas; some species attack ventral areas only and cause ventral dermatitis. Not all hypersensitivity is due to *Culicoides* spp. alone and it can be complicated by sensitivity to other flies, e.g. *Tabanus* spp. (horse flies), *Stomoxys* spp. (stable flies) and *Haematobia* spp. (buffalo flies).

Treatment

Individual horses can be treated daily with antihistamines such as tripelennamine or phenothiazine drugs which have antihistamine effects as well as sedation effects. However, results are disappointing. For longer-lasting effect in seriously affected horses, methylprednisolone acetate or betamethasone can be administered intramuscularly at 3–4 week (or sometimes lesser) intervals. Prolonged usage is not advisable as they have significant but small risks.

Daily oral prednisolone during the high-risk season can reduce pruritus to a minimal amount, but secondary effects from prolonged corticosteroid medication must be constantly considered.

Fly repellents Treatment of unrugged, grazing horses is extremely difficult but application of light-oil dressing to the dorsum of the horse gives some relief. Success has been claimed with 0.5% fenvalerate (200 g/l) at the rate of 200 ml per horse to the horse's backline, or alternatively 0.1% fenvalerate (200 g/l) is applied as a backline and body spray at the rate of 1 litre per horse every 7 days. Up to four applications are claimed to be curative, with hair regrowth and cessation of pruritus.[106] Insect repellents, such as dibutyl phthalate and benzyl benzoate applied to the rugs and/or the head, back and base of the tail of individual horses have been marginally effective in some cases. Permethrin fly repellents are sometimes useful.

Fly control The most important control measure is the protection of the horse against further contact with *Culicoides*. Unless this can be accomplished, all other measures are likely to be unsuccessful. Stabling in a protective environment between dawn and mid-morning and mid-afternoon and dusk combined with rugging with sheets and hoods may prevent serious skin damage. The use of insect-proof stables is certainly the ultimate method of prevention, but is rarely achievable; a very fine screen mesh must be used. *Culicoides* spp. midges seem less able to cope with air speeds over 10 km/h so moving the affected horse to a windy area away from river courses, woodlands and standing water is sometimes effective. Individual animals may be particularly sensitive to individual species of *Culicoides* and so may be moved away from the area.

CONTACT HYPERSENSITIVITY

Profile

Rare and poorly proven problem related to contact with soaps, blankets and rugs, bedding, medication, insect repellents and pasture plants. Simply, it is a type IV hypersensitivity reaction.

Clinical signs

Transient vesicles and papules over the contact area (seldom generalized). Contact areas of suspect material show greatest reaction. Vesicles rupture leaving an erythematous oozing and crusting on the skin surface (**Fig. 12.30**). There is variable pruritus but little pain.

Differential diagnosis

- Ectoparasites

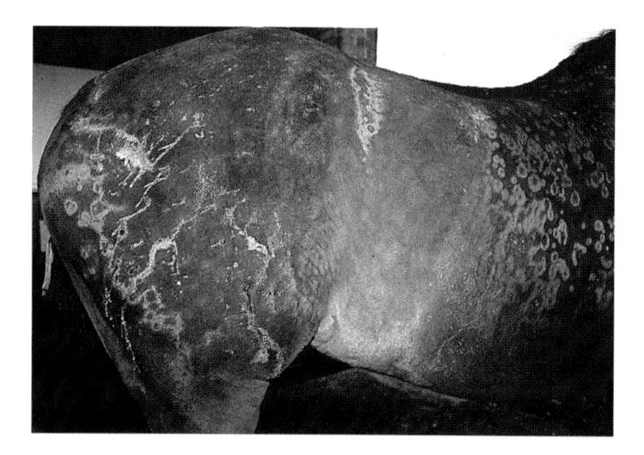

Figure 12.30 Contact hypersensitivity (severe). The areas affected corresponded to contact with a jute rug. Removal of the rug resulted in resolution and test contact again caused a more severe reaction over the contact area. Other fibres had no effect.

- Parasitic hypersensitivity (including sweet itch)
- Pastern folliculitis
- Other hypersensitivity (including food)
- Drug eruptions

Diagnostic confirmation

- Remove all suspected material for 7–10 days and then allow direct contact and observe for recurrence of signs. Owners may be reluctant to allow this.
- Patch testing involving the application of suspected substance(s) placed on cloth and fastened to the skin with adhesive tape (beware of possible reaction to the tape itself) for 48 hours. This is difficult owing to the difficulty of adhesion to skin, but a marked reaction is strongly suggestive. Using a blank as a negative control is a wise precaution.

Treatment

Wash affected area and remove the horse to different environment. Administer oral corticosteroids or if localized use topically at affected site.

DRUG ERUPTION

Profile

Drugs, including most antibiotics and many vaccines, given by any route, may cause significant skin eruptions. The reaction to a drug can be delayed for weeks or months and typically represents a type IV hypersensitivity reaction.

Clinical signs

Nonspecific skin eruption(s) which may show variable urticarial plaques, papules, and/or generalized pruritus. Mucocutaneous junctions may exhibit the earliest signs including vesicles, ulceration and scaling (**Fig. 12.31**) and so a history of initial involvement of these sites may be suggestive of a drug eruption. Long delays have no material influence on the severity of clinical signs but clearly make diagnosis more difficult.

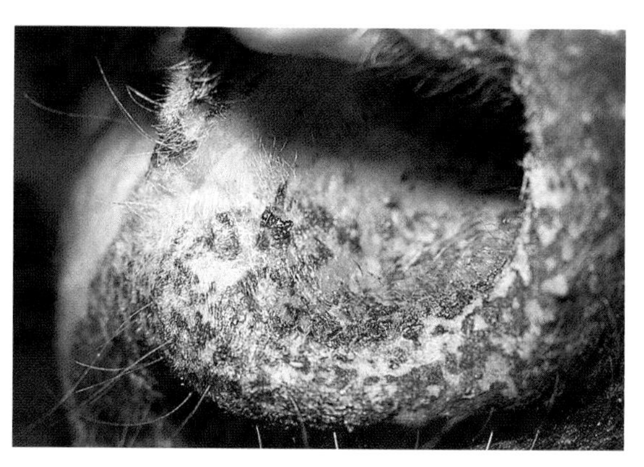

Figure 12.31 Drug eruption. Ulceration, exudation, scaling and crusting due to a drug eruption attributed to oral potentiated sulphonamide therapy.

Differential diagnosis

- Urticaria (particularly the gyrate or oozing forms)
- Systemic lupus erythematosus-like syndrome
- Food allergy
- Drug allergy
- Erythema multiforme
- Insect hypersensitivity (*Culicoides* spp. (sweet itch))
- Pemphigus foliaceus
- Bullous pemphigoid/pemphigus vulgaris

Diagnostic confirmation

- Very difficult unless the onset occurs immediately after the drug has been given. There are probably no pathognomonic signs associated with drug eruptions and any unexplained cutaneous lesions should be considered as drug eruptions. There is always a history of drug administration (even ivermectin anthelmintics have been implicated in the aetiology of variegated hyperaesthetic leukotrichia). Delayed drug reactions may not easily be attributable to the drug. No drug is more or less liable to induce the changes. Confirmed diagnosis of acute cases can be made if the drug(s) is withdrawn and signs disappear, and then reappear with re-introduction of the suspect drug. Even this may only provide a presumptive diagnosis since the drug is usually administered because the animal has an illness. Carriers and preservatives in drugs can also be responsible, so changing the specific brand may help.

Treatment

Discontinue suspected drugs immediately. If severe, acute reaction is present, administer high doses of systemic corticosteroids. Response may be poor.

LYMPHOEDEMA

Profile

Diffuse oedematous swelling of the limbs and the prepucial area may be primary due to a lymphatic system disorder or may be secondary to injury, infection or neoplasia. Significant oedema can also arise from lack of natural movement of one or more limbs or general body movement. The condition is best regarded as a sign of disease rather than a diagnosis in itself.

Clinical signs

Primary form Painless nodules and enlarged lymphatics involving prepuce which show little 'pitting on pressure'.

Secondary form Often painful and obvious pitting on pressure (**Fig. 12.32a,b**).

Differential diagnosis

- Oedema due to lack of movement (for whatever reason)
- Causes of lymphatic obstruction (haemangioma, lymphangioma, lymphosarcoma, other tumours or inflammatory lymphadenopathy, etc.)
- Low blood protein
  - primary due to starvation
  - secondary due to protein loss (via skin, gut or kidney), failure of absorption, hepatic failure or physiological or pathological consumption of protein
- Injury, post-castration swelling (preputial and scrotal forms)
- Lymphangitis and cellulitis
- Infection including 'schirrous cord' (staphylococcal granuloma of the spermatic cord and scrotum)

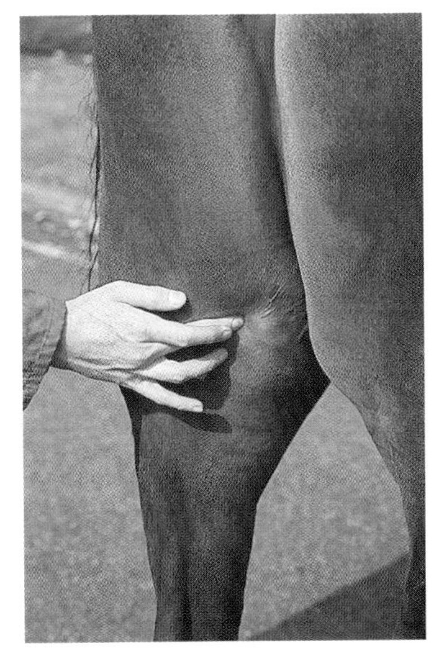

a

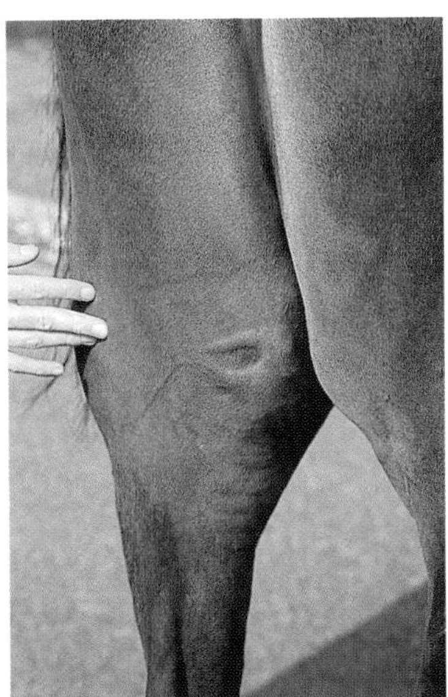

b

Figure 12.32 Lymphoedema. The oedema is diffuse and showed no evidence of inflammation. The pictures illustrate the 'pitting on pressure' test for oedema of any kind.

Diagnostic confirmation

- Characteristic lymphatic disorder of prepuce, inguinal region and limbs in particular

Treatment
Treatment options vary with primary cause. Any interference with oedematous skin carries a poor healing prospect.

(STERILE, NODULAR) PANNICULITIS/STEATITIS

Profile
Rare, multifactorial inflammatory condition of the subcutaneous fat of horses. Aetiology is obscure but a complex of vitamin E and selenium deficiency have been suspected in some cases and particularly in foals of the Fell Pony breed.

Clinical signs
Multiple, deep-seated, subcutaneous nodules affecting the trunk, neck and proximal limbs. Nodules may or may not be painful on palpation[61] and may be firm or soft. Initially, subcutaneous but in time will become fixed to the skin. Cystic lesions lead to ulceration and draining tracts which discharge an oily yellow/brown or bloody discharge.

Concurrent systemic effects include diarrhoea, anaemia, weakness and failure to thrive.

Differential diagnosis
- Granuloma
- Neoplasia including cutaneous lymphosarcoma and lymphoma
- Cysts

Diagnostic confirmation
- History
- Clinical examination
- Excisional biopsy

Treatment
Good results have been reported with high levels of systemic prednisolone or dexamethasone, but overall results are variable.[107] Correction of vitamin E/selenium status is helpful but may be disappointing.

EQUINE CUTANEOUS AMYLOIDOSIS

Profile
A rare papulonodular disorder of skin and upper respiratory tract mucosa. It usually occurs in older horses as a result of continuous immune stimulation of the reticuloendothelial system and the deposit of amyloid in various sites.[108,109]

Clinical signs
Nonpainful, nonpruritic nodules and plaques in skin and in mucous membrane of upper respiratory tract (**Fig. 12.33**). They may appear suddenly then regress and slowly reappear. Disease usually becomes chronic and progressive. A seropurulent nasal discharge containing flecks of blood or episodes of mild epistaxis may be reported. The nasal lesions are easily traumatized and even mild damage (e.g. passage of a nasogastric tube or endoscope) can cause alarming (though seldom life-threatening) bleeding.

Differential diagnosis
- Eosinophilic granuloma
- Mastocytoma and other nonspecific granuloma
- Cutaneous histiocytic lymphosarcoma
- Ethmoid haematoma/other neoplasia (respiratory signs)
- Squamous cell carcinoma
- Other causes of epistaxis (various)

Diagnostic confirmation
- History of prolonged immune stimulation
- Nodules in skin and nodular thickening of nasal mucosa and occasional nasal bleeding
- Biopsy using special stains to demonstrate amyloid in sections

Treatment
No effective treatment. Reductions in the demands on the reticuloendothelial system may be feasible (e.g. withdrawal from hyperimmune serum pro-

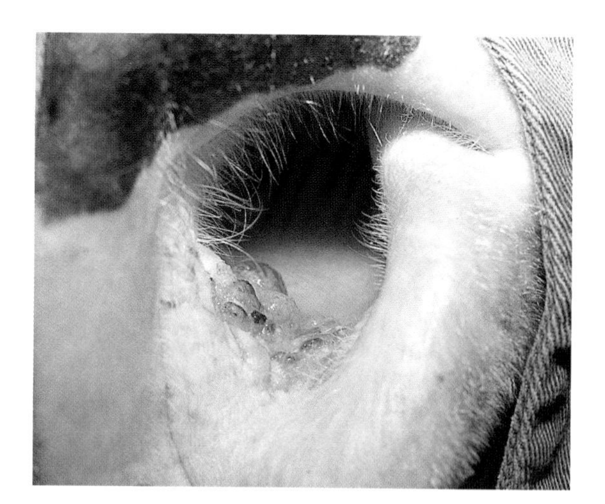

Figure 12.33 Nasal/cutaneous amyloidosis. The nasal lesions are the most easily recognized. Even minor trauma causes bleeding.

duction). The disease runs a long course and there are suggested inherited tendencies which should be considered with breeding horses. Nasal involvement and resultant dyspnoea are important considerations which may warrant supportive or even life-saving treatment.

AXILLARY NODULAR NECROSIS

Profile
Rare nodular skin condition of unknown aetiology. No breed, sex or age predisposition.

Clinical signs
One or two (occasionally many) firm, painless, well-circumscribed subcutaneous nodules (10–40 mm in diameter) near the girth or axilla (**Fig. 12.34**). No pruritus or pain associated with the nodules and no overlying alopecia. Affected horses are otherwise healthy. The nodules are of no material consequence but may resemble some other more significant diseases.

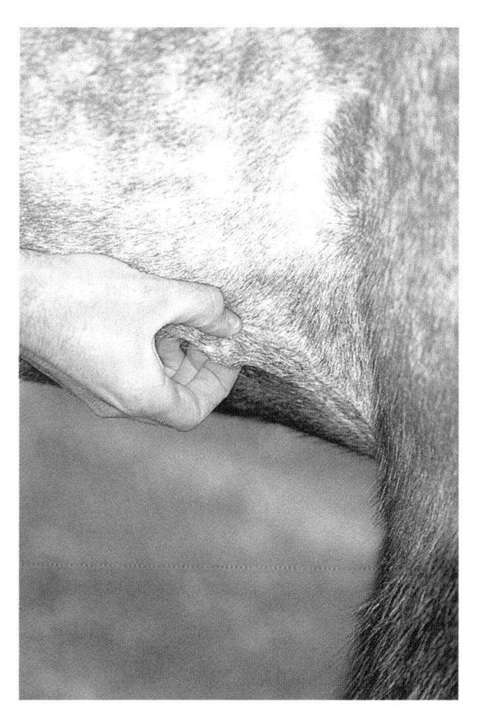

Figure 12.34 Axillary nodular necrosis. A single (or few), nonpainful solid nodule at this site is characteristic but not diagnostic.

Differential diagnosis
- Traumatic damage/scarring
- Mastocytoma
- Epidermoid and dermoid cysts
- (Eosinophilic) collagen necrosis
- Nodular sarcoid
- Lymphosarcoma/lymphoma
- Insect bites
- Hypodermiasis (*Hypoderma bovis*)
- Amyloidosis
- Nodular panniculitis

Diagnostic confirmation
- Clinical signs are almost characteristic.
- Biopsy is distinctive (focal dermal necrosis without collagen degeneration).
- Cultures for bacteria and fungi are negative.

Treatment
Surgical removal is possible and usually successful. Sublesional injection of small doses of methylprednisolone (5–10 mg/lesion) is usually successful also.

EOSINOPHILIC COLLAGEN NECROSIS/GRANULOMA

Profile
Probably one of the most common nodular skin conditions in the horse. Firm dermal nodules associated with degenerative collagen. It is possibly the result of local hypersensitivity reactions to insect bites. Some, however, have no insect contact history. Occurs primarily in spring and summer.

Clinical signs
One or more (occasionally many) firm, painless, well-circumscribed subcutaneous nodules 5–20 mm in diameter, usually but not always situated along the back and sides of the chest (**Fig. 12.35**). Chains and groups can occur, suggesting an insect-related aetiology in some cases (**Fig. 12.36**). The more mature lesions have a calcified, granular core which can be expressed from the open surface (**Fig. 12.37**). The condition is not usually pruritic and there is no overlying alopecia except at the centre of a degenerating lesion.

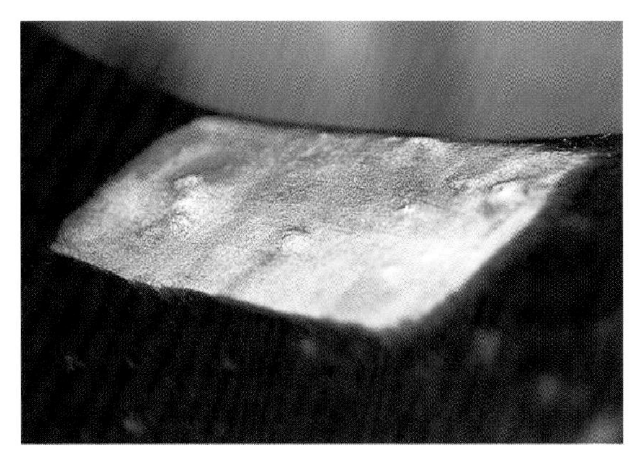

Figure 12.35 Eosinophilic collagen necrosis/granuloma lesions on the back. The firm, discrete, non-painful nodules are frequently more easily felt than seen, but erect hairs may be present.

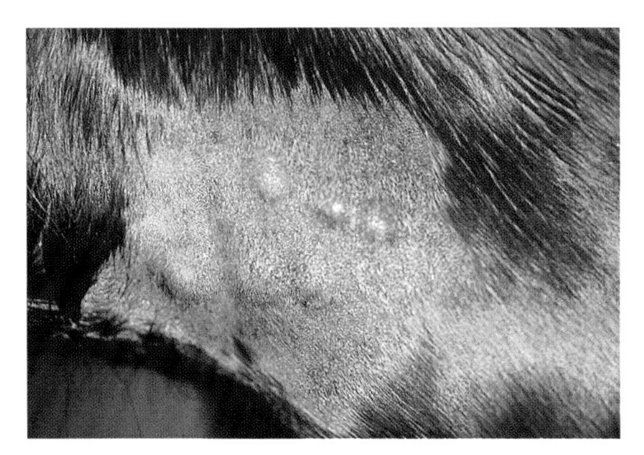

Figure 12.36 Eosinophilic collagen necrosis/granuloma lesions arranged in linear patterns in the throat region.

Differential diagnosis

- Axillary nodular necrosis
- Epidermoid and dermoid cysts
- Insect bites
- Hypodermiasis (*Hypoderma bovis)*
- Cutaneous lymphosarcoma
- Sarcoid (nodular)
- Amyloidosis
- Phaeohyphomycosis
- Panniculitis

Diagnostic confirmation

- Clinical signs are almost characteristic.
- Biopsy is distinctive (foci of necrobiosis of collagen fibres associated with heavy eosinophilic infiltration). Older lesions may mineralize.

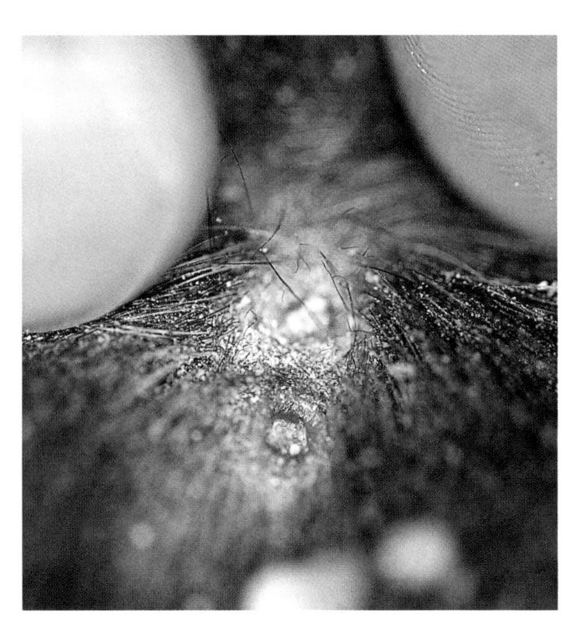

Figure 12.37 Eosinophilic collagen necrosis/granuloma lesion showing a calcified core under the firm cap.

Treatment

Intralesional injection of very small doses of triamcinolone (3–5 mg/lesion) or methylprednisolone (5–10 mg/lesion) is usually successful. Many nodules are dense and may require the use of a (Luer-lock) pressure syringe and a 25G needle. Systemic corticosteroids (prednisolone) can be helpful if many lesions are present, especially in early stages. Surgical removal is possible and usually successful, especially in older calcified lesions. However, some occur in difficult sites where surgery is difficult or may lead to behavioural problems (e.g. saddle area).

(GENERALIZED) GRANULOMATOUS (ENTERITIS) DISEASE (CHRONIC EOSINOPHILIC ENTERITIS)

Profile

Granulomatous enterocolitis affects small or large bowel or both resulting from specific defects in host defence mechanisms or dysfunction of local immune systems.[110] Very similar to sarcoidosis (or chronic granulomatous disease of horses) but tends to produce less obvious cutaneous lesions (see p. 169). It is probably justified at present to group all these diseases into one as they are similar in clinical appearance and have a wide variety of signs.

Clinical signs

Skin lesions such as exudative and ulcerative coronitis, alopecia, hyperkeratosis and exudative dermatitis on muzzle, face and limbs. Lesions on the skin tend to be intensely pruritic and moderate or severe self-mutilation can arise (**Fig. 12.38**). Oral and lingual ulcers occur in some horses (these signs differentiate it from sarcoidosis).

Possible associated signs are described as the generalized granulomatous disease of horses. In this there is a more pronounced cutaneous involvement with multiple small pustules which are most obvious in the groin and the ventral abdomen (**Fig. 12.39**).

Generalized signs of systemic disease include chronic weight loss, poor bodily condition, variable appetite, normal to loose faeces (but rarely patent diarrhoea), dependent oedema, dullness and lethargy. Recurrent pyrexia of unknown origin can sometimes be the first sign which is identifiable. Rectal examination may indicate enlarged lymph nodes, thickened mesentery and thickened bowel wall.

Differential diagnosis

- Pemphigus foliaceus
- Bullous pemphigoid
- Systemic erythematosus-like syndrome
- Sarcoidosis

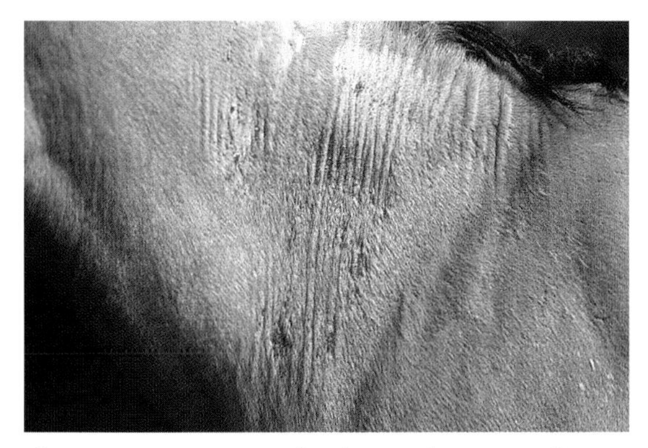

Figure 12.38 Generalized granulomatous disease. Notice the extensive inflamed and thinned skin which was intensely pruritic. Ulcerative lesions were also present from time to time in the mouth. The horse had recurrent bouts of diarrhoea and dullness.

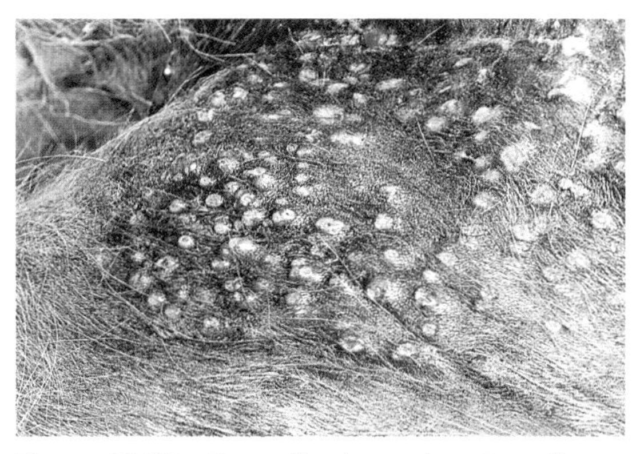

Figure 12.39 Generalized granulomatous disease with cutaneous pustules which extended over the whole ventral abdomen and flanks. Treatment failed to help.

- Cutaneous vasculitis
- Dermatophilosis (*Dermatophilus congolensis*)
- Dermatophytosis (*Trichophyton* spp.)
- Coronary band dystrophy
- Lymphosarcoma (cutaneous, intestinal and multicentric forms)
- Salmonellosis

Diagnostic confirmation

- Eliminate possibility of neoplasia (lymphosarcoma, adenocarcinoma) and hepatic failure.
- Rectal and intestinal biopsy may be needed to differentiate it from lymphosarcoma.
- Biochemical changes include low total plasma protein (and albumin in particular) with high plasma fibrinogen. Low glucose/xylose absorption test results suggestive of poor carbohydrate absorption.
- Haematology is usually unrewarding.
- Skin biopsy shows acanthosis, hyperkeratosis with foci of parakeratosis, crust and scale formation and eosinophilic infiltration of nonspecific nature.

Treatment

Unrewarding. Sustained (long-term) medication with corticosteroids may give temporary relief. Recovery has not been reported.

SEBORRHOEA

Profile

Primary sebaceous gland dysfunction is rare in horses. The disease seems more likely to be related to abnormal cornification resulting in scaling and

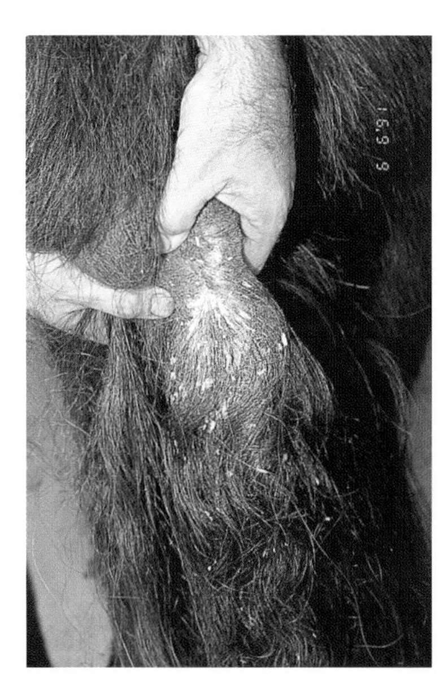

Figure 12.40 Seborrhoea showing extensive (greasy) scaling of the skin.

crusting than to sebaceous gland dysfunction. Secondary seborrhoea is usually related to a skin response from some other injury, e.g. 'greasy heel' in heavy horses.[111] An apparently identical appearance can be caused by secondary skin irritants (topical chemical or chronic urine scalding) or *Chorioptes equi* (primary dermatitis of limbs of heavy horses) and/or dermatophilosis (*Dermatophilus congolensis*).

Clinical signs

Matted, greasy hair coat with moderate to heavy scaling of mane, tail, limb (**Fig. 12.40**) and occasionally body skin. Patchy alopecia and hyperpigmentation (melanoderma) may occur.

Differential diagnosis

- Pemphigus foliaceus
- Other autoimmune complexes including systemic lupus erythematosus-like syndrome
- Cushing's disease
- Sarcoidosis
- Chorioptic mange (*Chorioptes equi*)
- Dermatophilosis (chronic) (*Dermatophilus congolensis*)
- Dermatophytosis (*Trichophyton* spp.)
- Iodine poisoning (iodism)
- Matted hair from heavy sweating with/without chorioptic mange in long-haired draught horses

Diagnostic confirmation

- Clinical appearance of hair full of 'dandruff' scales, particularly of the mane and tail.
- Biopsy is most often unrewarding.

Treatment

Close clipping of affected area(s). Antibacterial shampoos and parasiticides if necessary. Keep hair coat clean and shampoo as required with anti-seborrhoeic (selenium-based) shampoo every 2–3 days.

Ivermectin orally may be useful in controlling secondary chorioptic mange but may not always be effective.

PURPURA HAEMORRHAGICA (immune-mediated vasculitis)

Profile

An immune-mediated vasculitis commonly associated with the recovery phase of an upper respiratory infection (most often due to *Streptococcus equi equi* or *Streptococcus equi zooepidemicus*). Young and stressed horses are possibly more susceptible. Immune complexes are probably deposited on the walls of peripheral blood vessels, causing localized damage and increased vascular permeability. Leakage of proteins into the extravascular space causes severe oedema (which may initially present as discrete urticarial wheals).

Clinical signs

Initially urticarial wheals develop (mostly over the abdomen and thorax) and then severe diffuse oedema develops in the limbs characteristically with a clear demarcation at the elbow and stifle (i.e. level with the bottom of the heart) (**Fig. 12.41**). Oedema is severe with serum exudation from the skin (**Fig. 12.42**). Extensive skin erosions and exudation are sometimes encountered (**Fig. 12.43**). Marked or less obvious petechial or ecchymotic haemorrhages occur in the mucosae and the skin (especially in thin-skinned areas such as the muzzle and pinnae). Severe pulmonary oedema and central nervous signs arising from cerebral oedema may be life-threatening.

Differential diagnosis

- Bullous pemphigoid/pemphigus vulgaris
- Systemic lupus erythematosus-like syndrome
- Drug eruptions
- Actinic dermatoses

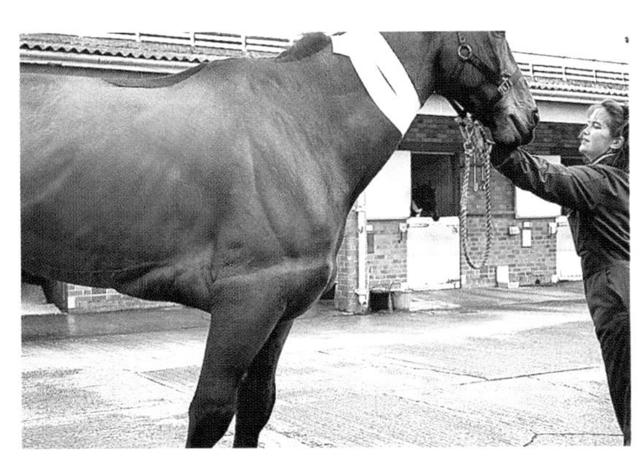

Figure 12.41 Purpura haemorrhagica showing the typical oedema pattern involving the limbs with a sharp demarcation level with the bottom of the thoracic cavity.

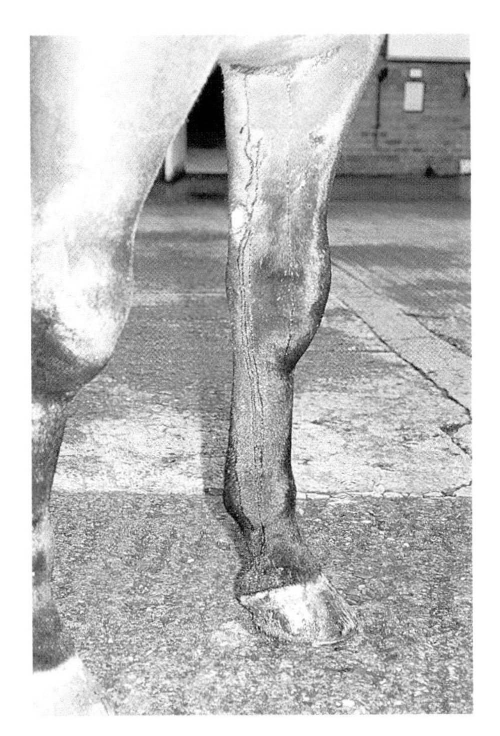

Figure 12.42 Purpura haemorrhagica showing oedema of the limb and severe plasma exudation as a result of plasma protein leakage into the extravascular space due to an immune-mediated vasculitis.

- Dermatophilosis (*Dermatophilus congolensis*)
- Infectious vasculitis (e.g. equine viral arteritis)
- Disseminated intravascular coagulopathy
- Lymphosarcoma

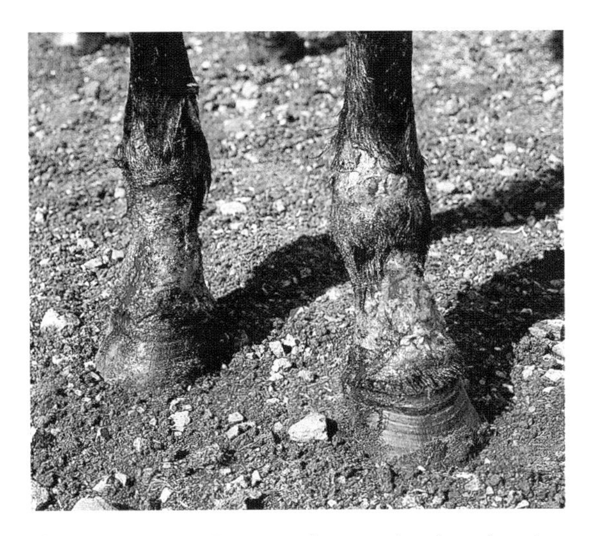

Figure 12.43 Purpura haemorrhagica showing extensive skin erosions with exudation on the distal limb.

Diagnostic confirmation

- History of respiratory disease some 2–4 weeks previously
- Characteristic clinical signs
- Nonthrombocytopenic purpura (normal platelet counts)

Treatment

High doses of systemic corticosteroids are indicated with aggressive antibiosis (high doses of penicillin and/or aminoglycosides). *Beware* of possible underlying drug sensitivity (drug eruption). Some cases of drug eruptions which look very similar may be the direct result of these drugs administered some weeks previously for the respiratory tract infection.

The prognosis is very guarded as some cases may respond initially only to relapse after some weeks. Recurrence carries a very poor prognosis.

chapter 13

CHEMICAL AND TOXIC DERMATOSES

Actinic dermatoses	183
Plant poisoning	185
Selenium poisoning	186
Arsenic poisoning (chronic)	187
Mercury poisoning	187

ACTINIC DERMATOSES

Profile

Caused by ultraviolet radiation. Facilitated by lack of pigment and hair. It may be acute or chronic and falls into two distinct categories:

1. Sunburn (excessive exposure to UV light) with *expected outcome*.
2. Photosensitization (normal exposure to UV light) with *unexpected* or *disproportionate response*.

Photosensitization requires three factors:

- presence of a photodynamic agent in the skin
- exposure to sunlight or certain wavelengths of ultraviolet light
- cutaneous absorption of ultraviolet light

Photosensitization occurs in two forms:

Primary photosensitization Encountered as a result of some plant and chemical poisonings (e.g. St John's Wort (*Hypericum perforatum*), other plant species and phenothiazine anthelmintic are regular causes). The ingested photodynamic agent is absorbed directly from the digestive tract and is delivered to the skin without any hepatic detoxification or alteration. The result is predictable in most horses and is seldom severe.

Secondary photosensitization Digestion of chlorophyll produces a potent photodynamic agent, phylloerythrin, which is normally detoxified and excreted by the liver. Severe liver failure allows the substance to pass into the bloodstream unchanged and it will accumulate in the skin. The aetiopathogenesis is related to concurrent hepatic failure and is therefore unpredictable. Severe actinic damage to the skin is common.

Most of the primary photosensitizing plants are only marginally palatable at best, but signs can be seen during periods of ingestion of the plant, i.e. during grazing in summer months. Ingestion of hepatotoxic plants such as *Senecio* spp. or *Lantana* spp. is unusual from grazing situations but horses are unable to identify and reject the plants in preserved forage (hay or silage). Thus, most cases develop in late winter and spring and manifest when the ultraviolet light levels increase in early summer.

Specific primary and hepatotoxic plants are probably well known to veterinarians practising in the areas concerned. Almost every country has examples of both types of plant.

Clinical signs

Cutaneous lesions usually obviously restricted to light skin or hairless areas.

(a) Simple sunburn (**Fig. 13.1**) can be difficult to differentiate from the more serious forms of actinic dermatitis but the horse is usually clinically normal and often has very pink skin with minimal hair cover over the muzzle and face. The extent of the damage is usually much less severe than in true photosensitization. Most prominent signs are found on the face, commonly around lips, nose and eyelids. If there is significant exudation there may be a complicating superficial infection with *Dermatophilus congolensis* (see Fig. 7.10).

(b) The more severe systemically mediated condition (either from direct photodynamic agents or hepatic failure) is usually much more serious and has a much more destructive nature. Again, the lesions are typically restricted to the white areas on the face and elsewhere (**Fig. 13.2**) and are always sharply restricted to the nonpigmented skin (**Fig. 13.3**). Severe cases may have lesions which just overlap into dark-skinned, well-haired areas. Conjunctivitis, skin oedema, erythema, pruritus and pain are usually present as the skin becomes necrotic. The perineum and coronary band region may be severely affected (see Fig. 13.2). Extensive

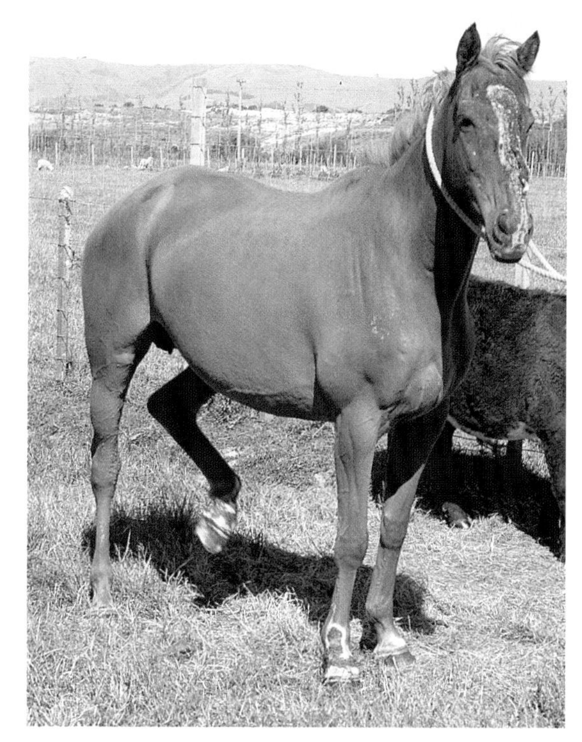

Figure 13.2 Actinic dermatitis (photosensitization) affecting the white facial stripe and the white digits in a mare with liver failure. The foot lesions affect the lateral aspects far more than the medial.

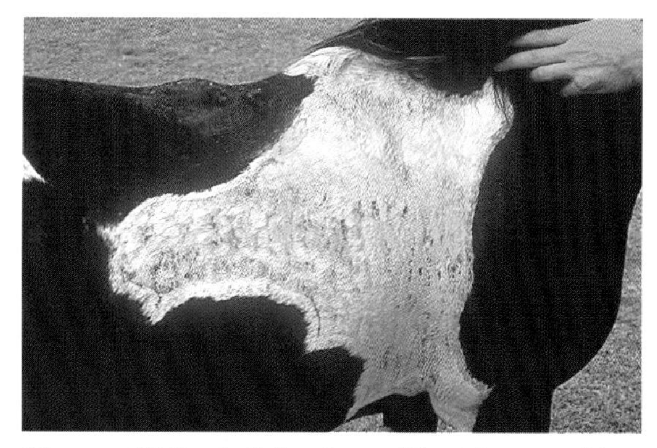

Figure 13.3 Actinic dermatitis (photosensitization) (severe) affecting the white areas of the skin in a piebald pony. Notice the sharp cut-off of the severe dermatitis at the margins of the white areas.

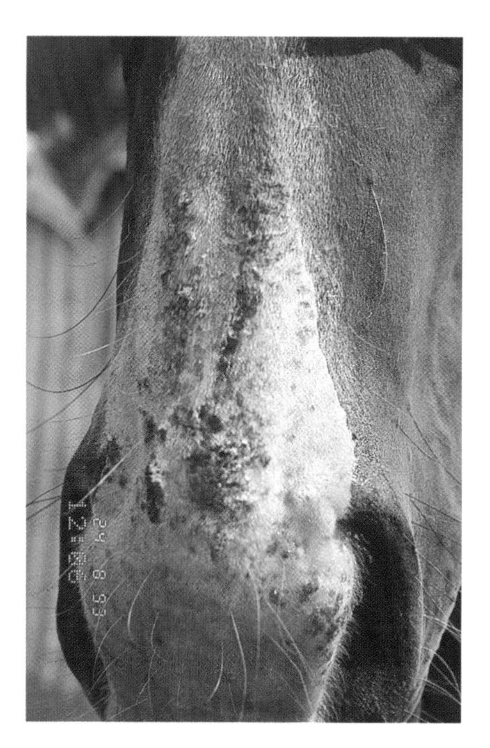

Figure 13.1 Sunburn on an unpigmented nose. No other areas affected and the animal was otherwise very healthy.

sloughing of skin occurs in most severe cases. Concurrent systemic signs of hepatic disease may be present (ventral oedema, hepatoencephalopathy, icterus and weight loss) with biochemical evidence of hepatic failure.

The role of plant or toxic chemicals and ultraviolet light in the pastern-related dermatoses (and pastern leukocytoclastic vasculitis in particular) is uncertain but the distribution of the lesions suggests in some cases that sunlight is involved (see Fig. 12.15, p. 165).

- Generalized lesions are suggestive of liver involvement.
- Localized lesions on lip and distal limb are suggestive of primary photosensitization (pasture plants, sprays or drugs).
- Involvement of the lateral aspects of pigmented digits only may suggest pastern leukocytoclastic vasculitis.
- Involvement of the face only in cream horses or those with lightly pigmented faces may suggest sunburn alone.
- ***All* horses showing any evidence of photosensitization *must* be investigated for possible hepatic damage using the full range of liver function tests (including bile acids, hepatic enzymes and possibly liver biopsy).**

The detection of pyrrolizidine alkaloids on erythrocytes has been described and is probably the definitive test for current ingestion of the plants.[112,113] Feeds can be closely examined for the plants themselves but this is not always easy and it may be better to analyse the feeds for the alkaloid.

Differential diagnosis
- Sunburn
- Dermatophilosis (*Dermatophilus congolensis*)
- Dermatophytosis (*Trichophyton* spp.)
- Pastern leukocytoclastic dermatitis
- Greasy heel syndrome

Diagnostic confirmation
- History and pasture content (or diet or drugs) for primary photosensitizing plants or hepatotoxic substances (including pyrrolizidine alkaloids).
- Physical examination with localized damage in non-pigmented parts.
- Blood sample for detection of alkaloid on red cells (lithium heparin anticoagulant) only effective during ingestion stages.
- Biopsy of skin is nonspecific with extensive necrosis and severe inflammation.

Treatment
Protect affected areas from direct or reflected sunlight by immediate stabling, use of hoods, rugs, etc. Apply emollient/soothing and local anaesthetic creams. Some protection can be provided by sunblock creams with factors greater than 20.

Glucocorticoids and non-steroidal anti-inflammatory drugs may be of assistance in reducing inflammation but may exacerbate hepatic failure and concurrent hepatoencephalopathy.

Eliminate all sources of photodynamic agents.

Symptomatic treatment of liver disease or other disorders should be instituted, but chronic severe liver failure is not usually treatable. Therefore, cases of true hepatic-related photosensitization carry a very poor prognosis.

PLANT POISONING

Profile
Ingestion of plants that cause hair loss including *Leucaena leucocephala* which is used as forage and shade trees and Mimosa (*Mimosa pudica*) which is the common 'sensitive' bush. The active principle in both these plants is mimosine, a toxic, non-protein amino acid.

Clinical signs
Alopecia, particularly affecting the mane, tail (**Fig. 13.4**) and around fetlock and coronary band. Severe cases may show chronic laminitis-like ringing to walls of all feet. Loss of appetite and weight loss are common.

Differential diagnosis
- Insect hypersensitivity (sweet itch)
- Selenosis (selenium poisoning)
- Iodine poisoning (iodism)
- Mercurial poison
- Arsenic ingestion
- Coronitis/coronary band dystrophy
- Anagen defluxion
- Malnutrition
- Mane and tail dystrophy (Appaloosa tail syndrome)

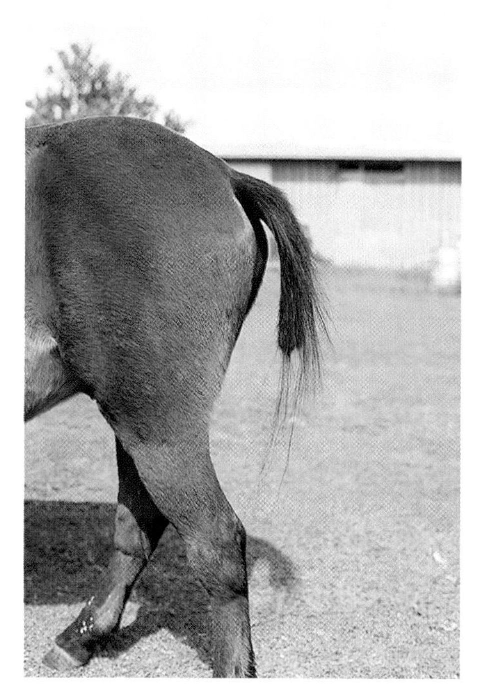

Figure 13.4 Specific *Leucena* spp./*Mimosa* spp. poisoning causing loss of tail (and mane) hairs but with no effect on body hair.

Diagnostic confirmation

- Access to *Leucaena* spp. or *Mimosa pudica*
- Elimination of other possibilities

Treatment

Remove source of plant material. Supportive multivitamin supplementation may help. Other remedies are anecdotal and unreliable.

SELENIUM POISONING

Profile

Selenium in plants is derived from soil, and some plants such as *Astragulus* spp. and *Oonopsis* spp. are capable of accumulating significant concentrations of selenium if the soil has an inherently high concentration. Examples of plants which actively concentrate/accumulate selenium are *Morinda reticulata*, *Neptunia amplexicaulis*, asters and *Senecio* spp.[114] Diseases associated with ingestion of seleniferous plants are geographically restricted to areas where the plants occur or where local conditions favour high dietary selenium. Unnecessary or excessive administration of selenium supplements may also be responsible for serious toxicity.

Clinical signs

The acute form of selenium poisoning shows no dermatological signs.

Chronic poisoning causes dramatic loss of mane and tail hairs in particular (**Fig. 13.5**). Body hair may become sparse with skin thin and fragile. Lameness may be severe with acute and/or chronic laminitis. Hoof slippering /sloughing may occur.

Differential diagnosis

- Mimosine toxicity
- Coronary band dystrophy
- Other causes of laminitis
- Other causes of mane and tail dystrophy
- Iodism

Diagnostic confirmation

- Assay of selenium in mane and tail hairs, hooves, liver and kidney.
- Affected animals usually have access to seleniferous plants
- Heavy dietary supplementation with selenium in animals which do not require it (iatrogenic selenosis).

Treatment

Remove source of selenium. Place affected horse on a high protein supplement and administer 2–3 g *d*,1-methionine orally per day. Feed additives such

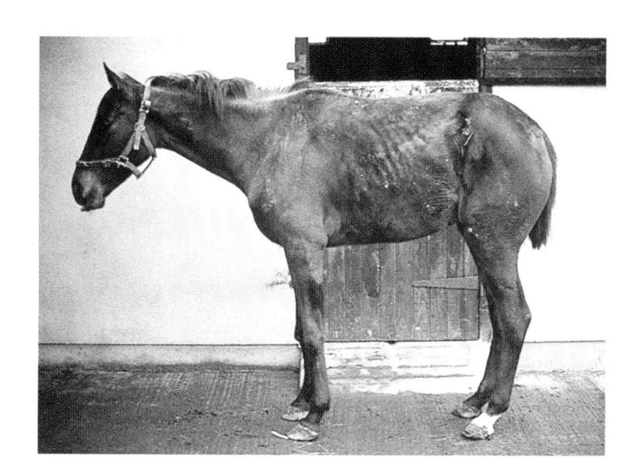

Figure 13.5 Selenium poisoning. Note the poor coat quality with generalized hair loss and a particularly severe depletion of the mane and tail hairs. The laminitic stance arose from severe 'slippering' of the hooves of all four feet.

as sodium arsenate, arsenilic acid and copper supplements have been reported as treatments.

ARSENIC POISONING (CHRONIC)

Profile

Arsenic compounds in minute amounts have historically been used as skin tonics and most cases are the result of excessive use of these. However, there is little doubt that arsenic can be beneficial in producing a shiny coat and so the use of the tonics is unfortunately still practised. Chronic poisoning can also be due to repeated contact with arsenical insecticidal dips (used in some parts for cattle and sheep) or from industrial pollution. Acute arsenic poisoning has no significant cutaneous signs. It is likely that arsenic poisoning will become less prevalent as compounds are removed from medications and industrial pollution.

Clinical signs

Chronic ingestion of arsenic compounds is associated with poor body condition and long hair growth, heavy scaling and scurf. Appetite may be near normal. There is loss of body condition when rested on basic rations. Mane and tail hair of poor density and irregular poor quality is a feature. Application of arsenic salts (particularly white arsenic trioxide) is commonly practised in treatment of the equine sarcoid. It is extremely caustic and indiscriminate in its destruction of tissue, causing extensive necrosis and sloughing. However, it is seldom used in sufficient quantity to cause systemic or chronic cutaneous signs.

Differential diagnosis

- Cushing's disease/syndrome (pituitary adenoma)
- Selenosis (selenium poisoning)
- Pediculosis (lice infestation)
- Plant poisoning (*Mimosa* spp., *Lucaena* spp.)
- Mane and tail dystrophy

Diagnostic confirmation

- History of feeding or ingestion of organic and inorganic arsenic compounds over long periods or in high dosage
- Acute poisoning in contact horses or other species
- Arsenic assay of hair

Treatment

Low and reducing (tapering) doses of an organic arsenical may quite rapidly reverse the horse's condition. Treatment doses must be tapered off gradually and may take a considerable time (10–16 weeks) before the horse starts to return to normal bodily condition.

MERCURY POISONING

Profile

Relates mainly to application of mercurial salts to the skin as counterirritants/therapeutic blisters (e.g. red mercuric chloride) or ingestion of dressed grain containing organic mercury compounds as antifungal agents. The latter are no longer used in most parts of the world, so systemic poisoning has largely disappeared.

Clinical signs

Acute mercurial poisoning from ingested organic or inorganic mercury compounds has no significant dermatological signs. Surface application of inorganic mercury salts (used as therapeutic blisters, etc.) causes vesicle formation with ulceration and inflammation (**Fig. 13.6**). Scabbing and scaling follow. The effects are localized to the treated areas of the limbs.

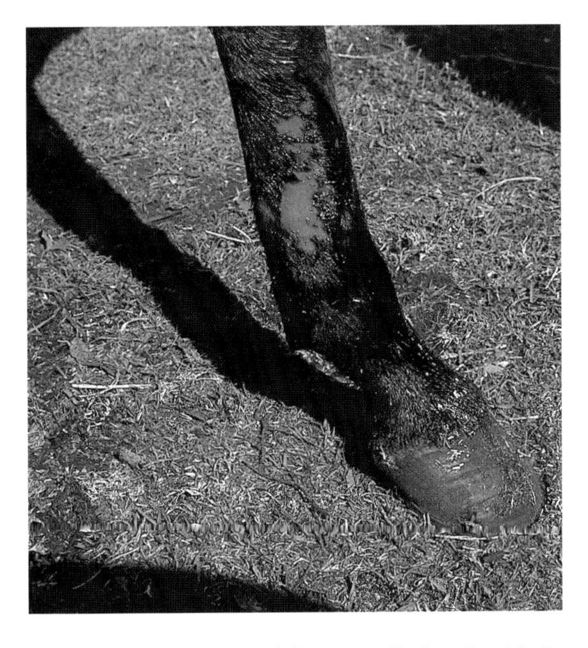

Figure 13.6 Mercuric blister, applied to the skin in expectation of a therapeutic benefit on the tendons below, resulted in severe dermatitis and extensive scaling over many months.

Prolonged overzealous topical applications (or ingestion) may produce systemic effects including loss of hair from head, neck, body and finally, legs. Mane, tail, forelock and fetlock hairs are least affected. Oral ulceration and corneal opacity with ocular pain may be present.

Differential diagnosis

- Dermatophytosis (*Trichophyton* spp.)
- Dermatophilosis (*Dermatophilus congolensis*)
- Pediculosis (lice) (*Damalinia equi*, *Haematopinus asini*)
- Trombiculidosis (*Trombicula* spp. mites)
- Occult sarcoid
- Anagen defluxion
- Plant poisoning (*Lucaena* spp., *Mimosa* spp.)

Diagnostic confirmation

- History of application or ingestion of mercury salts (usually some weeks previously).
- Severe/acute toxicity is unlikely to concern the dermatologist.

Treatment

Wash affected areas with warm soapy water or shampoo. Rinse, dry and apply emollient creams and lotions containing corticosteroids, antibiotics and possibly local anaesthetics. When corneal damage is evident, lavage eye with normal saline followed by antibiotics and corticosteroids applied every 2 hours.

chapter 14

ENDOCRINE DISORDERS

Hypothyroidism	189
Iodine poisoning (iodism)	189

HYPOTHYROIDISM

Profile

Uncommon disease in horses.[115] Foals born in areas where iodine deficiency occurs have been reported to have signs.

Note: Excessive feeding of kelp and high iodine levels can also be responsible for enlarged thyroids in newborn foals.[116]

Clinical signs

Enlarged thyroid (goitre) may or may not occur. Normal hair coat as a foal but abnormal hair coat develops as foal hair is shed. Skin may be thickened by myxoedema. Leg deformities (angular and flexural as well as arthrogryposis) may also occur in foals. Patchy hair loss over head, neck, forelimbs, hindquarters. Underlying skin is pigmented and the hair may be white in places.

No pruritus or ulceration.

Diagnostic confirmation

- Abnormally low levels of plasma T_3 and T_4.
- Confirmation is difficult as histopathology usually shows normal skin structure, but increased hair follicles and decreased sebaceous glands may be identified in the affected area. Hair shafts may be filled with irregular keratinized material.

Treatment

Oral L-triiodothyronine (4 mg/kg bodyweight) daily for at least 10 days. Treatment course may require months or years or may show no response at all.

IODINE POISONING (IODISM)

Profile

May occur as result of prolonged medication with oral potassium iodide or sodium iodide.[117] Significant iodism is very unlikely from ingestion of seaweed/kelp or iodine supplement, but foals delivered to mares being fed high levels may have obvious goitre with or without concurrent signs of hypothyroidism.

Clinical signs

Lacrimation is the earliest sign. Heavy scurf on neck, mane and body (**Fig. 14.1**). Alopecia has been reported.

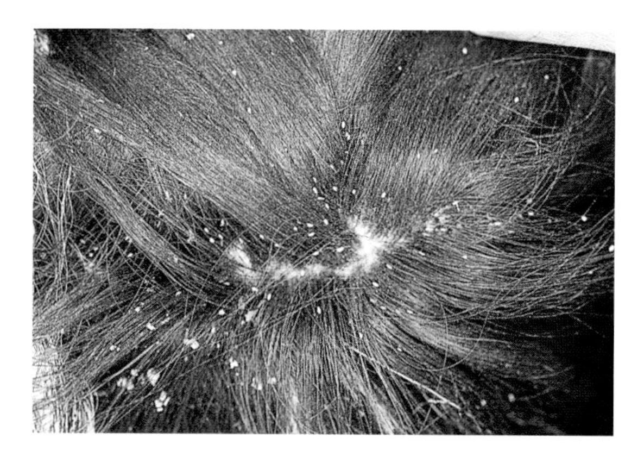

Figure 14.1 Iodism. Heavy scaling and flaking of the skin arising from persistent dietary supplementation with seaweed salts.

Differential diagnosis

- Seborrhoea
- Chorioptic mange (*Chorioptes equi*)
- Selenium toxicity
- Other causes of lacrimation

Diagnostic confirmation

- History of medication (usually with sodium or potassium iodide) or supplementation (often with sea-salt/sea-weed supplements)

Treatment

Reduce or stop intake of supplements or medication.

chapter 15

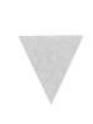

NUTRITIONAL DISORDERS

Energy deficits	191
Protein deficits	191
Dietary fats and oils	191
Dietary minerals	191
Vitamin A	192

It is easy to forget that the skin, like other organs, requires the normal nutrients if it is to behave in a normal fashion. Almost any inappropriate food material and any gross deficiency of the basic requirements can effect the skin to some extent.[118] However, even prolonged malnutrition may have surprisingly little material effect on the skin and hair.

Energy deficits (usually the result of starvation, malabsorption, parasites or concurrent disease) commonly induce a dry, scurfy, moth-eaten coat with poor skin elasticity. Normal hair shedding and regrowth can be impaired significantly with long coats and patchy moulting.

Protein deficits cause failure of hair growth and shaft weaknesses. Alopecia or poor coat density can develop but the status of the horse in other respects will probably command more attention.

Dietary fats and oils have been and are commonly added to feeds for horses (in particular linseed) and the use of these materials (including evening primrose oil) can have a dramatic improving effect on hair quality. Late winter coats are often improved significantly by dietary supplementation of a vegetable oil over 20–60 days. There are no known harmful effects of these on coat quality, but they may have some effects on fat-soluble vitamin absorption and some have significant metabolic/systemic effects when fed in excess (e.g. linseed).

Dietary minerals are known to affect coat and skin health as well as skin healing ability.

Zinc in particular appears to have a major influence on skin health and an adult horse requires a regular daily intake of around 500 mg of zinc. Deficiency of zinc develops within a short time as reserves are low and manifests as generalized alopecia with extensive surface scaling and flaking giving an appearance of severe dandruff.[119] Initially the lesions may appear on the thighs and ventral abdominal wall. Severe and prolonged deficiencies result in generalized exudation and flaking with extensive and severe loss of hair (**Fig. 15.1**). Any remaining hair is easily pulled out by light grooming. The histological appearance is characteristic (hyperkeratosis, acanthosis and parakeratosis). Daily dietary supplementation with zinc methionine or other zinc salts has a curative effect over some weeks.

Iodine deficiency during pregnancy has obvious effects on the hair coat of the foal at birth.

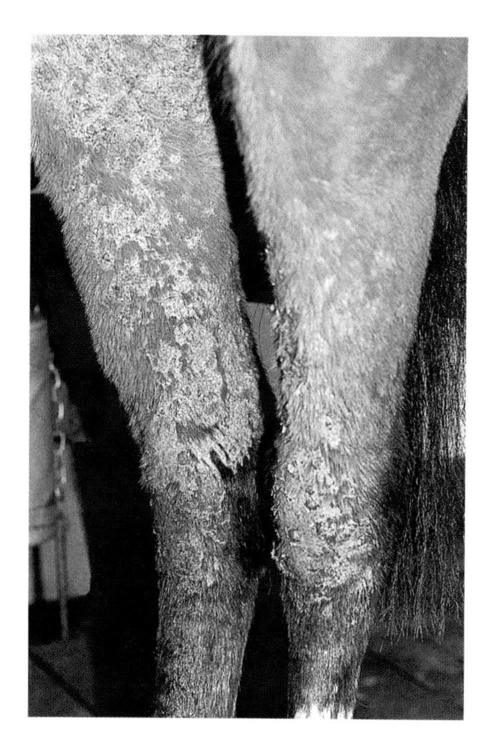

Figure 15.1 Zinc deficiency with severe exfoliative noninflammatory shedding of the hair and hyperkeratosis.

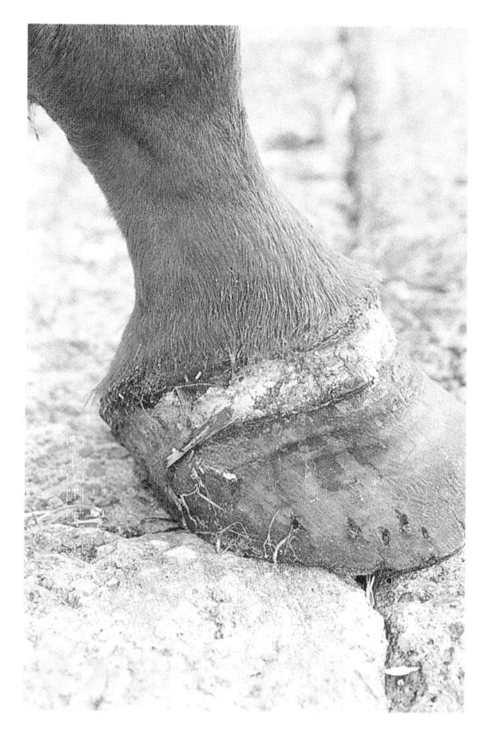

Figure 15.2 Vitamin A deficiency-related coronitis.

Affected foals have a sparse coat and an obvious goitre is often found at birth. Other deformities such as contracted tendons and fused joints (arthrogryposis) may be associated with iodine deficiency. Chronic excessive iodine fed to adult horses (often in the form of seaweed powder supplements, etc.) may be responsible for a sparse, short hair coat.[117] Iodism can also develop during treatment of fungal (and other) infections with potassium or sodium iodide. The earliest signs include lacrimation and a scurfy, dry coat quality (see Fig. 14.1).

Copper deficiency causes a loss of black pigment because it is essential for the production of melanin.[120] Affected horses develop a coarse, harsh hair quality and a russet-brown hue to the darker areas of the coat.

Alopecia and browning of the hair around the eyes gives the animal a 'spectacled' appearance, but these signs are not as prominent in the horse as in cattle and may easily be missed. Confirmation of the diagnosis can be made from blood and liver assays for copper, but response to careful supplementation may be as useful. A more serious tendency to arterial rupture and chronic anaemia is possibly associated with copper deficiency. Horses may be more resistant to copper deficiency than other domestic animals but there have been few studies on the status of horses grazed on known copper-deficient land.

Vitamin A dietary deficiency results in a rough, coarse and dull hair coat. Deficiencies of vitamin A are particularly rare in horses being maintained on normal feeding regimens, but prolonged deficiency may cause a mild or more severe inflammatory reaction at the coronary band (**Fig. 15.2**). Prolonged deficiency causes marked hyperkeratosis but this is very rare except in young growing horses maintained under prolonged extremely poor nutritional conditions (particularly if grains, which have a poor vitamin A concentration, are fed with very poor quality hay or straw).

Other nutritional elements are unlikely to cause dermatological problems but many which induce these signs in other species have not been

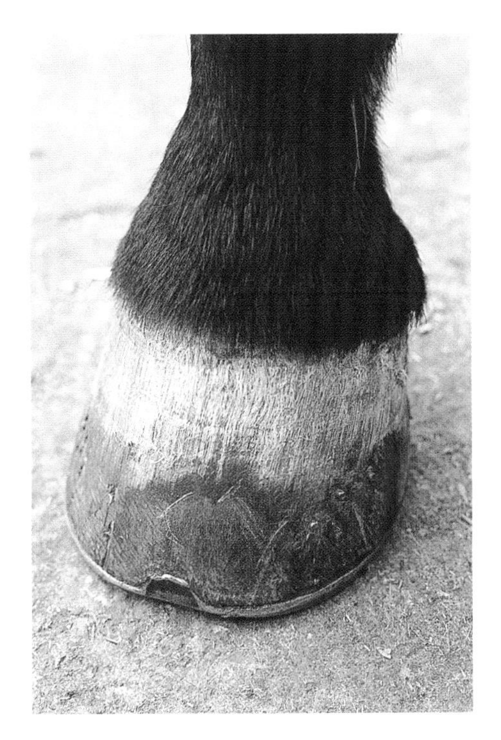

Figure 15.3 Biotin (and methionine) deficiency. The feeding regimen had changed drastically some 4–5 months previously and the deficiency is reflected in the poor quality of hoof periople. Correction resulted in a slow improvement with the damaged horn eventually growing out.

documented in the horse. Deficiencies of B and C vitamins are extremely unlikely in normal horses on normal feeding regimens or indeed even under conditions of moderate or severe deprivation/starvation. However, methionine and biotin (together or independently) have been used to improve hoof quality. Therefore, by inference, poor hoof quality may be associated with hoof walls which lack a normal periople (**Fig. 15.3**) or are subject to severe cracking and loss of normal hoof pliability. It is not always easy, however, to differentiate this from dryness and harsh underfoot conditions which cause break-back and alteration in hoof quality.

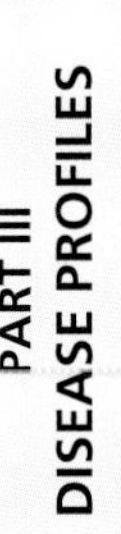

chapter 16

IATROGENIC AND IDIOPATHIC DISORDERS

Vitiligo	195
Leukoderma (acquired vitiligo)	196
Leukotrichia (tiger-stripe, variegated leukotrichia, reticulated leukotrichia)	197
Hyperaesthetic leuko(melano)trichia	198
Unilateral papular dermatosis	198
Anhidrosis	199
Anagen defluxion	199
Coronary band dystrophy	200
Idiopathic pastern dermatitis	201
'Greasy heel' syndrome	202

VITILIGO

Profile

Depigmented spots and larger, poorly defined areas appearing on the skin. They may be idiopathic or may follow primary damage to melanocytes.[121,122] They are usually restricted to horses over 4 years old. The condition may be heritable and is probably commonest in Shire and Arabian horses.

Clinical signs

Depigmented circular or irregular spots up to (or over) 1 cm diameter which increase in number rather than size (**Fig. 16.1**) are typical. On the body these seldom if ever cause alopecia, but around the eye where the hair coat is sparce in any case hair loss is sometimes very pronounced (**Fig. 16.2**). Leukoderma may or may not copy the associated leukotrichia. Owners often become very concerned but can easily be reassured of the benign nature of the condition, although the progressive nature of some cases makes certain uses of the horse unrewarding.

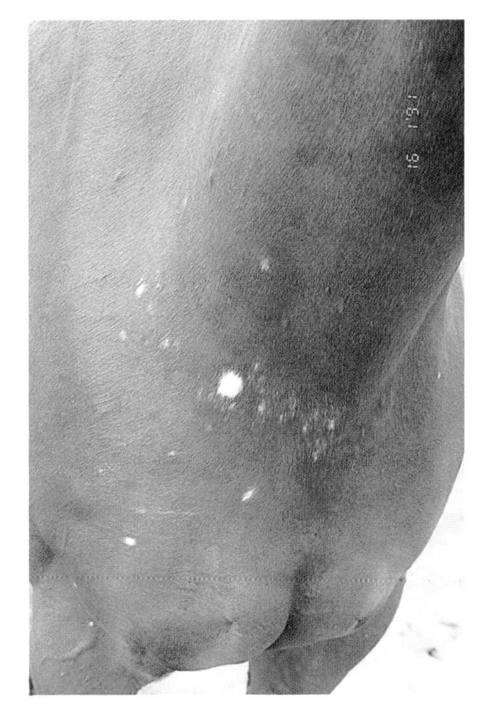

Figure 16.1 Vitiligo (idiopathic depigmentation): spotted, body form which caused changes in the hair colour.

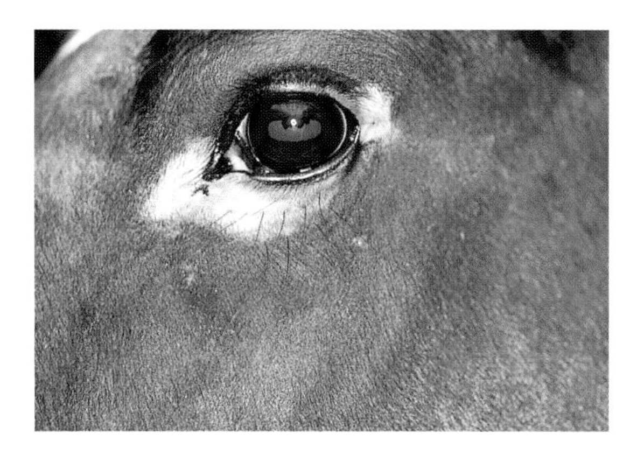

Figure 16.2 Vitiligo (idiopathic depigmentation) around the eye. Notice that the area has a naturally sparse hair coat but most of this was shed in the areas affected.

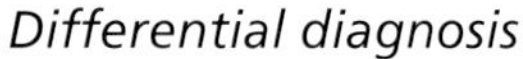

Differential diagnosis

- Acquired vitiligo (leukoderma/leukotrichia from skin injury such as cold, trauma, radiation etc.)
- Arabian fading syndrome

Diagnostic confirmation

- Absence of injury.
- Circular white spots which appear without reason and do not increase in size.

Treatment

There is no remedy. Surgical removal of 3–5 mm spots where only 2–3 areas occur may be feasible but may cause more extensive depigmentation. It is best left alone. Cosmetic coverage is possible in show horses by dyes or stains.

LEUKODERMA (aquired vitiligo)

Profile

Loss of pigment in hair and skin related to various factors such as pressure injury, cryosurgery, surgery, radiation or other skin disorders. The pathological consequence is exploited in freeze marking.

Clinical signs

Ill-defined, irregular white patches of hair and skin, developing after skin insult such as follows skin trauma and freeze branding (**Fig. 16.3**). Cryosurgery or normal sharp surgery, irradiation

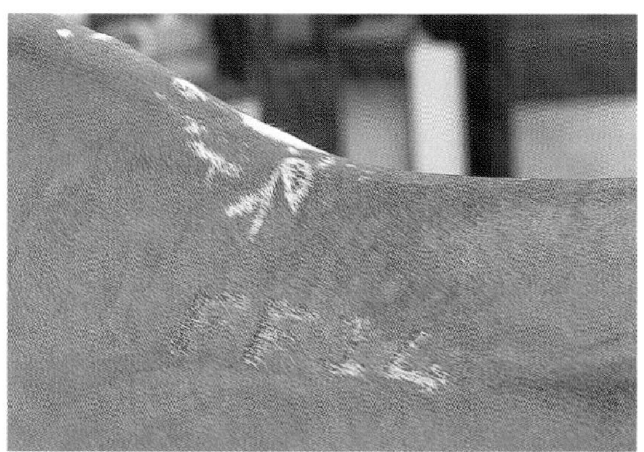

Figure 16.3 Leukoderma/leukotrichia (acquired vitiligo). Two forms of the condition are shown. Irregular 'saddle (and girth) marks' are usually accepted as being of traumatic origin. Freeze branding should result in a change in pigment without any other scarring, but in this case the 'burn' was less well judged and only limited pigment changes arose at the margins of the scars.

(X-ray or gamma) (**Fig. 16.4**), etc. can also cause changes in the melanocytes with local development of white hair. Melanocytes can be destroyed by contact with irritants, harness, rubber, bits, etc. Common sites include the saddle region and withers and girth where they arise from repeated minor or more severe trauma (see **Fig. 16.3**). There is often no apparent thickening or other cutaneous changes, but with injuries and surgical sites the skin is sometimes patently scarred and thickened.

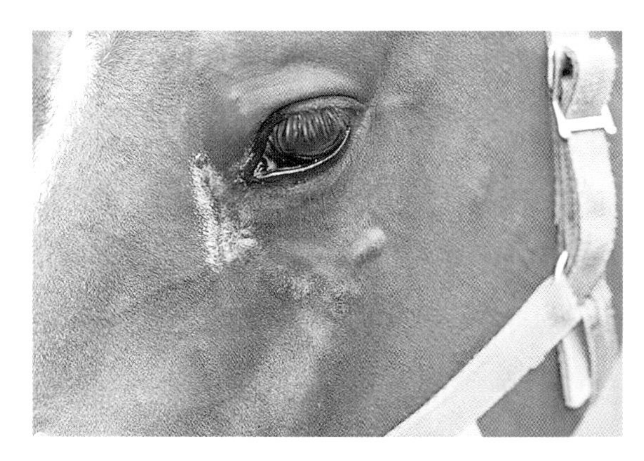

Figure 16.4 Acquired leukotrichia (without obvious leukoderma) as a result of γ-radiation brachytherapy successfully used to treat a periocular sarcoid.

Differential diagnosis

- Coital exanthema
- Arabian fading syndrome
- (Reticulated) Leukotrichia
- Systemic lupus erythematosus-like syndrome

Diagnostic confirmation

- History and physical appearance.
- Biopsy shows an abnormal lack of melanocytes but little else.

Treatment

There is no known treatment. Erasure of freeze branding is virtually impossible but can be attempted with laser surgery (however, it invariably leaves more white hairs and skin, but the number may be hidden).

LEUKOTRICHIA (tiger-stripe, variegated leukotrichia, reticulated leukotrichia)

NAm; Aus

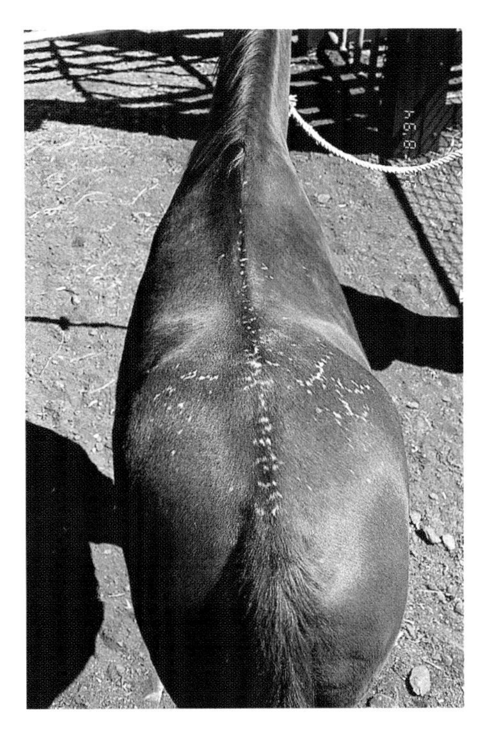

Figure 16.5 Leukotrichia (tiger-stripe, variegated leukotrichia, reticulated leukotrichia).

Profile

Dorsal, bilateral, reticulated, white hair-striping. May develop in yearlings but is most often seen in older horses with unknown earlier history. It has been suggested that it is a form of erythema multiforme. Mainly Standardbred, Thoroughbred and particularly Quarterhorses are affected. There is a suggested correlation between rhinopneumonitis (EHV) vaccine and the onset of the disease.

Clinical signs

Sudden onset of extreme cutaneous pain is associated with the development of small vesicles and crusts. Linear dorsal crusts arranged in a cross-hatched pattern across the back and rump (**Fig. 16.5**). Temporary alopecia follows shedding of crusts. New hair is white but the skin retains its original pigmentation. The condition has a course of about 3 months during which the horse will severely resent palpation of the affected areas. Repeated episodes have also been reported.[123]

Differential diagnosis

- Trauma-induced leukoderma/leukotrichia (e.g. saddle marks)
- Hyperaesthetic leukotrichia
- Iatrogenic (cryosurgery/freeze marking)
- Erythema multiforme
- Vitiligo
- Systemic lupus erythematosus-like syndrome of horses
- Appaloosa parentage

Diagnostic confirmation

- Absence of injury in clinical history.
- Clinical examination to eliminate any other causes: i.e., should check possibility of drug- or vaccine-related trigger mechanism.
- Biopsy of affected skin shows pronounced dermoepidermal inflammation (interface dermatitis).

Treatment

There is no known treatment; it is best left alone. Corticosteroids do not help even at high doses. Treatment with acyclovir has been suggested followed by administration of the post-herpes-zoster neuralgia drug amitryptiline. There are no reports of the results of this.

HYPERAESTHETIC LEUKO(MELANO)TRICHIA

NAm

Profile

Rare disease but highly characteristic disorder limited to the dorsum of horses and, as yet, only recognized in California, USA.[124]

Clinical signs

Single or multiple, *painful* crusts (1–4 mm diameter) along the dorsum of the back and over the saddle area. Obvious (sometimes extreme) pain is usually manifest – horses react violently if the lesions are handled. (Note: in some cases the pain may precede the development of overt lesions and the horse may be presented for a 'cold back' or saddle resentment.) Lesions remain for 1–3 months followed by spontaneous regression. Permanent white or dark/black markings and various degrees of alopecia develop at the affected sites (**Fig. 16.6**). Some cases will resolve completely (although some scarring usually remains), while in others it may recur or be persistent with variable degrees of hypersensitivity.

Differential diagnosis

- Dermatophilosis (*Dermatophilus congolensis*)
- Staphylococcal farunculosis (*Staphylococcus aureus/intermedius*)
- *Culicoides* spp. hypersensitivity (sweet itch)
- Dermoid cysts (single or few, nonpainful)
- Reticulated leukotrichia
- Idiopathic and trauma-induced leukotrichia
- Photosensitization

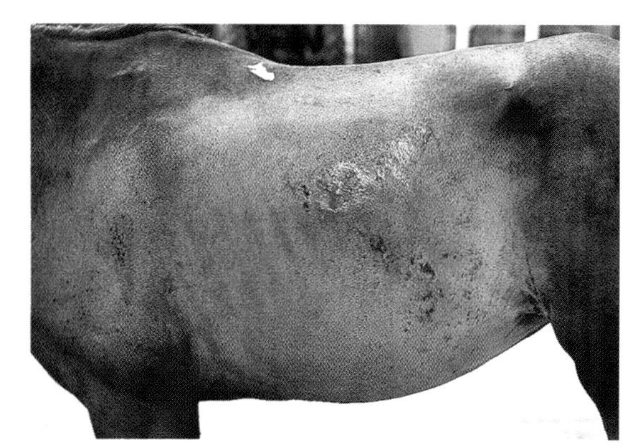

Figure 16.6 Hyperaesthetic melanotrichia. The sparsely haired pigmented areas were acutely painful and the hair colour changed to white over the following years.

- Sunburn
- Chemical burn/irritation
- Contact allergy

Diagnostic confirmation

- Clinical appearance.
- Biopsy shows a marked, chronic subepidermal and intra-epidermal oedema.

Treatment

There is no known treatment. Even high doses of corticosteroids and nonsteroidal anti-inflammatory drugs have no material effect. The course is usually some weeks with gradual remission, but some horses remain 'cold-backed' or 'saddle-shy'.

UNILATERAL PAPULAR DERMATOSIS

Profile

Uncommmon disorder of yearlings and 2-year-old Quarterhorses (and some Thoroughbreds). The aetiopathogenesis is unknown.[125] Most lesions develop in spring/summer, suggesting an insect-related aetiology.

Clinical signs

Acute appearance of nonulcerative, nonpainful multiple papules and nodules, usually in a loose group (30 to > 200 in number in a circular arrangement limited to one side of the body trunk (**Fig. 16.7**)). Older lesions may be obvious, even-sized, firm, round, well-circumscribed, nonulcerative and nonalopecic nodules. Fresh nodules may occur in almost concentric rings around the original lesions. There is no associated pruritus and horses are otherwise unaffected.

Differential diagnosis

- Dermatophytosis (*Trichophyton* spp.) (before hair is lost)
- *Stomoxys calcitrans* or other insect bites/reactions
- *Culicoides* spp. hypersensitivity (sweet itch)
- Nodular sarcoid
- Collagen necrosis/eosinophilic granuloma
- Axillary nodular necrosis
- *Onchocerca cervicalis* filariasis.

Diagnostic confirmation

- History and clinical appearance.
- Skin biopsy shows eosinophilic folliculitis/furun-

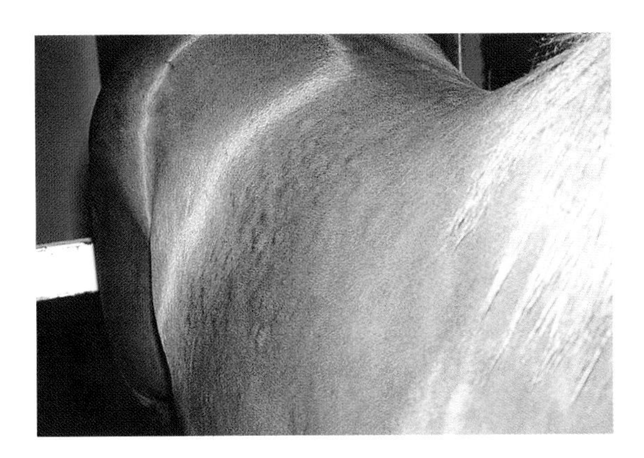

Figure 16.7 Unilateral papular dermatosis. About 30 nonulcerative, nonpainful papules and nodules in a loose group in a circular arrangement on one side of the body trunk.

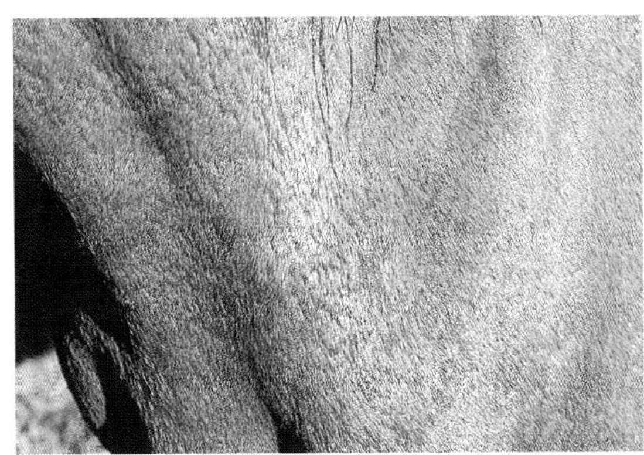

Figure 16.8 Anhidrosis. The coat is dull, dry, harsh and greasy.

culosis without any consistently recognizable microorganisms.

Treatment

Oral prednisolone daily[61] may produce a detectable benefit, but even prolonged courses of high doses do not always do so.[126] The nodules may persist and some become calcified.

ANHIDROSIS

Profile

Characteristic failure of sweating in horses which are subjected to movement from temperate to tropical climates, although not all cases have this history. Cases in temperate climates are uncommon.

Clinical signs

Loss of performance and/or exercise intolerance with an inordinately high respiratory rate after relatively minor exertion. Inability to sweat. Longer-term cases show patchy alopecia with a harsh, dry coat (often with a tessellated appearance and a seborrhoeic/greasy feel) (**Fig. 16.8**).

Differential diagnosis

- *Culicoides* spp. hypersensitivity (sweet itch)
- Dermatophilosis (*Dermatophilus congolensis*) (particularly the generalized, summer form)
- Dermatophytosis (*Trichophyton* spp.)
- Sarcoidosis
- Pemphigus foliaceus
- Other systemic illnesses with poor or restrictive performance and high respiratory rates

Diagnostic confirmation

- History of a move from temperate to tropical climate and loss of performance.
- Diagnostic confirmation by intradermal adrenaline injections of several dilutions of adrenaline. Usually 0.5 ml of dilutions of $1{:}10^3$, $1{:}10^4$, $1{:}10^5$, $1{:}10^6$ are injected some distance from each other on the side of the neck. Anhidrotic horses have reduced sensitivity and prolonged response time (some may not sweat at all), while normal horses sweat noticeably at all dilutions.

Treatment

Some cases fail to respond to anything other than return to a temperate climate. Moving to a colder climate for the summer months may not be a practical option and then air conditioning in the stables over summer can be used. Reduced stress and rest for an extended period sometimes helps but may not do so. Adrenocorticotrophic hormone (ACTH) in long-acting gel form by daily intramuscular injection may give some relief in very early cases.

ANAGEN DEFLUXION

Profile

Secondary acute hair loss associated with high fevers, illness or malnutrition in which affected hairs break easily during the growth (anagen) phase. Antimitotic drugs such as cyclophosphamide can be responsible for an identical syndrome.

Clinical signs

Acute onset of excessive, often extreme, hair shedding following systemic disease with an elevated body temperature and/or severe malnutrition over a short time span (**Fig. 16.9**). Administration of systemic antimitotic or cytotoxic medications can cause similar dramatic moulting.

Differential diagnosis

- Seasonal moulting
- Dermatophilosis (*Dermatophilus congolensis*) (generalized)
- Dermatophytosis (*Trichophyton* spp.) (generalized)
- Generalized granulomatous enteritis syndrome
- Sarcoidosis
- Pemphigus foliaceus
- Anhidrosis
- Mane and tail dystrophy
- Mercurial poisoning
- Telogen defluvium (stressful diseases)
- Selenium and seleniferous plant (*Lucaena* spp.) poisoning (tail/mane and hooves affected)
- Fulminating abscesses

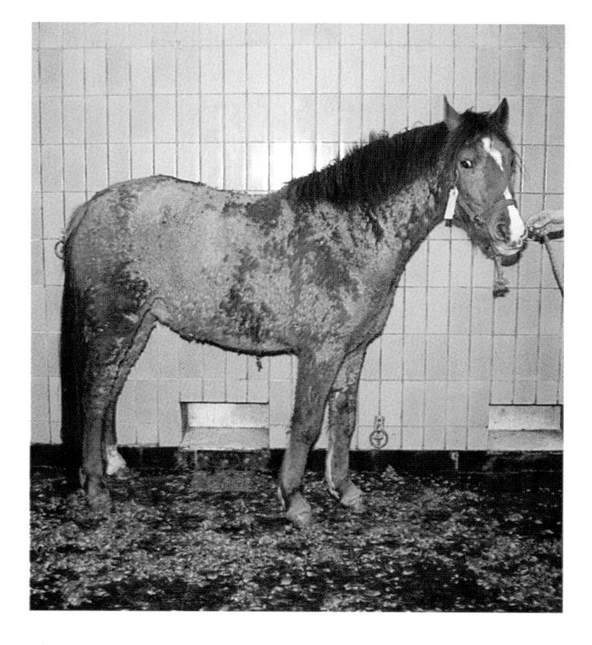

Figure 16.9 Anagen defluxion following an acute febrile disease.

Diagnostic confirmation

- Changes to hairs detectable microscopically as irregularities of shaft diameter with narrowing and deformity. Dysplastic changes such as ragged points in weakened areas. (Telogen hairs are normally of uniform shaft diameter and slightly clubbed with nonpigmented root ends and lack of root sheath.)

Treatment

Spontaneous resolution follows removal of the exciting cause of fever, etc. Withdraw any antimitotic drugs.

CORONARY BAND DYSTROPHY

Profile

An idiopathic defect in cornification of the coronary band which affects all four hooves simultaneously and equally. Mature horses of draught breeds seem most susceptible.

Clinical signs

All four coronary bands show progressive proliferation and hyperkeratotic changes with extensive scaling and have a greasy feel. There may be obvious hoof wall changes in severe or prolonged cases. Open lesions are often present with cracks and fissure which can bleed or ooze serum (**Fig. 16.10**). The ergot and chestnut may also be affected.

Differential diagnosis

- Laminitis (acute forms)
- Pemphigus foliaceus
- Dermatophilosis (*Dermatophilus congolensis*)
- Generalized granulomatous enteritis syndrome

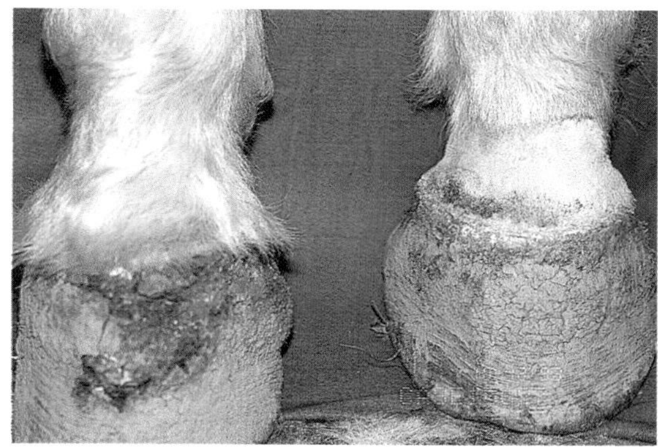

Figure 16.10 Coronary band dystrophy.

- Sarcoidosis
- Selenium toxicosis
- Verrucose sarcoid
- Pastern folliculitis

Diagnostic confirmation
- Clinical signs, elimination of all other causes
- Nonspecific poorly defined histopathology

Treatment
Palliative measures only with removal of excessive horn and application of emollient creams to affected tissues at coronet. Mild counterirritants applied to the coronet may be helpful in encouraging healthy coronary tissues but equally may make the condition worse. Dietary supplementation with evening primrose oil, biotin and methionine may be useful. Corticosteroids have no material effect.

IDIOPATHIC PASTERN DERMATITIS

Profile
Chronic disease possibly due to overtreatment, neglect, etc.

Clinical signs
Diffuse inflammatory dermatitis of the pastern. No apparent reason. Lesions are mainly found on the back of the pastern (**Fig. 16.11**). One or more legs may be involved with papular lesions which rapidly coalesce and produce large areas of ulceration and suppuration (**Fig. 16.12**). There is some tendency for the condition to occur more often on nonpigmented pasterns but this is not by any means invariable.

Differential diagnosis
- Pastern folliculitis (mixed *Staphylococcus* spp. infection)
- Photoactivated vasculitis
- Leukocytoclastic pastern vasculitis
- Dermatophilosis (*Dermatophilus congolensis*)
- Dermatophytosis (*Trichophyton* spp.)
- Pemphigus foliaceus
- Pemphigus vulgaris/bullous pemphigoid
- Coronary band dystrophy
- Contact with strong chemical irritant (disinfectants, etc.)

Diagnostic confirmation
- Complete history is important, including liver function tests if lesions are limited to nonpigmented skin.

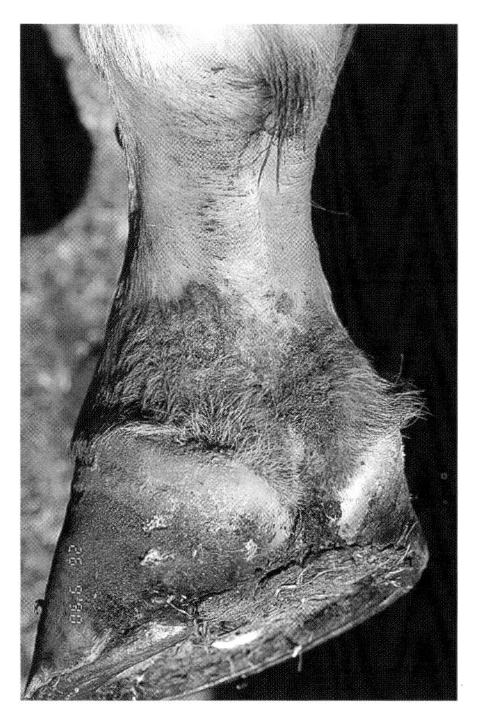

Figure 16.11 Idiopathic pastern dermatitis affecting the heels and distal pastern.

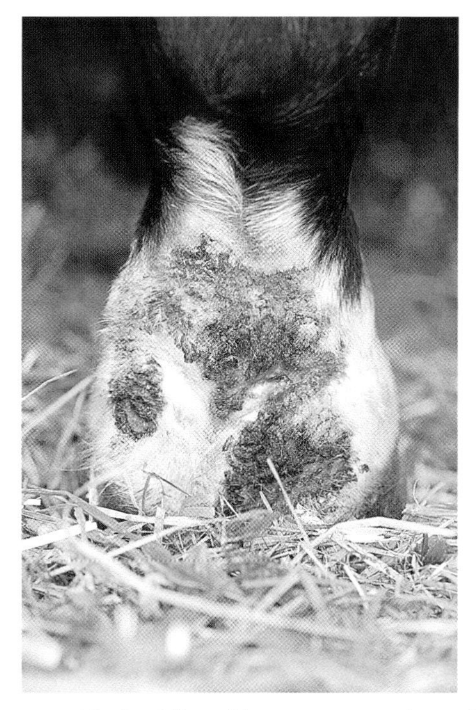

Figure 16.12 Idiopathic pastern dermatitis (chronic form) with adherent scabs and ulcerated areas.

- Biopsy with immunofluorescent studies.
- Bacterial and fungal culture. Check for dermatophytes such as *Trichophyton* spp. and dermatophilosis (*Dermatophilus congolensis*) in particular.

Treatment

Remove crusts, clip hair very thoroughly. Carefully clean the area with an antiseptic, soap-based surgical scrub. Protect the area from unhygienic conditions or contact with irritant chemicals and avoid high ultraviolet light conditions. *Do not use harsh remedies.* Emollients containing antifungal, anti-inflammatory and antibacterial lotions (triple anti-infective compounds) are commercially available. High doses of corticosteroid where immune complexes are involved.

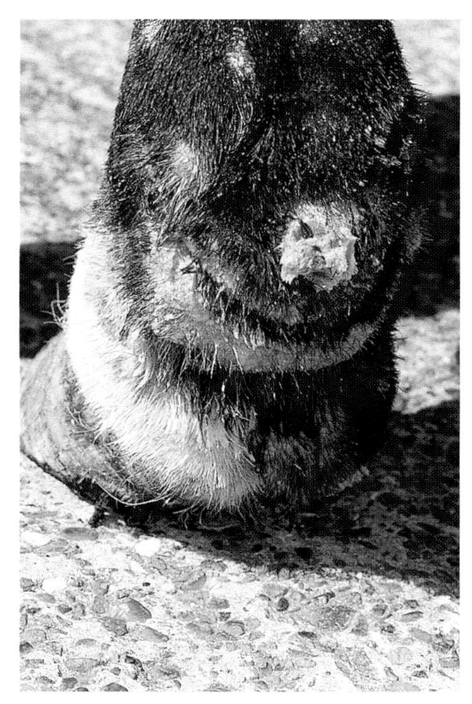

Figure 16.13 Greasy heel (chronic long-standing irritation of the skin of the pastern complicated by recurrent self-trauma and exudative dermatitis).

'GREASY HEEL' SYNDROME

Profile

This is a loose conglomeration of diseases which have similar clinical features including scaling, crusting, erosion, exudation and pyoderma of the pastern and heels of horses. It is not really a specific disease entity and can be due to a variety of inflammatory skin conditions. One pastern, frequently a hind leg, is often involved and may also be 'white socked', but it can affect all four legs and pigmented skin. It is probably more prevalent in long-haired (feathered) breeds and draught horses and has been described in these over many centuries.

Clinical signs

The clinical signs are common to the many aetiological factors. The condition usually starts at the posterior aspect of one (often white-skinned) pastern but, with time and inadequate therapy, may extend up to the fetlock and around the front of the leg. Erythema, oozing, crusting, alopecia, with vasculitis develop quickly. Erosion and ulceration of the skin with more serious exudation. In chronic (long-standing) cases the skin becomes thickened and may develop significant (often extreme) hypertrophy and deep fissures (**Fig. 16.13**). Secondary infections are common and some cases are pruritic in addition, which adds to the trauma of the skin. Severe chronic lesions may lead to chronic granulation tissue (so-called 'grapes') (**Fig. 16.14**). Lesions are characteristically painful and lameness occurs.

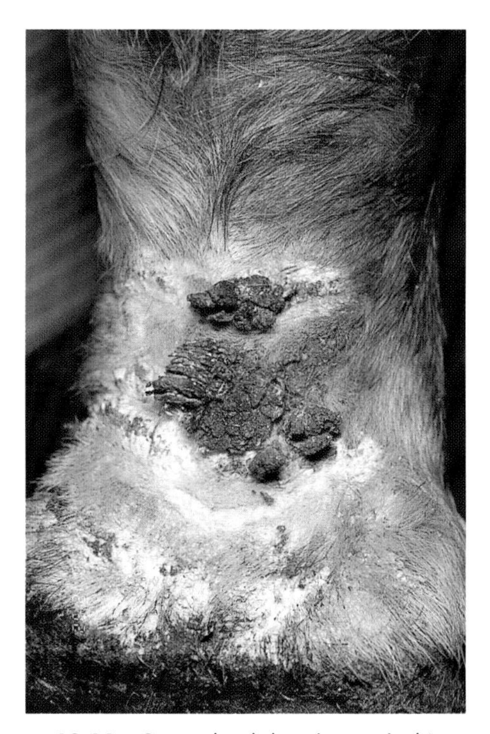

Figure 16.14 Greasy heel showing typical 'grapes', which are tightly adherent scabs and matted hair balled into small round clumps.

Differential diagnosis

- Contact dermatitis: primary irritant or allergic contact dermatitis; irritant substances on pastern; contact allergy (plants and other substances); chronic exposure to mud, unhygienic conditions (usually all four limbs are affected)
- Pastern folliculitis/pyoderma infections: staphylococcal infections/botryomycosis; dermatophilosis; fusiformis dermatitis
- Chorioptic mange (very pruritic and contagious)
- Photosensitization: systemic (phylloerythrin) involves white pasterns and other white areas (face, etc.).
- Idiopathic pastern dermatitis
- Vasculitis (pastern leukocytoclastic vasculitis/ immune-complex vasculitis/purpura haemorrhagica)
- Mycetoma
- Fibroblastic or verrucose sarcoid

Diagnostic confirmation

Diagnosis is difficult as secondary changes are often severe. The tests outlined below are all rather nonspecific and may not provide a positive diagnosis. Nevertheless negative results can also be useful.

- Swabs for culture to define infectious types and secondary bacterial contaminants.
- Scrapings for parasites (may be found but may be extensive secondary changes). Useful to look at other predilection sites.
- Biopsy (usually identifies nonspecific chronic dermatitis).
- Ultrasonographic and radiographic examination of the limb(s) may be useful if extensive thickening of the skin is present.
- Investigate systemic involvement by haematology and biochemistry.

Treatment

All possible causes should be eliminated as far as possible. The underlying cause should be treated, but realistically it is often impossible to establish this. Topical antiseptic washes are essential, initially with careful removal of all hair and necrotic tissue (this may require a general anaesthesia as it can be very painful and access to four feet may be difficult in the conscious horse). Once washed, the limb(s) should be kept dry as far as possible. Aluminium oxide powder and zinc sulphate and lead acetate solution BPC (White Lotion) have strong drying properties and reduce the extent of exudation. Nonsteroidal anti-inflammatory drugs and antibiotics (topical and systemic) may be indicated. Thick creams and lotions should not be applied if avoidable. Water-soluble-base steroid creams have been used but at least initially should probably be avoided. Many cases take years to recover fully and some have permanent skin thickening and a tendency to recurrence.

chapter 17

PHYSICAL AND TRAUMATIC DISORDERS

Traumatic skin injuries	**216**
Exuberant granulation tissue (proud flesh)	**217**
Burn/thermal/scald injuries	**218**
Pressure necrosis, rope/wire burns	**220**
Scar	**221**
Chemical trauma	**223**
Skin scalding (diarrhoea/urine or wound exudate)	**224**
Bursitis	**225**

Physical injury to the skin is very varied and the responses which are induced will reflect the wide range of direct and indirect consequences of skin injury.

TRAUMATIC INJURIES TO THE SKIN

The horse is very liable to skin injury and the full range of damage can be expected in normal practice. Bleeding into tissues can be extensive and abnormal blood clotting and high blood pressure (such as in an excited or exercising horse) can exaggerate the clinical appearance and consequences of skin injury. Wounds and wound management are described in detail in surgical texts. However, it is important for the dermatologist to appreciate the complexities of healing of skin. Skin repair occurs through the same mechanisms whether the injury is due to physical trauma or to damage through other disorders. A brief, simplistic summary of the process following a skin injury is shown in **Box 1** and a brief summary of the principles of wound management in the horse is shown in **Box 2**.

The healing process is a natural continuous process involving the control of bleeding and the development of an appropriate inflammatory response. The sequence of events involved in repair of damaged tissue can easily be disrupted by factors arising from the area and the general status of the patient but can also be significantly influenced by iatrogenic interference. Some of the most obvious factors which are responsible for the failure of a wound to heal are outlined below. With any of these factors the wound may either fail to heal or may show an inappropriate response with secondary consequences on adjacent tissues and structures. The primary objectives for the attending clinician should be to do no harm and to provide the best possible environment for wound healing.

The acute inflammatory response is critical to the process of healing and the rate of healing depends largely on the efficiency of this stage. Delays in the transition from acute inflammation to the repair phase results in an inevitable development of chronic inflammation. The longer the chronic phase is present, the greater will be the delay in healing and the more extensive the scarring and secondary consequences.

1. Wound healing – a summary of the physiological principles involved

NORMAL WOUND HEALING

1 Immediate response

Reflex vasoconstriction and tissue retraction effects early haemostasis

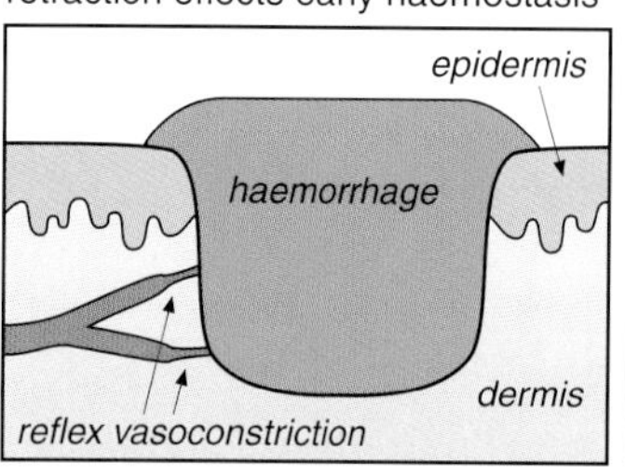

Coagulation cascade: exposed collagen triggers platelet aggregation

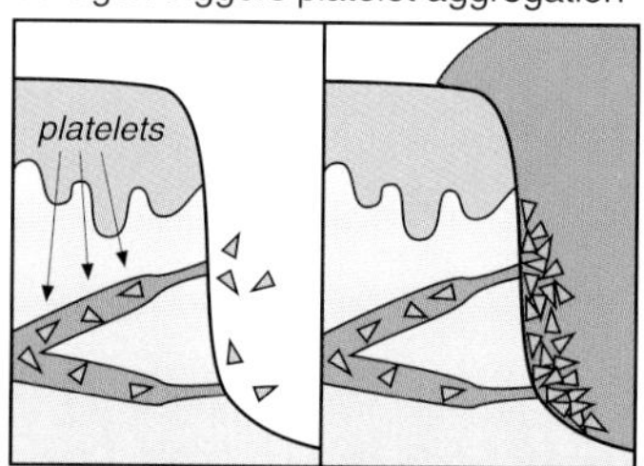

Released platelet factors result in formation of a fibrin network

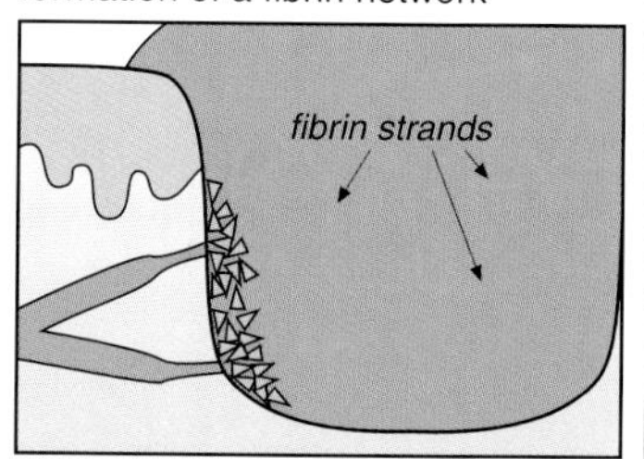

2 Inflammatory phase

Chemotaxis: neutrophils and macrophages enter the site and move along fibrin scaffolding

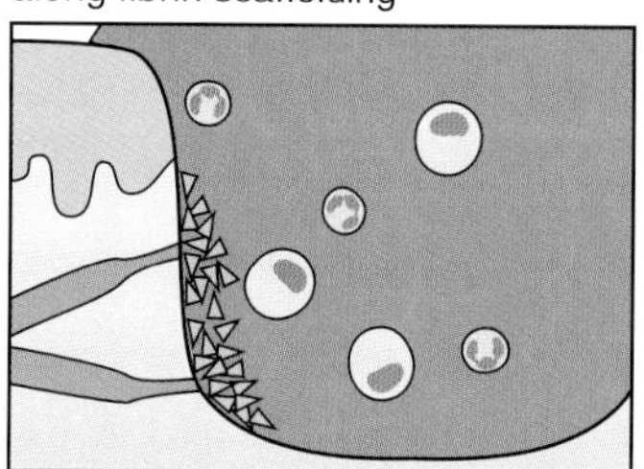

Phagocytosis: destruction of bacteria results in pus formation

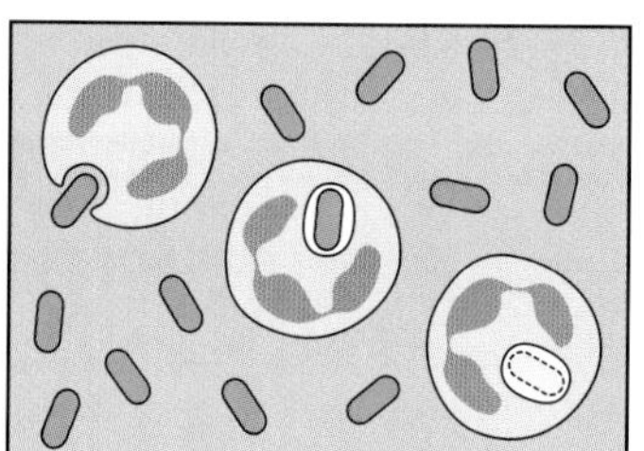

Wound debridement: proteolytic enzymes break down necrotic tissue

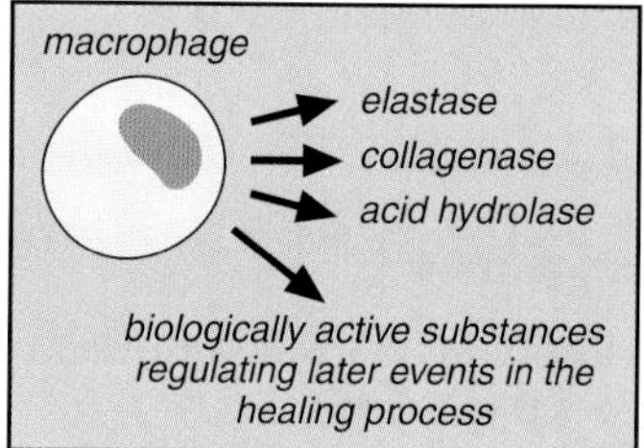

3 Proliferative phase

Granulation: neovascularization by capillary budding surrounded by fibroblasts which synthesize collagen

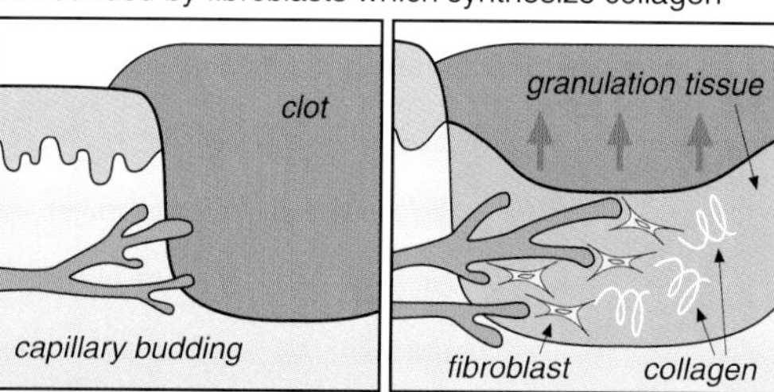

Epithelialization: a) loss of cell contact triggers cell migration; b) regeneration of normal epithelial layers

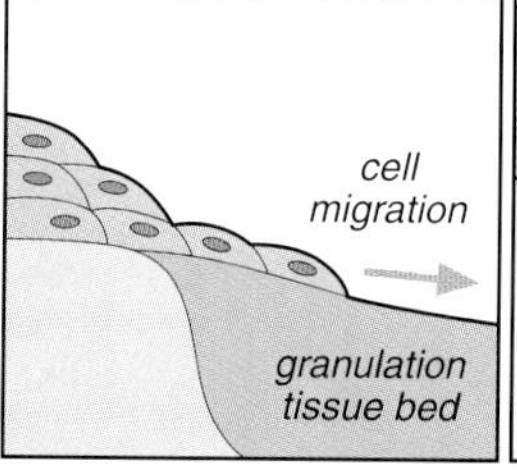

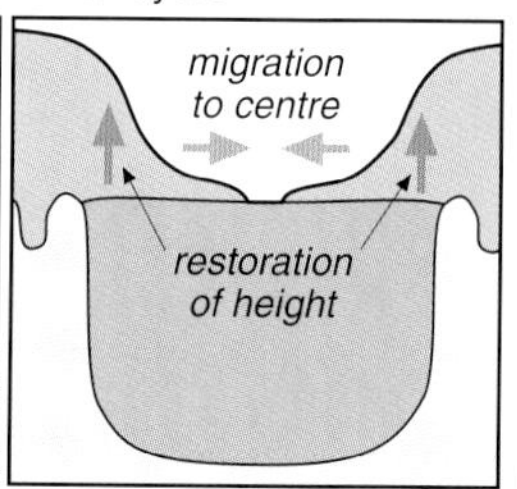

4 Maturation phase

Contraction and connective tissue reorganization: scar formation

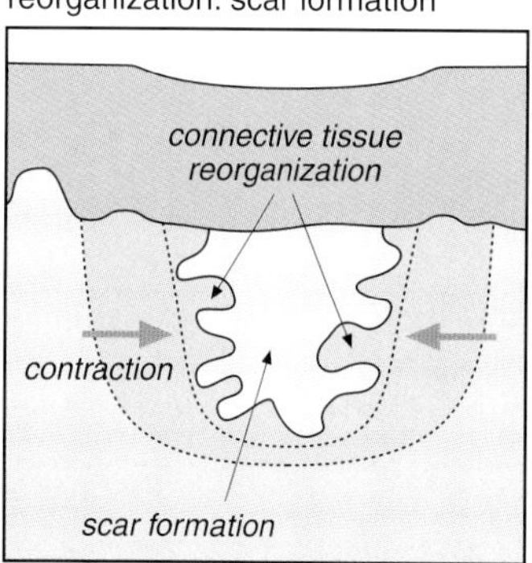

EXUBERANT GRANULATION

Uninhibited angiogenesis and fibroblast activity leads to excess production of collagen and blood vessels, over which epithelial cells are unable to migrate

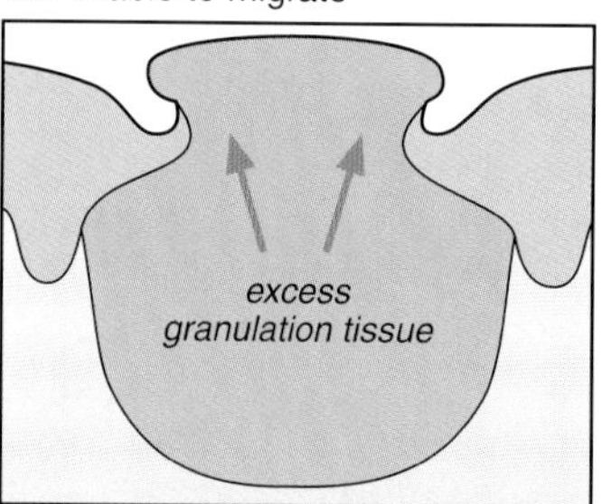

THE INDOLENT WOUND

Failure of angiogenesis results in poor or little epithelialization and ulcer formation; increased risk of infection may lead to further delay in healing

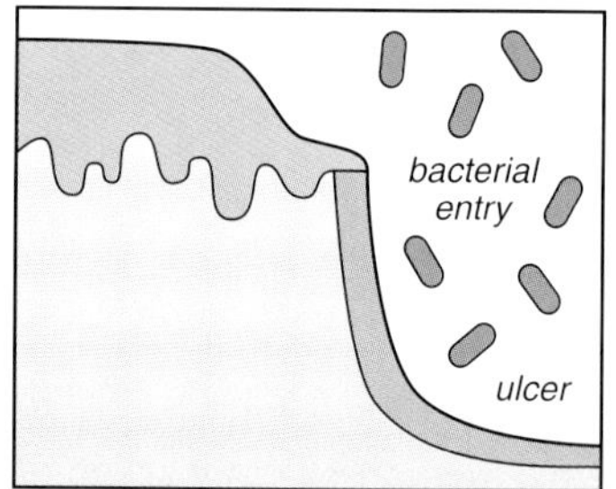

2: Summary of principles of wound healing as applied to horses

- Clean, fresh wounds are best treated to reduce the size of the deficit by reapposition of skin margins by sutures. Adhesive tabs and n-butyl cyanoacrylate adhesives or steel staples can be used in place of sutures where there is no (or little) tension on the wound margins. Moist wound healing principles employing collagen, hydrocolloids or hydrogels with an absorptive/protective pad are now accepted as being physiologically correct and encourage rapid healing. Dressings employing the same principles which are extremely adhesive even on haired areas can be used on the trunk and are becoming widely available.
- Bandaging aids healing; it promotes and maintains a moist environment, it may also control haemorrhage, oedema and excessive granulation tissue. It protects the wound from further trauma and contamination. Some areas are not amenable to bandaging, and badly applied bandages with excessive or inadequate tension are probably worse than none at all. Overtight bandages applied to the limbs can be particularly dangerous. Modern wound dressings mean that in many cases bandage changes can be made at intervals of up to 3–6 days, but each case needs to be managed individually.
- Often, horse leg wounds are severely traumatized and contaminated and they have the potential for extensive tissue necrosis. This necessitates degrees of compromise with some of the stages of healing; for example, bandaging to prevent further haemorrhage increases the risk of infection, reduces oxygenation and may seriously reduce dermal perfusion, etc. Consequently, all decisions made on the approach to a wound are a balance between good and bad effects on the healing process.
- Upper leg and body wounds can be massive, often with severe muscle damage/loss. They usually heal better by second intention than by primary union. Suturing cannot usually maintain closure where injury lies across muscle-plane movement. Where injury is parallel to movement then suturing with pressure relief sutures is possible and often helpful.
- Loose-skinned areas such as over the trunk and neck heal remarkably well by centripetal contraction and significant benefit can be gained by careful debridement and irrigation with normal saline only. Partial closure of such wounds may significantly reduce the time to repair.
- Wound breakdown due to contamination or suturing of old wounds often leads to slow second intention healing (with extensive chronic inflammation). This leads to the production of much fibrous tissue and scarring. Repeat surgery for cosmetic purposes should only be undertaken when all inflammation has settled and when/if the surgeon can be sure that matters will not be made worse by the surgery. Scars will inevitably contract with time and so an early decision on the ultimate cosmetic effects is unwarranted. If scarring and contraction have immediate secondary effects on adjacent structures (e.g. the eyelid, joints of the limb), early reparative surgery may be indicated.

Factors adversely affecting wound healing include the following:

- **Infection** Where tissue levels of bacteria are above 1×10^6 organisms, healing is inevitably delayed.[127] Some bacteria are liable to produce collagenases or other destructive enzymes and, in general, infected wounds are slower to heal than uninfected ones. Chronic infection with *Staphylococcus aureus* can result in a proliferative fibrogranulomatous mass of tumour-like tissue known as botryomycosis (see p. 101).
- **Movement** Movement at the site or in the attached tissues, e.g. the tendon in the palmar cannon area, results in marked disruptive forces within the wound and delays in wound closure due to a chronic inflammatory status. Lack of all movement is supportive of healing but in some cases can also be counterproductive to strong healing owing to the lack of arrangement of collagen along stress lines.
- **Foreign body and necrotic tissue** Foreign bodies embedded in the wound (sand or grit particles, wood or other plant matter, or metal/glass, etc.) or necrotic tissue (bone, tendon, skin, etc.) also cause delayed healing. Certain foreign bodies are more or less inert in tissue – organic materials tend to inhibit healing while metallic objects and glass tend to have less effect. Healing fails until the causative factor has been addressed.

- **Blood supply** Ischaemia, anaemia or a delay in capillary formation through tissue disruption or indirectly by thrombosis, oedema, contusion and overtight bandaging are common causes of failed healing. Even the limited-duration vasoconstriction caused by the adrenaline commonly included in local anaesthetic agents may have an adverse influence on healing. From a more general perspective, heavy blood loss and conditions associated with clotting disorders or serious anaemia are also capable of retarding healing significantly.
- **Oxygenation** Adequate oxygenation of tissue in the immediate vicinity of the lesion is important for normal healing. Anaerobic conditions in a wound can be conducive to the development of some of the most serious clostridial infections including *Clostridium tetani* (tetanus) and *Clostridium welchii* (gas gangrene).
- **pH of wound site** Changes in local acidity of the wound have a significant bearing on cell behaviour and ideally the pH should be slightly acid. Iatrogenic factors (including wound irrigation fluids and dressings) affecting the local (surface) pH can have a markedly deleterious effect on healing.
- **Local factors (dead-space/tension/body fluids)** Local factors such as tension on the skin (possibly through swelling or sutures or both) and excessive dead space result in retarded healing. The local temperature of the wound site can also influence the healing process. Cold may be a significant factor in the healing of wounds on extremities.
- **Cell transformation** Transformation of a normal, healing wound site to neoplastic (tumour) tissue is probably the preserve of the equine sarcoid. Wounds on the distal limb are particularly liable to develop fibroblastic sarcoid at the site (this may be highly suggestive of exuberant granulation tissue). Sarcoid transformations at wound sites on the head and body are more likely to be verrucose in nature and are slower growing. They are not usually ulcerative in character.[19] It is clear that there are regional differences in the character and rate of growth of sarcoids developing at the site of wounds.[128]
- **Systemic or nutritional disease** Debilitated and/or old horses heal much more slowly than healthy, young ones. Concurrent disease may have profound harmful effects on wound healing. For example, a horse with Cushing's syndrome due to a pituitary tumour may have excessive circulating corticosteroids and so even small wounds may fail to heal. Hypoalbuminaemia with serum albumin below 30 g/l will have a significant retarding effect on healing and will encourage chronic inflammation. Vitamin A and C deficiency can retard healing: topical dressing with these vitamins has been shown to improve healing rates. Zinc deficiency causes delay in healing and clinically significant loss of zinc can occur from exudative open wounds. Zinc is an important component of metalloproteinase enzymes which are responsible for some of the natural breakdown of the extracellular matrix during normal healing.
- **Iatrogenic factors** The clinician or owners may introduce many harmful factors, including excessive pressure by dressings, noxious chemicals and overstrength or inappropriate antiseptics, etc., which can damage or harm tissue repair mechanisms.

THE APPROACH TO A SKIN WOUND[129]

After any emergency treatment, such as arresting serious haemorrhage, the horse should, if possible and practical, be moved to a suitable environment for assessment and further treatment. It may be necessary at this point to protect the wound so as to avoid further contamination. All wounds should be routinely subjected to prompt and thorough examination to determine from the site, depth and direction which tissues and structures have been, or are likely to have been, involved. In assessing the likelihood of secondary complications, a knowledge of anatomy cannot be overemphasized. It is important to determine whether significant structures, e.g. joints, tendons, nerves or blood vessels, have been damaged, so that the risk of complications may be minimized. It is most unwise to assume all wounds will heal rapidly or at all. Some of the smallest, most innocuous-looking wounds are extremely serious and some dramatic and extensive ones heal remarkably quickly without complication. The owner should be warned at an early stage that wound management can be one of the most expensive veterinary procedures. Treatment can be prolonged and drugs and dressings rapidly become a significant investment. However, failure to provide the best immediate treatment is frequently even more expensive in the long term.

History

As much information as possible should be sought regarding how and when the injury occurred. In many cases this information is readily available, but in others it can only be deduced from the appearance of the wound and circumstantial evidence such as broken glass or blood or hair caught on barbed wire or fence posts. In some cases no specific cause can be found. If the injury is known to have resulted from a stake wound, the possibility of fragments of wood remaining buried deep in the tissues must be considered.

Up to 4 hours after the injury was sustained, a wound can be considered to be merely contaminated (the so called 'golden period'). Beyond that time, bacteria will have become established in the damaged tissues and the wound is then justifiably classified as infected.

The rate and efficiency of healing are largely dictated by the care with which the wound is managed initially.

Restraint and anaesthesia

Quiet, well-mannered horses may require no more than a foreleg raised or a twitch applied to allow the preliminary examination to be carried out. Newer sedative drugs (romifidine, detomidine, etc.) combined with narcotic analgesics (e.g. butorphanol) have made examination of even young, fractious horses much simpler and safer. As the extent of analgesia may be limited, wounds should not be handled extensively without regional or local anaesthesia. General anaesthesia may be required for large and/or complicated wounds or those in difficult sites.

As far as possible, infiltration of local anaesthetic agents should not be made into the wound itself. Every effort should be made to use remote regional blocks to avoid any additional tissue damage either directly from the agent (most local anaesthetic agents are highly acidic) or secondarily from the vasoconstrictive effects of added adrenaline.

Preparation and preliminary exploration

Prior to clipping of the hair, the wound should be packed with a water-soluble inert jelly or preferably a hydrocolloid or collagen wound dressing gel (a saline-soaked sterile gauze swab is not ideal but can be used as a protective plug). Open joints or tendon sheaths should be plugged for later attention. All gross contamination can then be removed. The area surrounding the wound should then be clipped and washed with a mild antiseptic soap/scrub solution. The wound edges are clipped or shaved to effectively expose the full extent of skin damage. The gel will prevent the clipped hairs and other contamination from entering the wound during this procedure. Suitable local anaesthetic can now be used to provide analgesia (see above).

Careful irrigation with warm normal saline (only) using a syringe (50 ml syringe with an 18G needle with firm applied pressure) or a Mills wound irrigator (**Fig. 17.1**) can then be performed. The pressure of irrigation should be restricted to between 0.5 and 1.0 bar (7–10 lb/in^2) to ensure that it is effective in washing away bacteria, particles and the protective gel while not driving these into the tissues still further or opening cleavage lines in the depths of the wound. The deeper parts of the wound can be exposed for exploration during this procedure. Although water can be very harmful to tissues, it can be used if saline is not available – the benefits of irrigation far exceed the risk of cell damage by water. However, this cannot be said for the application of chemicals to the fresh wound. This may have a significant harmful effect and is therefore unnecessarily harsh in fresh wounds. Under no circumstances should acidic solutions or other noxious chemicals be applied to a fresh wound. Time spent on this stage

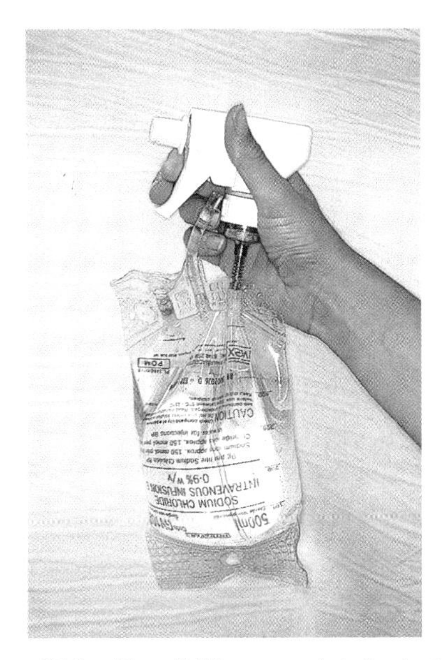

Figure 17.1 The 'Mills wound irrigator' which conveniently connects to standard fluid bags and delivers the correct pressures for wound irrigation. Horticultural sprayers can also be used.

far outweighs the risk of further contamination of the wound, although contamination can be minimized by covering the exposed tissues with a wound-healing hydrogel or hydrocolloid (or even a lubricant gel) or, less ideally, a clean swab or cotton wool soaked in saline.

All surgical equipment should be sterile and antiseptic technique should be followed. Using a sterile gloved finger, the wound should be explored thoroughly to establish the extent of complications and to ensure that no pockets of contamination or damage remain undisclosed. Careful simultaneous irrigation is often helpful. Preliminary exploration of the wound should be undertaken to establish:

(a) The extent of the wound and the degree of damage or loss of skin. This is of particular importance in wounds of the lower parts of the limbs because at these sites wounds are notorious for prolonged healing and any inhibiting factors must be eliminated as soon as possible. In the case of lacerated barbed-wire wounds the edges are often ragged and there may be several cuts in close proximity to one another. At this stage it may not be possible to decide exactly which parts are viable.

(b) The direction and depth of the wound (in relation to other anatomical structures) and the extent of complicating factors involved (joints, tendons, nerves, etc.). Ultrasonographic examination of a wound site is extremely useful and can quickly and easily identify damaged or inflamed tendons (and/or synovial structures).

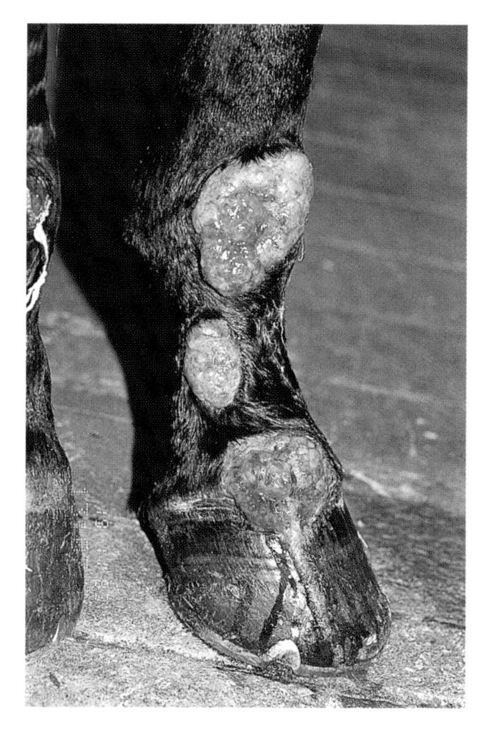

Figure 17.2 Multiple wounds of 2 weeks' duration on the distal limb with joint involvement of the distal interphalangeal joint (coffin joint). Synovial fluid issued freely from the wound as the horse moved. It was extremely painful.

Septic arthritis is one of the most serious complications which may follow accidental wounds and it is essential that involvement of a joint be recognized immediately (**Fig. 17.2**). The location and direction of the wound are important but the skin wound may not directly overlie a joint. During the incident the skin may have been stretched so that the damage may be remote from the site of the skin wound. The tibiotarsal (hock) and metacarpophalangeal (fetlock) joints, which have only limited protection, are particularly prone to penetration even with very small skin wounds. In severe lacerations the articular cartilage may be exposed and even damaged. In the majority of cases evidence of joint involvement is much less obvious. The elbow joint, for example, can be opened via a very small wound on the proximal lateral radius just below the radiohumoral joint. Clear, yellow, somewhat oily fluid exuding from the depth of the wound could be joint fluid, but it can be difficult to distinguish it clinically from drops of serum which exude from lacerated wounds. Probing with a scrubbed finger after thoroughly cleaning the wound is often helpful. A finger is preferable to a rigid probe for exploring wounds and is able to detect roughened bone surfaces, fragments of bone and foreign bodies. Small wounds may require enlargement to allow this examination, but it is probably worth it in many cases. Some wounds are not amenable to exploration in this way and require other techniques. Solar penetration of the middle third of the frog with a nail is dangerous because if the nail is withdrawn the fibrocartilage may close the tract, which may lead directly to the digital sheath, the navicular bone and/or its bursa or the distal interphalangeal joint. Radiographic (plain and contrast) studies, synoviocentesis and flushing from a proximal site towards the suspected problem area are possible ways of testing the integrity of a synovial structure, but in many cases the first sign of a problem is severe lameness some hours or even days after the event. Arthroscopic examinations are particularly helpful as the joint can be visualized directly and flushed via large portals.

Where any doubt exists about possible joint penetration, synoviocentesis, heavy parenteral antibiotic cover and a close daily examination for evidence of joint swelling, heat and increased lameness are essential. Repeated samples of joint fluid should be avoided – it is too easy to introduce infection. However, if there is evidence of joint involvement, the treatment may need to be adjusted significantly.

Tendon damage Damage to tendons is a common feature of wounds of the distal limbs. Extensor tendons are particularly prone to traumatic injury (see Fig. 17.3). Although disruption of the tendon initially results in knuckling over at the fetlock, the horse adapts and normal function is usually restored. It is unnecessary, therefore, to attempt surgical repair of this tendon. By contrast, wounds involving the flexor tendons in the cannon, fetlock or pastern regions are very serious. The skin wound often belies the severity of the underlying tendon damage. Close observation of the posture of the foot and fetlock when the horse is made to take full weight on the leg will help to identify both the structures involved and the severity of the injury.

- Severance of the superficial digital flexor produces slight lack of support to the fetlock.
- Severance of the deep digital flexor results in the toe lifting from the ground and is extremely serious. While palpation with a finger may help to confirm tendon damage, its full extent is often not apparent until an exploratory incision is made under general anaesthesia. Gross contamination and severe fibrillation of the severed ends necessitate extensive debridement and an inevitable gap in the tendon. This then has to be bridged with a prosthesis if the animal is to be salvaged.
- Severance of all the supportive structures of the foot results in a completely collapsed fetlock with an upturned toe and represents the most serious complication of these injuries.

Tendon sheaths Penetration of tendon sheaths can be life-threatening or can result in chronic lameness. Immediate flushing from a proximal site towards the injury or via the open wound with copious warm saline solution under pressure will improve the very poor prognosis somewhat. Sampling of synovial fluid may be helpful, but if the sheath is widely open this may be impossible. One of the most serious such injuries is laceration of the palmar pastern with a flint or metal in the ground. Opening of the digital sheath at this site seems to be particularly dangerous. These injuries all require hospital attention and emergency aggressive flushing and antibiosis. Even under the best conditions failure is still frequent.

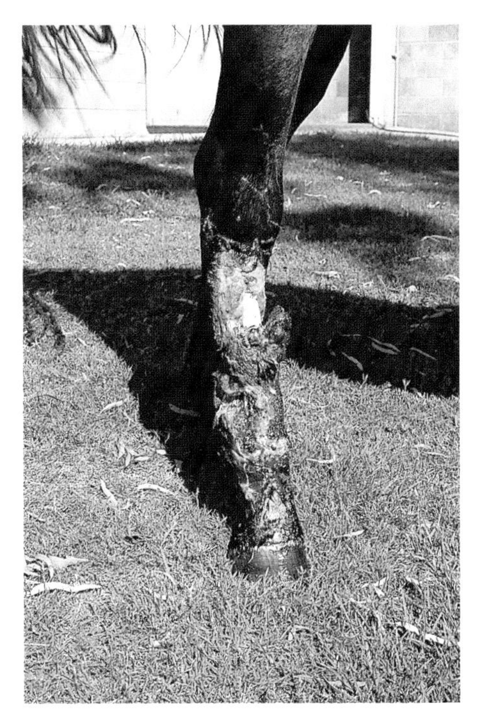

Figure 17.3 Extensive laceration of the distal limb involving several different complications. These include extensor tendon laceration, periosteal exposure, drying and damage, downward flap displacement of the skin (degloving injury), extensive bruising and tearing, blood vessel and nerve damage.

Periosteal damage Exposure, stripping, damage or drying of the periosteum (**Fig. 17.3**) may, with or without infection, lead to the development of a sequestrum. The outer one-third of the cortex derives its blood supply from the periosteum and this becomes necrotic, separating from the underlying healthy bone. The process takes several weeks or even months, by which time the bone is often obscured by unhealthy granulation tissue. The necrotic bone sequestrum is effectively a foreign body and may be walled off by granulation and fibrous tissues or it may gradually be sloughed. The sequestrum can often be clearly recognized radiographically provided the beam is angled appropriately. A note of the site of periosteal damage made at the time of the initial examination will enable the correct view to be taken. Once confirmed, the sequestrum can be surgically removed along with any unhealthy granulation tissue.

Blood vessel and nerve damage Damage to blood vessels (often with accompanying nerves) is of major importance in wounds of the lower limbs. Loss of blood supply is of course most important when there is limited or no collateral circulation (such as the distal limb). Spiral or extensive wounds may involve both the medial and lateral palmar (plantar) digital vessels. Comparison of the surface temperature below the injury, particularly of the foot, with that of the other limbs will help to assess the extent of vascular impairment. Angiography or laser Doppler ultrasonography may establish the viability of blood supply. Although surgical re-anastomosis of major arteries of the limb is an attractive prospect, most such wounds are badly contaminated or neglected and failures are common.

WOUND LAVAGE

Following careful exploration, all wounds must be thoroughly cleaned and foreign bodies and any obviously dead or bloodless tissue must be removed. This frequently involves excision of contaminated or damaged tissues using a scalpel and dissecting forceps. Extensive debridement of this nature is often best performed under general anaesthesia. It is, however, very important to preserve as much skin as possible; even if the skin is badly damaged and plainly compromised it should be retained (even if only as temporary biological cover for the defect). The advantage gained from optimum conditions for surgery far outweighs the initial additional cost and effort.

Swabs are not ideal for wiping the surface of fresh or healing wounds; they merely succeed in redistributing bacteria and driving foreign particles into the tissue. Lavage is superior to swabbing techniques. Lavage pressure is as important as the use of a suitable physiological fluid such as saline or Ringer's lactate (Hartmann's solution). Pressures between 0.5 and 1.0 bar (7–10 lb/in^2) are ideal and are conveniently achieved by the commercially available 'Mills Wound Lavage System' (see Fig. 17.1). This apparatus is a hand-held spray pump which is simply connected into a fluid administration bag, thereby avoiding complications from the use of tap water or crude saline solutions, needles and syringes. A similar pressure can be obtained using a 35/50 ml syringe with an 18G needle attached.

Lavage fluids

Water Effective and available in large volumes. However, it does cause significant (harmful) cell swelling if used for long periods. Cell bursting can take place within seconds of application and release of cell breakdown products may then seriously influence subsequent healing.

Saline/balanced electrolyte solutions These are physiologically sound and, if used immediately after water, may overcome some of the criticism above. Warming the solution minimizes reflex vasoconstriction. An approximate physiological saline can be made using a flat teaspoonful of salt (approximately 5 g) in 450–500 ml of warm, boiled water.

Povidone-iodine Commonly supplied as a 10% solution or scrub soap. The active ingredient is free iodine. Povidone-iodine can be detrimental to healing; most authors recommend a 0.1–0.5% solution for lavage purposes and this is conveniently made by adding 1–2 ml of the concentrate to 10 l of water. The solution should be virtually colourless. Dilute (0.1–0.5%) solutions have greater bactericidal activity than the full-strength product owing to release of bound iodine. Serum can reduce the antibacterial activity (by binding free iodine). Povidone-iodine has only a short-lived residual effect and so 4- to 6-hourly repetitions may be necessary.

Chlorhexidine Lavage with a concentration of 0.05% produces fewer adverse effects on the tissues and fewer infections when compared to 0.1–0.5% povidone-iodine. A suitable solution can be made by adding 2 ml of the concentrate to a 10-litre bucket of water. It also has a useful residual antibacterial activity. However, it also causes the cells to shrink and cell multiplication is strongly inhibited for several hours.

Note: 0.5% solutions of both povidone-iodine and chlorhexidine cause joint pain, severe lameness, limb oedema, increased synovial fluid protein levels and a moderate-to-severe neutrophilic synovitis if used for lavage or irrigation of closed joints. They are therefore contraindicated for this purpose or where a wound involves an open joint.

Hydrogen peroxide This is generally considered unsuitable as lavage fluid. It causes impressive frothing but it is tissue toxic! Its use should be limited to circumstances when anaerobic conditions are likely (e.g. irrigation of a deep wound which might be infected with *Clostridium tetani*). It does have a significant (and sometimes helpful) debriding effect. Solutions of less than 5 volumes concentration have limited tissue toxicity and stronger solutions should not be used on tissues at all.

Acetic acid/malic acid These solutions are markedly tissue toxic and should never be applied to fresh wounds. They do, however, have useful activity against *Pseudomonas* spp. and also have a strong debriding effect. The circumstances for their use are therefore very limited in the horse.

Soluble antibiotics (e.g. **penicillin, ampicillin, neomycin, kanamycin and gentamicin**) These may be beneficial when added to lavage solutions. Direct application of powdered antibiotics is probably not helpful overall, and they often have acidic properties. Bovine intramammary preparations are not suitable for wounds at all and should be reserved for their intended purpose.

DEBRIDEMENT OF THE WOUND

Grossly contaminated areas should be meticulously and systematically cleaned by sharp debridement. A scalpel rather than blunt instruments such as scissors should be used in order to minimize trauma and immediate and subsequent tissue loss. The ideal objective is to convert an accidental, contaminated wound to a surgical one.

With the exception of the skin, all damaged or compromised tissue and contamination should be removed. The area should be repeatedly lavaged with normal saline. A thorough approach should then be made to any complicating factors. Open joints or tendon sheaths are particularly dangerous and should be attended to before closure of the wound. Soluble antibiotic may be applied to the wound if infection is thought to be significant. Other wound sprays, powders and ointments should be used with caution. Dressings using moist wound-healing principles with hydrogels/hydrocolloids or collagen based, nonadherent, absorptive pads should be applied to the wound after appropriate surgical procedures (sutures, staples, tissue repair, drain insertion, etc.) have been completed. Suitable antibiotics and tetanus prophylaxis may be administered parenterally.

Every effort must be taken to preserve as much skin as possible. Even damaged skin which is not viable may provide a helpful if temporary biological cover for a wound. In particular, skin which still has a viable blood supply should be managed with great care and must be preserved almost at any cost. This particularly applies to degloving injuries (see Fig. 17.3).

In some cases it may be necessary to delay debridement for several days until it is possible to differentiate between viable and devitalized tissue.

Whether lacerated wounds should be sutured is a topic of much debate. There may be strong pressure from owners to suture wounds. Suturing should only be carried out if it is certain that it will help rather than hinder healing. Incised wounds frequently enable primary union to be achieved by suturing. It must always be performed carefully and precisely, paying attention to meticulous cleaning of the wound to avoid trapping infection and excessive tension on the wound margins or the sutures themselves. No wound should be completely closed unless the deeper tissues are effectively sterile. Gross contamination, infection, significant skin loss or marked swelling are factors which are likely to result in wound dehiscence. Sutures tear out, tissues slough, or the closed wound provides an ideal environment for bacterial multiplication. As a result, the healing time is prolonged and in some cases the animal's life may be endangered owing to spread of infection to adjacent structures. However, if the margins of the wound can be approximated, it might serve to reduce the overall size of a wound which has to heal by second intention. This effectively reduces the extent of granulation tissue and the distance over which keratinocytes have to migrate to close the wound. It also serves to provide a biological cover for the wound site. Scarring may also be reduced.

Inability to create a completely sterile wound by debridement and lavage can be partially compensated by adequate drainage through *partial* suturing, the use of supported, tension sutures, counterincisions where necessary and the use of drains (Penrose, vacuum or other) (**Fig. 17.4**).

Drains are inserted with the ends exiting remotely from the wound and should lie deep within the wound so as to provide an effective means of reducing the build-up of tissue fluids. A drain should not be placed directly under the skin. The stab incision through which the drain exits should be of sufficient size to allow drainage to occur around it. Daily cleansing of the drain and protection by bandaging will

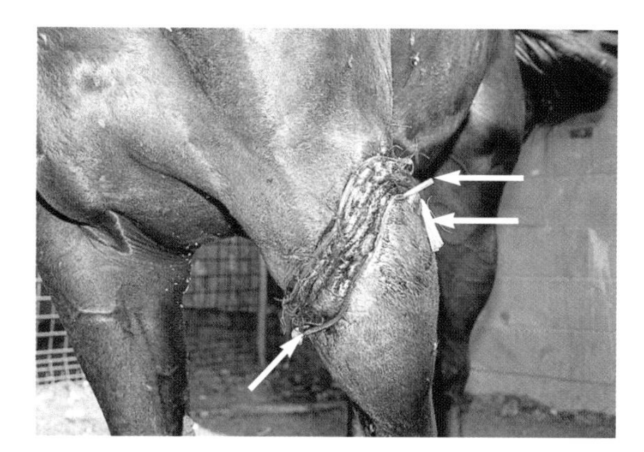

Figure 17.4 An extensive wound repaired with the help of supported quill and mattress sutures and a Penrose drain (arrows). The wound healed without significant problems.

minimize the risk of retrograde infection, which is time related. The drain should be removed as soon as it has ceased to function. The drain itself can act as a foreign body and daily drainage of less than 50 ml/day may be purely drain induced.

EXUBERANT GRANULATION TISSUE

Wounds involving the lower parts of the limbs present the greatest problems. The nature of the wound may make suturing impossible or unwise. Provided there is no specific reason for healing failure, the wound should fill with healthy granulation tissue. Possibly because of the absence of significant subcutaneous connective tissue, significant contraction does not occur on the limbs and skin deficits have to be resolved by centripetal epithelialization. This is a relatively slow process – under optimum conditions it proceeds at only around 0.5 mm/day. Granulation tissue can become exuberant long before significant epithelialization has taken place (**Fig. 17.2**).

In addition to absence of wound contraction, bacterial infection and movement at the site play important roles in the development of exuberant granulation tissue ('proud flesh'; see p. 217). Control of infection, local corticosteroid therapy and the application of a pressure bandage, together with movement restriction (by rigid limb casting and/or by confining the horse to a loosebox), help to slow down the rate of production of granulation tissue. Despite these measures it often becomes exuberant and, if allowed to proliferate unrestricted, will come to overlie the boundary of the wound, preventing ingrowth of epithelium. Furthermore, it sometimes results in further epithelial loss from pressure and bacterial necrosis and such a wound may appear to expand rather than contract.

In large wounds, the excess granulation tissue may require cutting back to skin level on a number of occasions before epithelium completely covers the wound.[130] As this tissue has no significant sensory nerves, this can usually be done without recourse to anaesthesia. The resulting haemorrhage can be very severe and can usually be controlled by pressure bandaging. This is much better practice than using caustics, such as copper sulphate, nitric acid or malic/salycilic acids. These are not physiologically sound and are nonselective in their action – they will destroy the delicate epithelium at the periphery of the wound just as readily as the granulation tissue.

Large masses of exuberant granulation tissue are best excised under general anaesthesia. It should be removed to 0.5 cm below skin level. Because the epithelium at the periphery of the wound in these chronic cases is usually keratinized and totally quiescent (see Fig. 17.5), a 2 mm wide strip should be

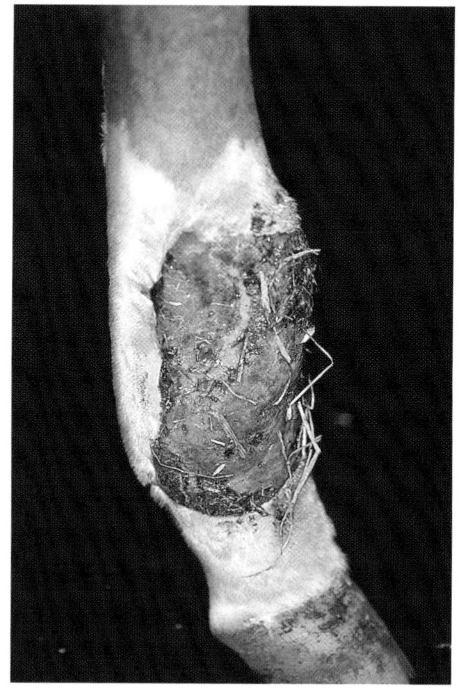

Figure 17.5 A long-standing, nonhealing wound with unhealthy, infected exuberant granulation tissue. Notice the general thickening of the limb in the area of the wound and the hypertrophic margin to the wound. There is a singular lack of contraction.

removed to stimulate resumption of mitotic division. Within 7–10 days, fresh granulation tissue will usually have developed up to skin level. Early skin grafting should always be considered as this will usually result in a dramatic reduction in closure time and an earlier return to normal use with reduced scarring.

CLOSURE OF WOUNDS

The goal of suture repair is to achieve first intention healing with both functional and cosmetic restoration.[131] With wounds having significant crushing injury, primary closure with an aggressive approach may give poor results. Loss of local blood supply and contamination are further reasons to delay suturing. Primary closure of limb wounds is unlikely to be successful if favourable criteria cannot be met (**Fig. 17.3**).

Dead space and drains

Where wound closure is likely to produce dead space, this should be countered by vertical sutures. Accumulation of fluid and dead space will delay healing as it acts as a medium for bacterial multiplication. Drains should be used if fluid is likely to accumulate and create dead space. Vacuum drains are preferred to Penrose drains but are more difficult to manage (**Fig. 17.4**). Where vacuum drains are used, they must be placed under at least two closing rows of sutures and the leg bandaged. Any break in the vacuum renders them valueless. They should be removed as soon as bleeding and/or exudation has ceased. Other tubing drains (such as fenestrated semirigid plastic tubes) can also be used to flush pocketed wounds and siphon off fluid. They must also be regarded as potentially dangerous as they can also introduce or harbour infections if left *in situ* for long periods.

Where bandaging is not possible, gentle pressure can be maintained over a potential or actual dead space by means of a 'stent' or tie-over bandage. Wounds of lower limbs are usually best managed by compression bandaging and avoiding sutures as far as possible. However, care should be exercised to avoid compromise of blood supply both to the area and to regions distal to the injury. Staples, adhesive suture tabs and n-butyl cyanoacrylate adhesives are potentially very useful. They have no significant inhibitory effects on healing but are less able to sustain high tensile forces across the wound. Swelling of the limb inside firm or tight bandages results in rapid compromise of the most superficial capillaries and those vessels which have been damaged in the injury. These may be occluded completely with resultant ischaemic necrosis (see Fig. 17.10).

Tension relief and suturing

Relief of tension on the primary skin sutures is essential, particularly if the skin has already contracted away from the margins of the wound. Excessive tension delays healing and often results in skin necrosis and dehiscence. Where this is likely to occur, primary closure is avoided as it will lead to failure in any event. Overtension on the primary row of sutures usually results in wound dehiscence around days 4 and 5.

Tension can be relieved in several ways.

- **Undermining** Sound tissue away from the wound edge is undermined with scissors to open up subcutaneous tissue, thereby allowing skin to slide toward the wound edge. Up to 4 cm can often be safely undermined even in such areas as the metacarpus and metatarsus.
- **Relief incision** Where tension is excessive after suture placement, relief incisions parallel to the wound may be used. Care must be taken that these are not placed too close to the original wound and that they are as small as is compatible with the relief of tension. Some relief incisions may require suturing after undermining adjacent subcutaneous tissues. Others can be treated as open wounds and left to heal by secondary intention.
- **Tension sutures** The placement of single interrupted, or vertical or horizontal mattress, or far-and-near tension sutures some 2–4 cm from the skin edge helps to draw the wound edges together to assist closure of the primary suture row (**Fig. 17.4**). Horizontal mattress sutures tend to be the least favourable as they have the potential to interfere with circulation to the wound area, while vertical mattress sutures provide the best compromise between tension and circulatory obstruction and may be regarded as a combination of two interrupted sutures laid over each other.

  Far-and-near sutures provide the greatest tension component and have been found to be ultimately stronger than other types of tension sutures.
- **Quilled or support sutures** Where tension is marked and some closure is essential, quilled sutures can be used to provide greater tension relief. Tubing or gauze may be placed on either

side of the wound with sutures passing over or through the tubing to spread the area of pressure (**Fig. 17.4**).

Most limb wounds are best closed with single interrupted patterns because loss of some sutures does not immediately endanger the whole wound as would occur if continuous sutures were used. Skin staples and adhesive tabs reinforced with *n*-butyl cyanoacrylate adhesives can be used but they are often not satisfactory in control of tension when used on limb wounds and in any case have less retention power to cope with tissue swelling.

Following suturing of a wound it should be covered with a collagen, hydrogel or hydrocolloid nonadhesive dressing. Suitable supportive bandaging may then be applied over this to minimize infection, movement and/or trauma.

Wounds should remain bandaged until wound stability is established. Sudden oedema due to early bandage removal can cause wound dehiscence. Tension applied to bandages must be sufficient to prevent slippage without compromising the superficial or deep circulation. Bandaging techniques require that all protruding bony prominences are well padded to prevent pressure necrosis. In particular the accessory carpal, the point of the hock and the region above the hock over the common calcanean tendon should as far as possible not be covered with any pressure bandage at all. It may be worth considering adhesive dressings, which avoid the need for any heavy dressings in these areas.

Dressing changes should be performed at reasonable intervals but overfrequent attention is probably unnecessary in most cases and positively harmful in some others. Excessive exudate or infection necessitate more frequent dressing changes than in a wound without these complications. In general bandages should be changed as soon as they appear to be 'wet'. Failure to change them frequently enough in severe contused wounds leads to skin maceration and suture line necrosis. If the area remains dry, then most dressings can remain unchanged initially for 4–5 days. Every case needs to be assessed individually with appropriate measures taken to ensure the continued health of the wound, so rigid rules cannot be applied to any type of wound.

Where rigid limb casts are used, particular care must be taken to ensure adequate protection of the coronet, all bony prominences, and all other likely pressure areas. The risks are minimized if the horse's leg is placed in either slight flexion or slight extension.

Horses with bandaged limbs should be confined to a stable or very small yard to allow limited exercise. All efforts must be made to prevent both bandage slippage and overcompression. The areas most at risk from movement of the bandage and consequent trauma are the front of the fetlock and pastern, the calcanean region and over bony prominences.

TRAUMATIC SKIN INJURIES

Clinical signs

Bruising shows as swelling and red/purple-brown discoloration of white skin. Pigmented skin, if shaved, has a shining appearance due to the turgidity of surface layers caused by extravasation of either blood or tissue fluid.

Haematoma is initially a firm subcutaneous swelling. As the blood clots and the clot retracts, the swelling becomes more fluid/fluctuant. Fibrin can be felt to 'crackle' if the haematoma is deeply palpated and squeezed gently. There is seldom marked increase in local skin temperature, and apart from the initial insult a haematoma is not often painful on palpation.

Laceration and other damage to the skin is usually obvious, but some very small injuries have potential to be extremely serious and no wound should be treated lightly.

Cellulitis is a painful oedematous swelling of the subcutaneous and connective tissues. The area becomes hot and obviously inflamed. Serum exudate may be present, often with secondary scalding dermatitis and lymphangitis. The skin may rarely 'pit on pressure' but then quickly regains its previous outline.

Differential diagnosis

- Urticaria – pressure pits remain longer and it is usually not painful or inflamed.
- Hot abscess – more painful, localized swelling.
- Cold abscess – does not pit on pressure. Aspiration is helpful.
- Snake, spider or insect bite.

Diagnostic confirmation

- Visual appearance of skin colour and its texture are characteristic.
- Ultrasonographic examination.
- Needle aspiration.

Treatment

All skin injuries should be very carefully assessed for complicating factors which might adversely influence the healing process. These are listed on p. 207.

Bruising can be reduced by using cold compresses, cold hosing or ice packs. Restriction of inflammatory response in this way limits the extent of secondary damage (to nerves or muscles, etc.) or the long-term complications and scarring.

Generally, a fresh haematoma should be left to clot. Drainage is probably not advisable as there is a risk of introducing infection, but in some cases it is necessary for cosmetic as well as medical reasons. Drainage should be by wide incision to ensure that all the clotted blood can be removed. Antibiotic therapy is important.

Cellulitis is particularly difficult to treat effectively (especially if on the limbs) and requires the use of hot and cold compresses and intensive antibiotic therapy with nonsteroidal anti-inflammatory medications to ease pain and encourage some movement. Some cases progress to chronic lymphangitis.

EXUBERANT GRANULATION TISSUE (proud flesh)

Profile

Overgrowth of normal granulation tissue which occurs particularly (but not exclusively) on lower limbs. Fresh cases may be crusted but are usually pink and moist and bleed easily if abraded. Chronic tissue is very firm, often dark red in colour and bleeds less easily than fresh granulation tissue.

Clinical signs

Overgrowth of normal granulation tissue above skin edges and failure of tissue to epithelialize (**Fig. 17.5**). Infection of the surface is common, with purulent exudate which may cause scalding below the wound site. The area is seldom painful but occasional horses will bite or chew at the site (particularly if there are complicating factors such as foreign bodies and *Habronema musca* larvae) (see Fig. 10.33). Exuberant granulation may reach enormous proportions. In some cases an explanation can be found (see above for factors influencing wound healing (**Fig. 17.2**).

Some wounds, however, fail to produce healthy granulation tissue and these usually show a hypertrophic fibrous scarring margin with a poorly vascularized and poor-quality granulation tissue (**Fig. 17.5**). These too will fail to epithelialize until a suitable basis is created. Indolent wounds are most often encountered on the dorsum or plantar regions of the hock (**Fig. 17.6**). Here the wound fails to produce any significant granulation tissue and is most often covered by a flaking thin layer of fibrin and purulent exudate. There is usually no evidence of epithelialization at all or it is very poor and has a hypertrophic appearance giving the margin of the wound a piled-up appearance.

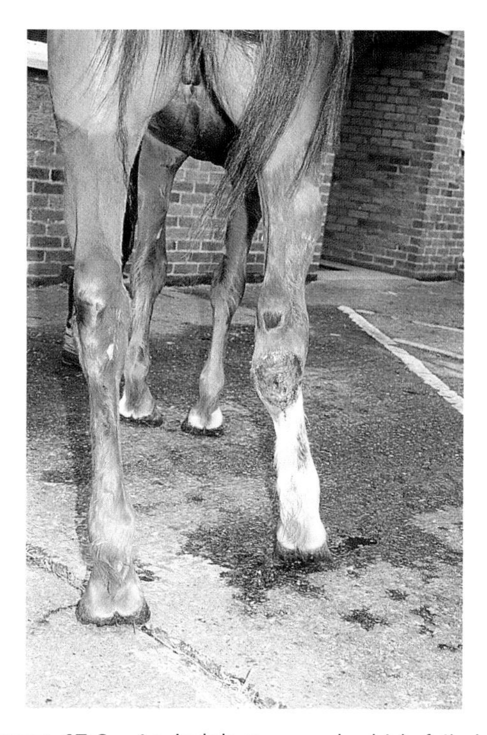

Figure 17.6 An indolent wound which failed to show any significant granulation tissue or any epithelialization for several months following an innocuous-looking cut.

Differential diagnosis

- Fibroblastic and malevolent sarcoid
- Botryomycosis (fibrogranuloma)
- Squamous cell carcinoma
- Foreign body
- Habronemiasis
- Pythiosis

Diagnostic confirmation

- Clinical appearance is characteristic.
- Biopsy of several sites should be taken to ensure

differentiation from fibroblastic sarcoids, botryomycosis and other proliferative masses arising secondarily to parasitic infestations in particular.
- Radiographic, ultrasonographic and vascular perfusion studies with laser flow Doppler may be performed to establish possible aetiological factors.

Treatment
Management of exuberant granulation tissue *must* always be preceded by a full investigation of the possible causes: without addressing the underlying problem, treatment is likely to fail. Under no circumstances should caustic materials (including copper sulphate, sulphuric acid, nitric acid, mercuric chloride, etc.) be applied to the tissues. While the initial effects may appear to be beneficial in reducing the bulk of the tissue, the long-term consequences are very harmful.

Medical management of exuberant granulation tissue should be directed towards reducing the extent of chronic inflammation. Thus, application of corticosteroid creams and nonsteroidal anti-inflammatory drugs is logical. However, they will also retard epithelialization and so may ultimately be of less value. They are indicated in the early management of granulation tissue prior to grafting but should not be applied for at least 6–7 days prior to grafting.

Surgical trimming of the exuberant tissue and careful management to produce a healthy granulating bed of well-vascularized tissue level with the epithelial margin should be followed as soon as practicable by suitable grafting techniques. The best granulation tissue quality is obtained by using a full moist wound-healing technique with application of hydrogels and hydrocolloids or collagen-based wound dressings. The best cosmetic effects are obtained with the use of split skin thickness grafts over the whole wound surface (with meshing techniques to enhance adhesion and graft take and minimize the donor site deficit), but good effects can also be obtained by the simpler pinch, punch or tunnel grafting methods which may not require general anaesthesia and sophisticated skin harvesting apparatus.

BURN/THERMAL/SCALD INJURIES

Profile
Although horses are seldom burned except in stable fires where escape is not possible, extensive body burns are encountered and life-threatening burns are common in stable fires. Burns are classified in terms of the depth of the burn and the extent of skin affected. The depth of burns is usually classified in three degrees.

- **First-degree burns:** erythema, pain and localized, transient oedema.
- **Second-degree burns:** vesicle formation, necrosis and sloughing of the epidermis with exposure of deeper dermal tissues.
- **Third-degree burns:** destruction of cells and blood vessels in the skin and hair follicles. Loss of cutaneous sensation. Sloughing and separation of all layers of the skin.

As the skin of horses has a much reduced tendency to blister (in comparison to the human), this classification is somewhat artificial. In horses first- and second-degree burns are probably best grouped together as partial-thickness burns and the third-degree burns as full-thickness burns.

The extent of the burn can also be described in terms of the percentage of total body surface which has been involved. Burns over greater than 10–15% of the body surface carry a particularly poor prognosis.

Accidental or deliberate application of heat to the skin causes burns. The severity of clinical signs varies with the length of contact time and the temperature. Hot branding and ‘pin’ and ‘line firing’ are the commonest iatrogenic causes of this type of burn.

Freeze burns are used to produce identification freeze brands which are visible in grey or cream horses (an identifiable scar is produced). Lesser skin injury is used in horses with brown or chestnut coats and here the ‘burn’ induces a change in melanocytes without scarring. Surprisingly, frost bite is particularly unusual in horses even under very adverse cold conditions.

Clinical signs
The initial injury almost always results in skin blistering and a progressive vasculitis, bruising, oedema and exudation. The latter can be very severe even from limited areas of skin damage. Clinically significant protein loss is common. Superficial blistering with hair loss (singeing) is the mildest consequence. More serious burns cause loss of hair and sloughing of the superficial layers of the dermis (or deeper in case of more severe burns) occurs, leaving large skin deficits (**Fig. 17.7**). Scalding injury may initially show various degrees of blistering without hair loss. The full

extent of a burn (however it is caused) is not always easy to establish at the first examination. Although a great deal of heat has to be applied to cause damage, once it is present, the heat dissipates slowly and so the extent of damage can be much greater than is first suspected. Progressive loss of hair, vasculitis, bruising and oedema of the area precede exudation (see **Fig. 17.7**). Death of the epidermis and dermis leads to drying of the skin and/or skin sloughing or the formation of an eschar (an extensive dry, leathery plaque of necrotic skin).

Sloughing of the skin leaves a raw, bleeding, ulcerated area with extensive exudation of plasma. Pathologically significant (and detectable) protein loss can occur with even minor burn injuries. Full-depth burns heal very slowly with extensive scarring and local tissue distortions.

Second- and third-degree burns covering over 10–15% of the body surface are almost impossible to manage. Burns to the limbs (as occurs in grass fires) are also very difficult and commonly fail to heal acceptably within a reasonable time.

A potentially dangerous skin burn can arise in foals which are recumbent on electrically heated pads. Foals in intensive care often have complications of compromised blood pressure and the skin in contact with the pad can easily be burned even if the pad is thermostatically controlled. The true extent of the damage can take days or even weeks to develop (or become apparent).

Iatrogenic burns such as 'pin' and 'line' firing (**Fig. 17.8**) and hot branding follow a predictable course with initial acute inflammation accompanied by pain and gradual healing with scar formation. The 'firing' of horses for musculoskeletal disease has disputed therapeutic benefits but the chronological course of the cutaneous repair mechanism is predictable. The scar is permanent but its ultimate extent often belies the extent of the initial insult as contraction of the wound site makes the scar smaller than might be expected.

Differential diagnosis

- Chemical burns (from overstrength therapeutics or errors of application)
- Iatrogenic spirit or antiseptic contact (especially in anaesthetized horses and those with compromised blood pressure)

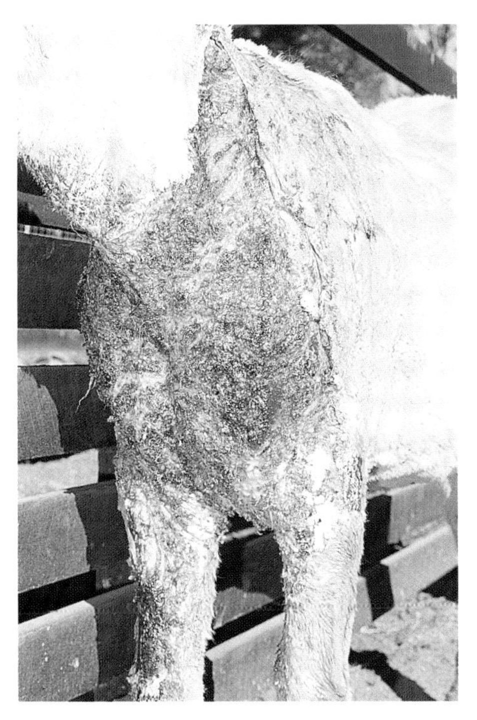

Figure 17.7 Thermal burn showing extensive blistering and sloughing of the skin. Plasma loss can be very significant and such wounds can take a long time to resolve. Skin grafting is often needed.

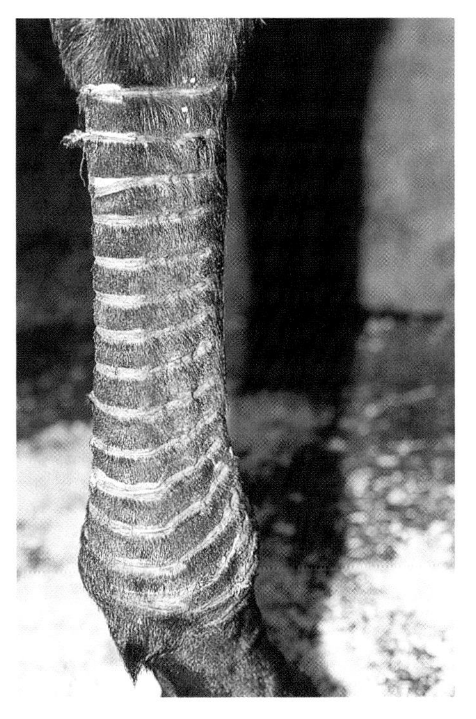

Figure 17.8 Iatrogenic thermal burns caused by a line firing iron used in an attempt to treat a sprained tendon. The eventual scars were insignificant.

- Decubitus (pressure) sores (recumbent horses)
- Pemphigus vulgaris (bullous pemphigoid)
- Generalized dermatophilosis (*Dermatophilus congolensis*)
- Arsenic or mercury poisoning/caustic effects

Diagnostic confirmation

- History of burn or scalding contact is usually available.

Treatment

Emergency measures should be taken to save the life first and to relieve pain. Immediate cold water lavage for 20–30 minutes after the burn helps to reduce the extent of scarring and damage. This has a marked effect on the future healing and scarring. Wrapping or covering the burnt area in domestic cling-film is helpful in reducing the immediate extent of plasma/serum loss and controlling shock. Immediate fluid therapy and plasma should be given if indicated. Protection of the burn site can also be provided by silver sulphadiazine cream. Do not attempt to wipe the site with gauze swabs, etc. Do not apply grease-based emollient creams or lotions as they retain heat and may exacerbate the problem. Partial-thickness burns usually heel well, but deeper burns require intensive therapy to debride all dead tissue and encourage healing. Sustained nonsteroidal anti-inflammatory drugs such as phenylbutazone and antibiotics may be required. Self-trauma can be severe and so cross-ties and cradles may be needed.

Scarring is often extensive and the wounds may require cosmetic surgery to speed closure and limit the physical problems associated with prolonged healing.

PRESSURE NECROSIS, ROPE/WIRE BURNS

Profile

Rope burns and pressure necrosis are common consequences of tethering or other method of restraint. Pressure necrosis (decubitus ulcers) results from prolonged recumbency or from destruction of the skin blood supply from applied pressure (bandages, plaster casts and other over-restrictive equipment.

Clinical signs

Rope burns are commonly encountered on the distal limb and initially cause hair loss and exudation. The extent of skin damage is variable with the type of rope, diameter and extent of rub/contact as well as the pressure applied to it. Recurrent injury tends to induce chronic thickening and extensive scar formation with extensive often movement-limiting scarring.

Pressure sores (decubitus ulcers) arise from interference to blood supply and subsequent necrosis of the overlying skin during prolonged recumbency. Some decubitus/pressure wounds are slow to appear. They may show an area of pain, heat and swelling some days or weeks before the skin is obviously identifiable as dead.

Bandaging injuries are common on the distal limb and vary widely in extent from mild surface epidermal damage and erythema to extensive necrosis involving the underlying structures (**Fig. 17.9**). Commonly the dead overlying skin forms an eschar (sitfast) of dry, leathery, coagulated skin (**Fig. 17.10**). In some cases the underlying tissue is severely compromised and may serve to delay healing still further. The secondary consequences of this type of injury are often even more serious than the prolonged healing and extensive scarring which are characteristic of the condition. Healing by granulation and eventual epithelialization is particularly slow. Scarring in either case can be severe and may be limiting to function.

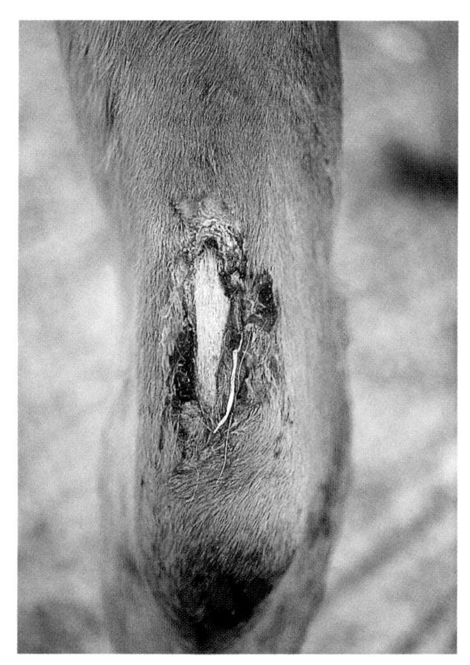

Figure 17.9 Dermal ischaemia caused by bandaging of this difficult site. The exposed fibres of the Achilles tendon were necrotic and the wound only healed after a prolonged nursing period during which no further bandages were used.

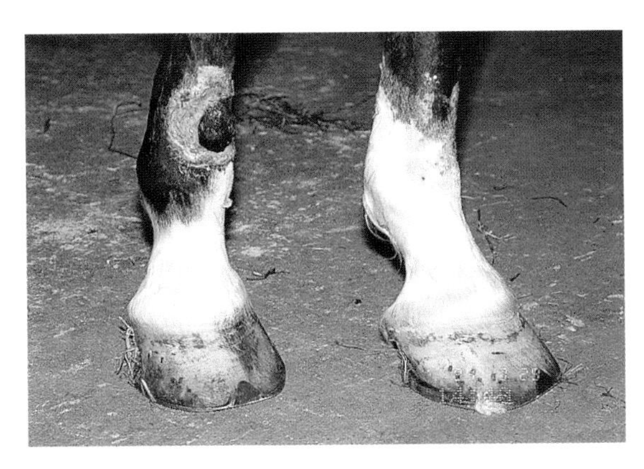

Figure 17.10 Cutaneous ischaemia caused by overtight bandages applied for an unrelated problem resulted in the formation of an eschar. The black necrotic area of dried leathery skin can be seen on the wound.

Differential diagnosis

- Dermatophilosis
- Greasy heel syndrome
- Mercurial blisters
- Pemphigus foliaceus
- Vasculitis
- Thrombosis (particularly if arterial)/thrombophlebitis
- Pastern and cannon leukocytoclastic vasculitis
- Chemical burns

Diagnostic confirmation

- Clinical examination and history are almost always clear.
- Overtight bandages are commonly involved in limb pressure necrosis wounds.

Treatment

Restoration of blood supply by hot and cold compresses and local application of soothing emollient creams is required. Normal wound management procedures should be followed to encourage rapid healing, but such wounds are often very refractory to healing and become a chronic problem. Surgical debridement and grafting may speed the repair and limit the scarring.

SCAR

Profile

Scarring is the inevitable result of full skin thickness injury. The character of the scar can vary widely. Scarring is minimal in wounds which heal by primary intention (e.g. surgical wounds), but prolonged healing results in larger scars. Hypertrophic or cheloid scars are the result of abnormal cell behaviour in the healing process.

Clinical signs

Scarring is minimal in surgical wounds which heal by first intention – the site of a Mackay–Marks laryngeal prosthesis or a digital neurectomy, for example, may be impossible to feel and may be visible only with difficulty in the clipped/shaved skin; **Fig. 17.11**). Some injuries which heal by secondary intention may also leave a very small scar and may be difficult to identify, e.g. the site of a lateral ventriculectomy (Hobday) incision. The latter is usually the case where wound contraction is most effective, i.e. on the body and head/neck regions. Scarring on the limbs associated with wounds which heal by secondary intention in particular is often severe and reflects the early transition of the wound to a state of chronic inflammation. Prolonged healing on the distal limb is frequently associated with exuberant granulation tissue (see Figs 17.2 and 17.5) or an indolent nongranulating, nonhealing wound (see Fig. 17.6).

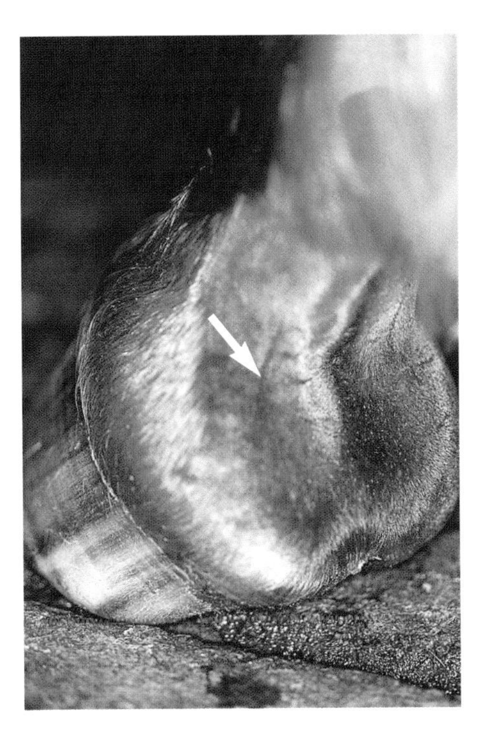

Figure 17.11 A surgical scar at a palmar digital neurectomy site showing minimal scar formation (arrow) typical of first-intention healing. Such scars are often very difficult to detect.

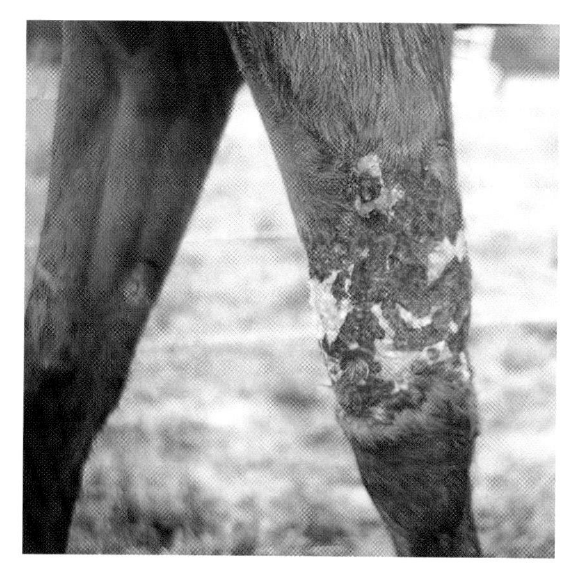

Figure 17.12 Dense fibrotic scarring typical of a slow healing wound.

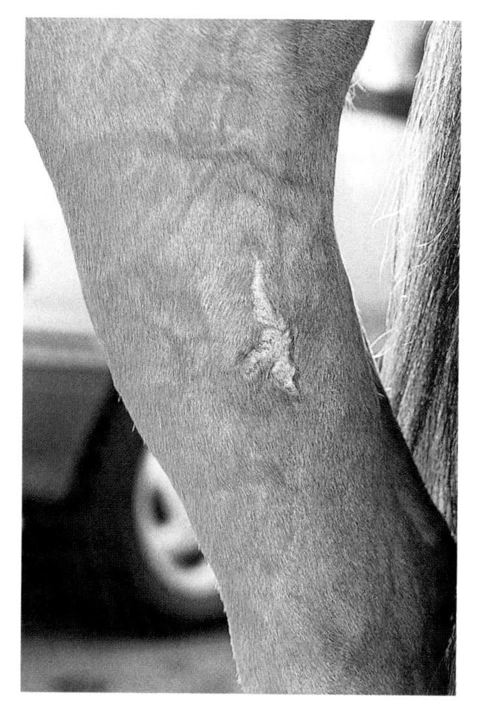

Figure 17.13 Hypertrophic scar developing at the site of a small surgical wound some 12 months previously which appeared at first to heal normally.

Most scars show loss of hair (absence of hair follicles) and presence of modified skin. The area is fibrosed and dense with limited elasticity and often with an altered hair growth pattern (**Fig. 17.12**).

Some scars induce leukoderma and/or leukotrichia (e.g. saddle marks and girth marks) (see Fig. 16.3). Freeze branding causes alteration in hair follicle structure and loss of melanocytes without significant scar, while hot branding or repeated freeze brands cause hair loss and scarring. Normal scar tissue contracts markedly over years.

Hypertrophic scarring is an uncommon potential problem of wound healing in the horse. Here the ultimate size and depth of the scar are inappropriate to the original size and severity of the wound (**Fig. 17.13**). A relatively small injury can sometimes result in an extensive scar which can have serious effects on the adjacent tissue. There are few circumstances when such a response can be predicted.

Cheloid scar occurs when the character of the scar is irregular and the surface is roughened, giving a reptilian look to the wound site (**Fig. 17.14**). Again there are no predictable types or location of a wound which predispose to the problem.

Differential diagnosis

- Sarcoid (verrucose, fibroblastic and mixed forms)
- Recurrent abrasions from harness or other conditions
- Self-inflicted bites
- Thermal injury/burns and scalds
- Frost bite
- Chemical injury

Diagnostic confirmation

- Clinical history of wounds is almost always present. Some result from application of strong chemicals, blisters, insecticides, hot or cold thermal injuries.
- Biopsy shows absence of hair follicles and structureless hyaline connective tissue. Hypertrophic scars are densely packed with fibrocytes which have little or no contractility and so these scars do not alter with time. Cheloid scars have dense granulation tissue with a rough irregular epithelial surface which produces excessive and irregular hyperkeratosis.

Treatment

Scarring can be minimized by careful wound management directed at reducing the extent of chronic inflammation. The longer a wound takes to heal,

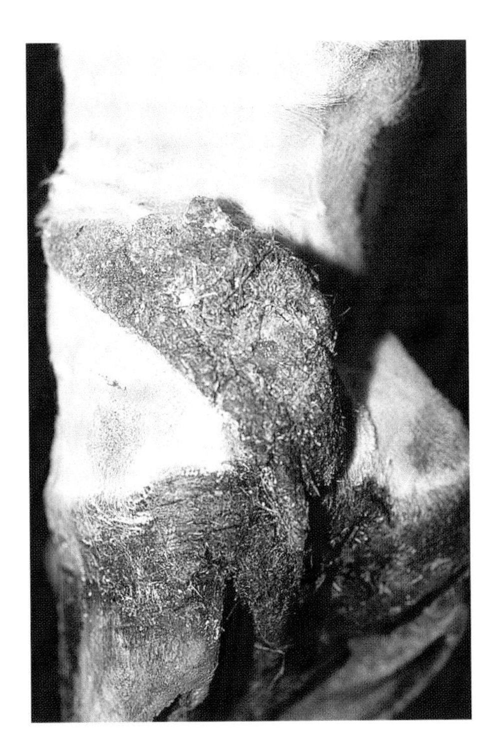

Figure 17.14 Cheloid scar with a typical reptilian appearance.

the more extensive is likely to be the scarring. Scars may be surgically removed, but there is a risk of further (sometimes worse) scarring after surgery. Daily application of keratolytic agents followed by vitamin E cream may soften the skin and allow contraction of the scar. Where scarring causes limiting distortion of tissue such as the eyelids or over joints, skin grafting and other reconstructive measures may be applicable.

CHEMICAL TRAUMA

Profile

History of application of 'pour-on' or topical medications such as antiseptics, insecticides or fungicides (or other materials) is usually obtained. Application of overstrength medication or of normal strength medication on an oversensitive skin. Application of blisters, counterirritants and vesicants is a common iatrogenic cause of this response, where it is regarded as a good therapeutic effect (see Fig. 13.6). Prolonged skin contact with surgical spirit or other chemicals may arise during general anaesthesia (recumbency) and can cause serious problems which are actually 'chemical burns'. Historically, old/used engine oil has been used to treat lice and culicoides hypersensitivity (sweet itch) and this can cause extensive and severe damage to skin and has serious potential systemic toxicity.

Clinical signs

Acute cases show marked moist, exudative dermatitis with matting of hair (**Fig. 17.15**). Extensive generalized dermatitis such as is caused by application of engine oil causes severe hair loss and a fragile skin which is easily traumatized. Hair loss (**Fig. 17.16**) and sometimes even open wounds are common consequences. Scarring is often extensive when deeper damage has been caused by prolonged contact with chemical substances. Chronic or mild recurrent skin insult causes fine

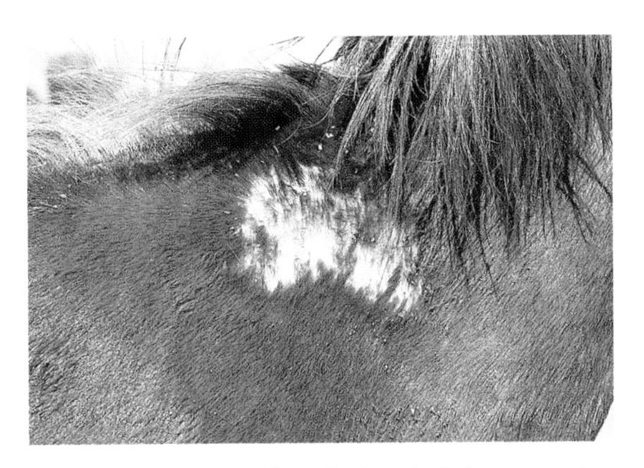

Figure 17.15 Accidental chemical burn causing matting and exudation of the skin.

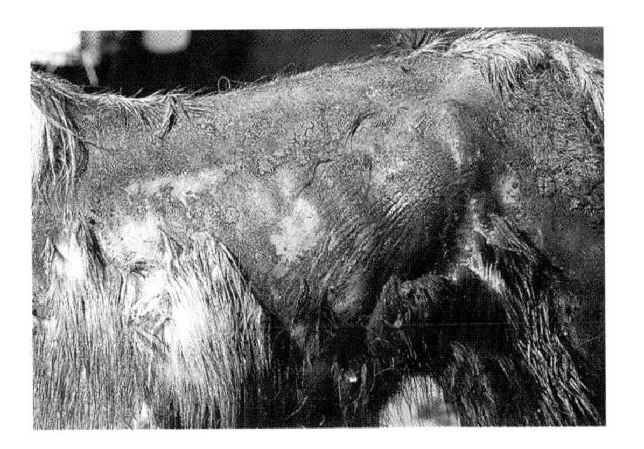

Figure 17.16 Extensive hair loss and generalized dermatitis arising from the ill-advised application of hot engine oil in a misguided attempt to treat louse infestation.

to coarse scaling and (temporary) loss of hair (alopecia) over the affected area, often well-demarcated over the area of application (e.g. following therapeutic blisters). Pruritus and self-inflicted trauma may be marked. Longer-term effects include skin thickening with lichenification and rugae formation.

Focal application of strong chemicals, focal burns or physical cautery to the skin may result in a dense, coagulated slough (eschar) which may remain *in situ* for prolonged periods (a 'sitfast') (**Fig. 17.17**) and inevitably leave a scar.

Differential diagnosis

- *Culicoides* spp. or other insect hypersensitivity (sweet itch, etc.).
- Louse infestation (*Damalinia equi*, *Haematopinus asini*)
- Insect bites with secondary self-inflicted trauma
- Dermatophytosis (*Trichophyton* spp.)
- Dermatophilosis (*Dermatophilus congolensis*)
- Chorioptic/psoroptic/poultry red mite mange
- Linear keratosis
- Scars
- Wounds
- Scalding

Diagnostic confirmation

- History of application of pour-on insecticides, blisters or other overstrength medication/applications. Owners, however, may deny having used anything at all.

Treatment

Acute cases should be washed with warm soapy water and dried and an emollient cream applied.

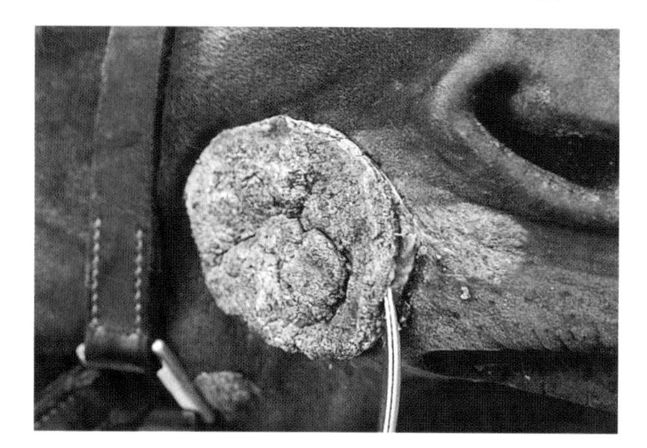

Figure 17.17 Application of a strong arsenic powder caused cutaneous coagulative necrosis. The large eschar sloughed slowly leaving a large cicatrized scar.

The chronic or severe forms often resolutely fail to heal and/or leave extensive unsightly scars which may require corrective surgery with skin grafting. Healing is often very difficult in damaged skin so surgical interference should be considered very carefully before embarking on prolonged and extensive conservative treatments.

SKIN SCALDING (diarrhoea/urine or wound exudate)

Profile

Prolonged diarrhoea, urine contamination or wound exudate lead to scalding and hair loss in the affected skin. These conditions are usually secondary to other pathological disorders. Wound fluids may cause serious excoriation and loss of hair.

Clinical signs

Temporary loss of hair around anal and perineal regions if of diarrhoeic origin (**Fig. 17.18**). Urine scalding usually occurs around caudal area of hind legs of mares or the lower regions of the hind legs in geldings with urinary incontinence (**Fig. 17.19**). Where urine is responsible an obvious stale, ammoniacal, urinary smell on legs can be detected. Urine and faeces may contain blood and this can be obvious. Skin may be extensively damaged and exudative.

Hair matting is more obvious with wound fluids; and serum exudate appears to induce a moderate or severe dermatitis and this also seems to encourage the development of skin infections.

A similar diffuse excoriation of the perineum with diffuse dermatitis can be caused by repeated rectal

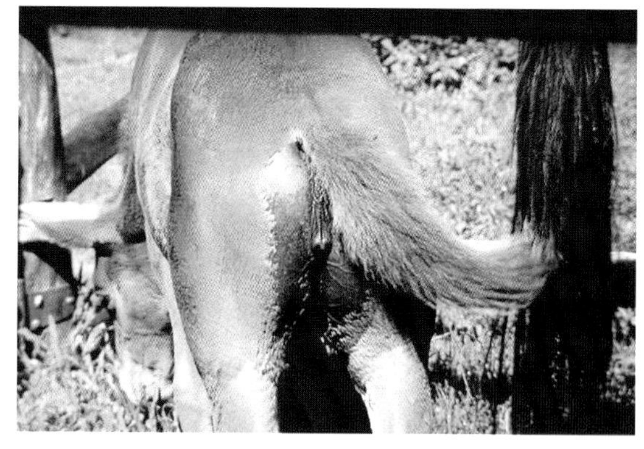

Figure 17.18 Diarrhoea-induced skin scalding with temporary hair loss.

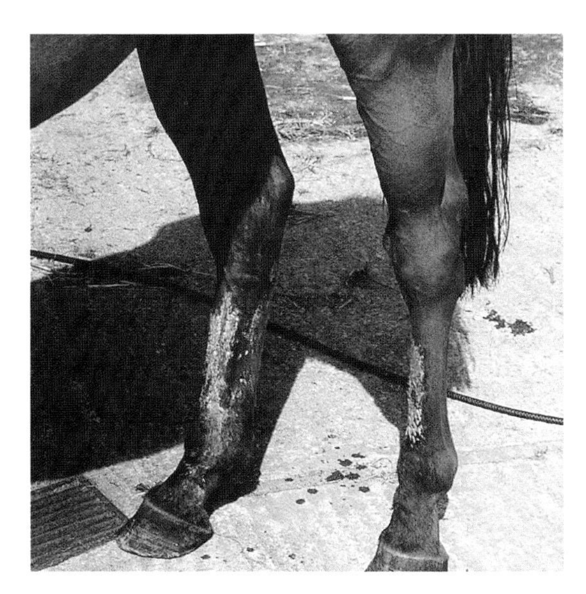

Figure 17.19 Urine scalding dermatitis affecting the dorsal aspects of the hind cannons in a gelding with urinary incontinence.

examinations and other procedures involving repeated superficial trauma to delicate skin areas.

Differential diagnosis

- Lice infestation
- Dermatophilosis
- Dermatophytosis
- Chemical irritants (e.g. strong iodine/disinfectants, mercurial blister)
- Allergic dermatitis

Diagnostic confirmation

- Almost all cases are secondary to other pathology. Full history and clinical assessment may establish the primary cause.
- If urinary problems are suspected, examine the entire urinary tract to determine whether retention with overflow or cystic calculi is the primary cause.
    - Urinary incontinence can be due to feed sorghum poisoning, cauda equina neuritis, rabies, sacral or spinal fracture or the neurological form of equine herpesvirus 1 (EHV1) infection.
- History of foaling accident, trauma to hindquarters, e.g. rearing over backward and landing on sacrum or spontaneous sacral fractures in racing horses.
- Primary diarrhoea from any cause (especially in foals).

Treatment

Control or treat the cause of the exudate, diarrhoea or urinary scalding problem. Where the cause is related to nerve damage, treatment is unlikely to be effective. Once the primary cause is controlled, hair and skin return to normal rapidly. If treatment is ineffective, local protectants are helpful, e.g. petroleum jelly or waterproof barrier creams with antiseptic and soothing properties (emollient creams, zinc oxide cream). Corticosteroid and local anaesthetic creams can be helpful.

BURSITIS

Profile

Change in size of an internal or external bursa overlying a bony prominence joint or tendon caused by acute or chronic/recurrent trauma. Excessive (abnormal) secretion of fluid of non-inflammatory or inflammatory nature within the bursa. Chronic trauma over bony prominences may result in acquired bursa such as capped elbow or hock.

Clinical signs

Enlarged soft (or occasionally firm) fluctuant swelling in an anatomical area where natural or acquired bursae occur such as the hock (**Fig. 17.20**) or the withers (**Fig. 17.21**) and the poll. They are usually distinctive, being of body warmth and non-painful. Once they become infected and can discharge onto the body surface they create serious problems both for the surgeon (in treatment of the disorder) and the dermatologist (in the management of the secondary scalding dermatitis which is the consequence of profuse discharges running over the adjacent skin).

Differential diagnosis

- Inclusion cysts (atheroma)
- Haematoma
- Calcinosis circumscripta
- Enlarged joint capsule
- Abscess
- Melanoma in grey horses
- Nodular sarcoid
- Tendon sheath fibrous enlargement

Diagnostic confirmation

- Needle aspiration for analysis of content leads to local collapse unassociated with joint.
- Ultrasonography is a useful way of establishing

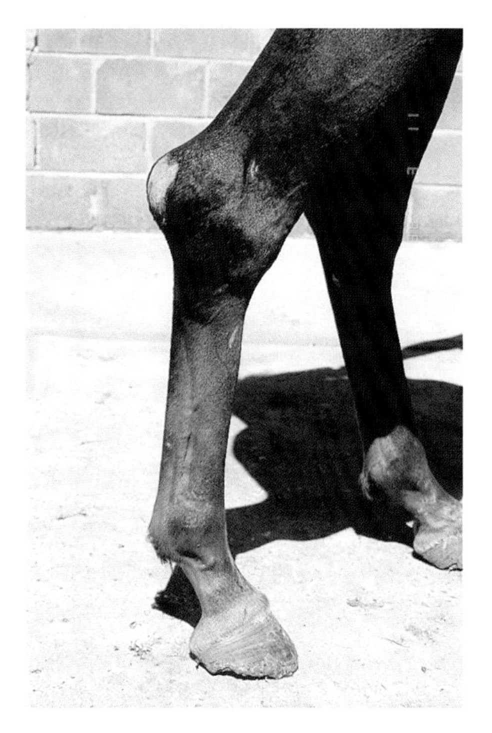

Figure 17.20 Bursitis of the hock bursa ('capped hock').

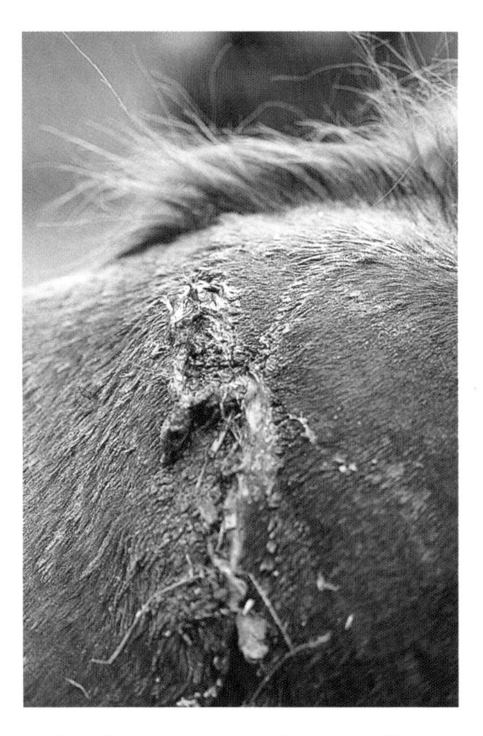

Figure 17.21 Infected bursitis of the withers bursa ('fistulous withers').

the true nature of the structure, its contents and its anatomical relations.

Treatment

Treatment of noninfected enlarged bursae is often unrewarding/disappointing with rapid recurrences and possibility of infection following attempts to aspirate contents and injection of corticosteroids. If the bursa is not infected and sterility can be assured, an attempt can be made to drain the bursa followed by intrabursal injection of corticosteroids and pressure bandaging. Recently there has been some suggestion that very small doses of atropine injected with or without corticosteroids have some benefit. This has not yet been critically evaluated. Surgical removal of the whole structure is very difficult and often leaves a defect larger than the original. Most acquired, noninfected bursae are therefore best left as cosmetic blemishes.

Infected bursae (such as 'poll evil' and 'fistulous withers') create serious problems and extensive surgical interference is usually required. Many of the cases presented as fistulous withers do not, however, involve the bursa and are the result of extensive subcutaneous tracking of infection from injury to underlying bone or ligaments.

chapter 18

INJURIES AND DISEASES OF THE HOOF

Genetic defects of the hoof: thin walls and soles; flat soles	228
Physical disorders and injuries of the hoof: Wall/toe/quarter/heel/vertical or transverse hoof-wall cracks	228
Coronary band injuries (wire and overreach wounds)	230
Puncture wounds of the sole	232
Haematoma of heels	233
Sole bruising and haematoma	234
Wall break-back	234
Hoof wall rings/laminitis	234
Canker	235
Thrush	236
Lateral cartilage necrosis (quittor)	236
Seedy toe/white line disease	237
Corns	238
Tumours of the foot	238

The hoof and its components can be regarded as special appendages of the skin. Various conditions caused by environment, injury, neglect or poor farriery practices may cause changes to the wall, sole, frog and/or coronary tissues. These changes may also be related to physical, infectious, neoplastic or genetic factors. It is difficult to categorize the various conditions as they often co-exist and many have a common aetiology. For example, a sole crack may lead to an abscess with an underrun sole or wall and then break out at the coronet, thereby involving at least three different hoof structures in different ways.

Clinical examination

The horse may be presented for lameness or for an actual foot condition, so it is necessary, as for any other skin condition, to carry out a full clinical examination of the patient before a detailed examination of the foot. Before the foot can be examined it must be thoroughly cleaned and the shoe may have to be removed. A full set of sharp hoof knives, a hoof pick and a wire or stiff bristle brush capable of penetrating the cleft of the frog should always be available. In any event, the wall, sole and frog should be scrubbed clean and all dead, discoloured and damaged horn and frog material should be removed from the sole in particular. However, if the tissue is patently normal it is unwise to remove excessive sole, wall or frog. The periople or outer waterproof surface of the wall should be interfered with as little as possible as it may result in drying and cracking.

The sole should be palpated using digital pressure and hoof testers, starting at the toe and working laterally and medially. Pressure can be applied to the frog and across the heels from frog to wall. Squeezing gently across the heels (medial and lateral) from the back of the foot applies pressure to the plantar/palmar structures. The wall should be palpated carefully and its temperature assessed in comparison with the contralateral limb. Gentle tapping with a small round hammer is a good test of wall pain, particularly over shoe nails which might be causing problems. Evidence of bruising, haemorrhage or abnormal tissues (both in appearance and texture) in the sole wall or frog should be noted. The white line should be carefully examined for breadth, normality of horn tubules and bruising/haemorrhage.

GENETIC DEFECTS OF THE HOOF

THIN WALLS AND SOLES

These are characteristic of certain breeds and genetic lines of horse. They usually appear together and create difficulty in shoeing. Thin walls often lead to pricking, nail binds and wall-breakout during shoeing which make successive shoeing increasingly difficult. Thin soles are more liable to bruising and concussive injuries such as haematoma formation. Repeated bruising of the soles increases the opportunities for foot infections and corns. This has been blamed for some cases of pedal osteitis. While horses are in training, great care has to be given to the method of shoeing and the placement of the nails.

Treatment

Whilst resting the horses in rocky, rough hill country may produce a harder foot, it seldom corrects the original defect – indeed it may sometimes cause serious break-back of the wall. Thin-soled horses benefit from polypropylene pads or a thin 2–3 mm layer of acrylic filler applied over the whole solar surface. Chrome-treated leather has also been glued with contact adhesive to the soles under the shoes. Glue-on plastic shoes help considerably by avoiding the need for any nails at all but they are not as durable and the methacrylate adhesive often loses its strength if allowed to get wet for long periods. Acrylic hoof support bandages applied around the wall before shoeing assist some horses and can be used to provide extra hoof strength. Daily supplementation with biotin and methionine may improve the quality of the hoof structure but it is not usually curative on its own.

FLAT SOLES

Horses which do not have normal concavity of the sole without any pathological reason are classified as having flat feet. This can be described as a developmental/genetic condition. It occurs more often in some lines of Thoroughbred horses in particular.

Treatment

There is no effective medical option and therapy is limited to placement of well-seated shoes and avoidance of hard or rough going. Polypropylene or leather anti-concussion pads can be applied to help cushion foot impact.

PHYSICAL DISORDERS AND INJURIES OF THE HOOF

WALL/TOE/QUARTER/HEEL/VERTICAL OR TRANSVERSE HOOF-WALL CRACKS

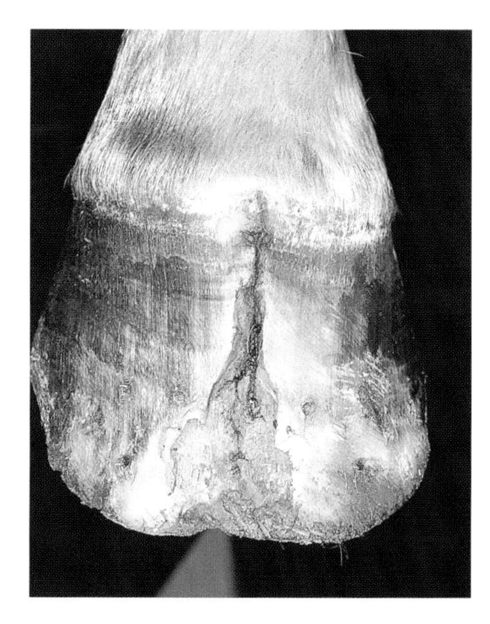

Figure 18.1 Deep toe crack extending from solar margin to coronary band and down to sensitive tissue.

Profile

These are characterized by fissures in the wall. Wall, toe and quarter cracks have a defect which is parallel to the laminae, while transverse cracks are at right angles to the laminae. Most cracks of the former type are superficial and due to prolonged desiccation. Deep cracks may extend into the sensitive laminae (**Fig. 18.1**). Coronary band injuries are a common cause of clinically significant secondary cracks and horn defects.

Toe and quarter cracks These are mostly due to neglect from allowing the hoof to dry out, or improper dressing to reduce 'winging' of the quarters and heels. They may also arise from sudden turns on rough ground or injuries to the coronary band (**Fig. 18.2**).

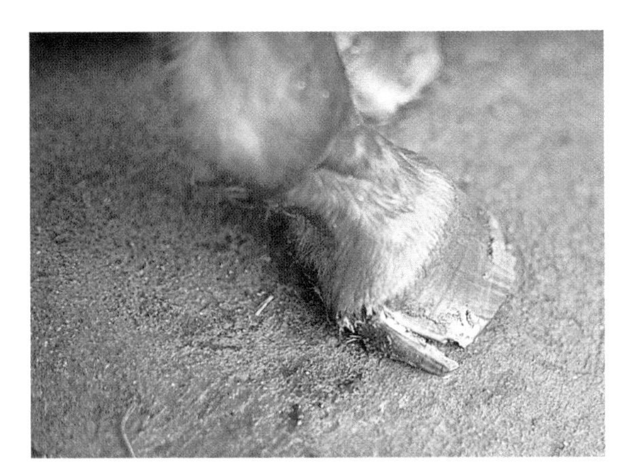

Figure 18.2 Quarter crack extending from solar margin to coronary band.

Transverse cracks Coronary band injuries or infections spreading up the white line from sole abscesses are usually responsible for these. They only become serious if they are extensive and when they have nearly grown out at the solar margin (**Fig. 18.3**).

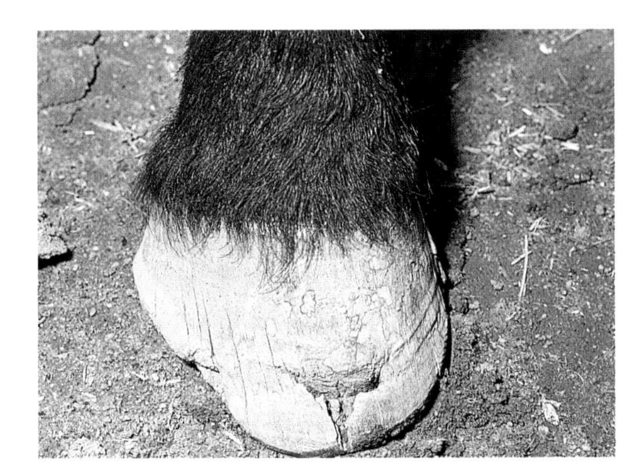

Figure 18.3 Transverse crack.

Sole cracks These are caused by a combination of excessive drying of the sole and standing on rocks or other hard objects in paddock/grazing horses (**Fig. 18.4**). They are not commonly observed in shod horses.

Heel cracks Cracks in the wall of the heel usually have two fairly distinct causes: (a) coronet injury leading to a persistent defect in the coronary band and so to a wall deficit; (b) bearing-surface injuries which seem to occur more frequently from poor heel support. This is encountered where the angle of the heel becomes more and more acute, leading to tearing of the laminae (**Fig. 18.5**).

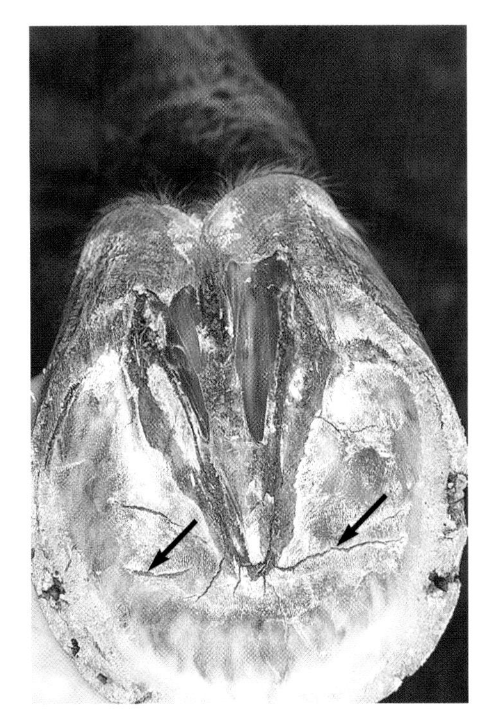

Figure 18.4 Sole crack (arrows).

Clinical features

Superficial cracks are not often associated with lameness. Deep cracks with pressure on the sensitive laminae may cause lameness. Haemorrhage or purulent discharging sinuses and foci with movement of the wall have serious implications.

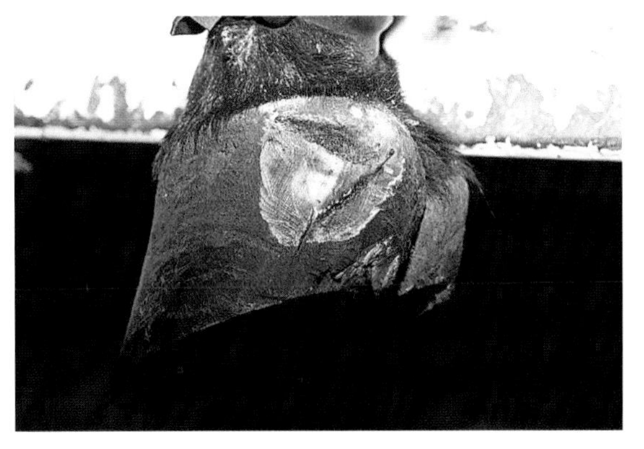

Figure 18.5 Heel crack due to poor hoof conformation and lack of corrective farriery. The true extent may be visible only after careful dressing.

Working the horse may cause bleeding from the area and, in paddock/grazing horses, pus is often associated with neglected hoof injuries.

Heel cracks are often painful and contact with the ground is too far forward compared with the horn at the coronary band. The cracks are often deep and easily bleed and/or become infected.

Diagnostic confirmation

- Clinical appearance is typical. The extent of crack and/or depth may be determined with a hoof tester applied before and after work.
- Diagnosis of sole cracks is sometimes more demanding. Discoloured horn and the actual line of the crack may only be visible after careful paring of the entire sole surface.
- Long-standing dorsopalmar or mediolateral imbalances which lead to heel cracks are usually easily appreciated.

Treatment

The first objective is to address the underlying cause. Brittle horn and weak horn have both been improved by prolonged feeding of gelatin at 30 g per day or by continuous feeding of biotin at 15–20 mg per day. Foot balance and regular farriery are very important at any stage in the development of a crack. It is important to ensure that the crack is not a secondary manifestation of a seedy toe area.

Uncomplicated superficial cracks These should be treated early by dressing the feet with 50% Neatsfoot (or horse foot) oil and 50% Stockholm tar. Deeper cracks on the toe or quarter are treated by several methods depending on the availability of shoes, farrier and severity of the injury.

Wall, quarter or heel cracks Treatment of cracks which involve sensitive laminae often requires regional anaesthesia. The wall of the fissure should be gently debrided using an electric burr and very sharp, fine hoof knives. Tight wire sutures can be placed through the hoof wall to limit movement and the whole area can then be filled with synthetic resin hoof-filling compounds. Alternatively, the debrided fissure can be treated with undiluted metacresolsulphonic acid and formaldehyde solution and dried before a synthetic filler is placed in the groove and allowed to set. The surface is then rasped to give a rough 'key' level with the wall. Self-tapping screws (4–5 mm or shorter) are set in the wall through several layers of fibreglass cloth and this is then covered completely with a synthetic filler or fibreglass car-body material. The fibreglass acts as a stable bridge between the self-tapping screws. It is important that any haemorrhage occurring in the fissure is cauterized or allowed to seal over for 24–48 hours before filling and sealing is attempted.

Heel cracks The damaged horn can be stripped off with shoeing pincers. The loosened wall is torn upwards, outwards and backwards. Tranquillizer and digital nerve blocks can be used but are often unnecessary; a twitch is usually the only restraint needed. Antibiotic powder is applied to any area showing excessive haemorrhage and the hoof is bandaged. With larger cracks, or with horses in training, a bar shoe may be used to protect the remaining wall from further injury after removal of the quarter. Alternatively, the stripped area can be repaired with a synthetic filler once it has dried out and is free of infection or necrotic tissue.

Transverse cracks The weakened wall should be removed and a shoe with side clips each side of the area of horn removal is prepared. An old piece of X-ray film is placed between the foot and lightly nailed shoe to prevent the filler adhering to the shoe. The defect is then repaired using synthetic resin filler. Once the filler has hardened, the shoe can then be removed to allow resetting and final attachment.

Sole cracks Carefully pare out all discoloured horn until pin-point haemorrhage appears. Dress the region with undiluted metacresolsulphonic acid and formaldehyde liquid, or 5% phenol. The area is covered with a steel or polypropylene treatment plate bolted onto the shoe. Modern strong plastic overboots make repeated treatments simpler. Leather pads/soles can be used in stabled horses and, if a shoe is unavailable, leather can be glued onto the sole and wall of the foot. Leather is not suitable under wet, boggy conditions or if exercise is allowed on a hard surface.

More severely infected cases can be difficult to treat. The entire sole area may have to be stripped. Where this has occurred, the foot should be examined and dressed daily with antibiotic and metronidazole (or 4% povidone-iodine-soaked swabs) to control infection.

CORONARY BAND INJURIES (wire and overreach wounds)

Profile

Injuries which physically damage or permanently disrupt the continuity of the corium almost all cause persistent hoof growth abnormalities (**Fig. 18.6**).

Wire cuts or overreaching injuries are probably the commonest causes. Horses paw at fences, hook the heel over wire, and either pull back or saw the leg sideways, often causing extensive damage to the skin, lateral cartilage, tendons and coronary band (**Fig. 18.7**).

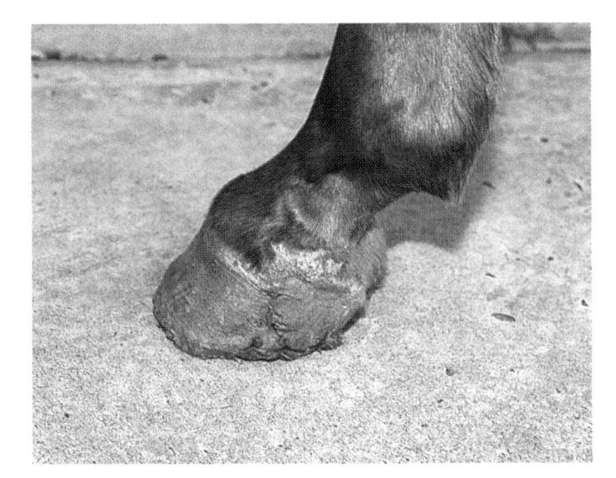

Figure 18.6 A permanent hoof defect as a result of a coronary band injury.

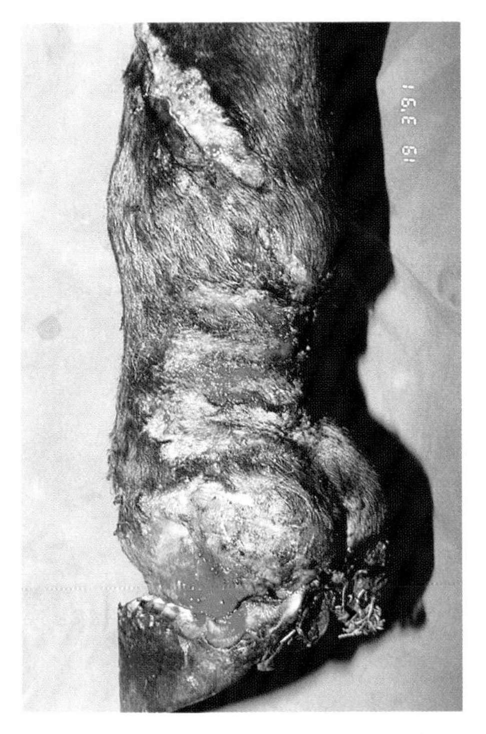

Figure 18.7 Extensive wire injuries involving the hoof, coronary band and deeper tissues of the foot and the pastern and fetlock.

Clinical signs

Obvious injury involving the coronary band or abnormality of the coronary band caused by previous injury. Acute injuries *must* be assessed carefully to establish extent of damage to vascular and nervous supply to foot and damage to heel tissues and lateral cartilage.

Secondary defects in horn growth are very variable and depend largely on the extent of treatment applied at the acute stage. Cracks in the hoof wall commencing at the coronary band and extending distally are common.

Diagnostic confirmation

- Visual inspection is simple but establishing the extent of the original injury may not be simple.
- Radiography should be used to establish the extent of underlying damage to structures of the foot.

Treatment

Very careful assessment of the wound is essential: most are heavily contaminated and/or infected. Prompt, careful debridement using a scalpel (not scissors) of all dead or compromised or contaminated tissues is an essential first step. It is very rare that wounds of this type can be sutured and most attempts to do so result in failure or worse. The wound should be allowed to heal by delayed union. Initially the debrided and cleaned wound should be irrigated carefully and packed with a hydrogel wound dressing material and a cavity absorbent dressing should be inserted into any defect to minimize dead space and to remove wound exudate. This dressing should be replaced at 48-hour intervals (or more frequently if exudate is excessive or patently infected) until granulation tissue is obvious and the wound bed is healthy.

Application of rigid limb casts over a suitable dressing is a rewarding procedure which has been made simpler and safer by synthetic polypropylene or polyurethane resin bandage casting materials. These are light, strong and easy to apply but the cast should always be applied (and removed) strictly according to the manufacturer's instructions. Cast management is vitally important. Unless complications develop, the cast can be left for 3–4 weeks. In the event of any complication (pain is often the earliest evidence of something going wrong) it must be removed immediately and if necessary replaced. Suitable antibiotic and tetanus prophylaxis should be given. Casting often reduces healing time by up to 50% or more. Casts should be used until healing is well advanced. Early removal of support can lead to the wound splitting open over the original wound site. With complicated wounds, appropriate other measures will be required.

Chronic secondary defects can be treated by several different methods:

- The horn can be grooved out to create a dove-tail-type groove (as for the toe crack) extending from the coronary band to the solar surface or the most distal extent of the crack. The two sides can be wired or laced and reconstructed with acrylic filler using screws or lacing methods in which holes are drilled in the insensitive horn on either side of the defect.
- A groove can be cut down either side of the crack using a vibrating plaster saw or air drill circular saw at low speed. The whole defect is then stripped out and haemorrhage is controlled by pressure bandages for 10 minutes. A bar shoe using wall clips either side of the defect is then applied to restrict spreading and movement of the healing site. When infection and necrotic tissue are absent the defect can be reconstructed using acrylic filler compounds.

PUNCTURE WOUNDS OF THE SOLE

Profile

These result from penetration of the solar surface of the hoof by foreign bodies such as sharp stones, sticks, glass, nails, etc. Deep punctures (street nail) can be catastrophic and are outside the scope of this text. Punctures in the middle third of the sole are likely to be the most serious. However, serious damage can be done both to the sole itself and to the other structures of the hoof from any solar injury.

Clinical signs

Acute onset of a progressively severe lameness is characteristic. Toe-pointing, reluctance to bear weight on the leg and swelling of the back of the pastern and fetlock are present in some cases. Swelling as high as the knee may develop.

Penetration of the synovial structures (navicular bursa, distal interphalangeal joint or deep digital flexor tendon sheath) gives extreme acute lameness with swelling of the flexor sheath behind the pastern and fetlock.

Diagnostic confirmation

- Thorough cleaning of the foot with a hoof knife to remove all loose or scaly sole, dirt, etc., should be carried out immediately. Hoof testers are then used to carefully press the entire white line, the entire sole and seat of the corn, the entire frog and bars area and, if shod, all the nails.
- If the testers locate a painful area in the foot, the shoe should be removed. Careful examination of the nails should be made to see whether any are blackened or discoloured or set higher than normal in the wall. Re-testing with testers over the white line and nail holes is then carried out.
- Localized painful area(s) should be pared with a hoof knife until the solar horn is shown to be free of cracks or punctures. The hard, horny layer of the frog is carefully pared with a very sharp knife or scalpel and the sulci are likewise carefully investigated with a fine seeker knife.
- All black, cracked puncture marked or necrotic areas should be very carefully, lightly pared away until normal horn shows underneath or the actual damaged or infected area has been found (**Fig. 18.8**). Test the foot again for pain response to the hoof tester. Should this fail to locate an infection or injury site, careful deep palpation of the coronary band may show a small sore area to correspond to a very small 'pipe' of infection leading up a single lamina interface from an infection of the white line in the sole – so called 'gravel' infection.

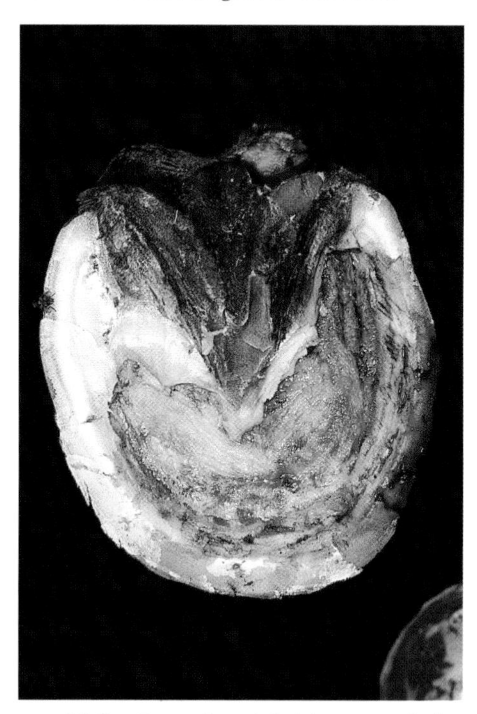

Figure 18.8 Extensive debridement of the sole following a puncture wound and sepsis with under-running.

- If a lesion cannot be found with paring, nerve blocks should be used to ensure the lameness is in fact in the foot. A posterior digital nerve block will desensitize the posterior third of the foot and a low '6-point' block will desensitize the foot.
- Radiological examination may be necessary for differential diagnosis of fracture of the pedal bone, pedal osteitis, navicular disease and septic laminitis. Contrast medium can be introduced into the penetration tract to describe its true extent.
- Synoviocentesis of the various synovial structures of the foot can be used to establish their involvement. Lavage from these structures may identify that the injury has penetrated them (lavage fluid will be seen issuing from the tract during pressure irrigation of the relevant synovial structure).

Treatment

Nail pricks, and nail-binds of recent origin, are treated by cleaning out the nail hole and packing with povidone-iodine or 5% phenol solution. Antibiotics maintained daily for 4 days and analgesics (such as phenylbutazone) are also commonly beneficial. Some cases recover without further development of infection. Infected nail pricks, nail holes and puncture wounds of medium duration require that a 1 cm diameter hole with sloping sides be created around the wound to relieve pressure on the sole. This defect can be packed with an antiseptic-soaked swab or cotton wool and a shoe with treatment plate or a plastic boot can be applied to facilitate treatment and provide protection for the injury. The dressings should be replaced daily until a pad can be fastened under the shoe for more permanent protection.

Underrun frogs are treated in a similar manner. In severe case, the entire frog may have to be removed.

Deep punctures of the middle third of the sole in the frog region often penetrate the deep flexor tendon and/or navicular bursa. These injuries require specialist attention under general anaesthesia and should be referred accordingly as a matter of extreme urgency. They all carry a grave prognosis.

HAEMATOMA OF HEELS

Profile

Subcutaneous blood is present in the bulb of the heel(s). In the front feet, it is usually due to overreaching by the hind foot; in the hind feet, it may be due to being galloped on, or kicking at walls or rails. Overtired horses at the end of a race are more likely to receive this type of injury. The injury can also be due to badly balanced feet and occasionally it occurs after a rough journey in a transporter.

Clinical signs

Obvious acute onset of foot pain with pointing of the toe in the absence of other more obvious causes for this. Discoloration (bruising) of the heels may be obvious in white-heeled legs (**Fig. 18.9**) but may be very difficult to confirm in brown- and black-haired heels.

Diagnostic confirmation

- Clinical examination.
- Needle puncture over the heel area reveals dark blood.

Treatment

Blood can be drained from the haematoma with a 16G needle. A pressure bandage is applied to prevent refilling. Analgesics such as phenylbutazone for 3–4 days are advisable. Correction of foot balance and particularly the provision of adequate heel support is important in cases where the dorsopalmar balance is incorrect (overlong toes with broken-back hoof pastern angles and forward-located shoes).

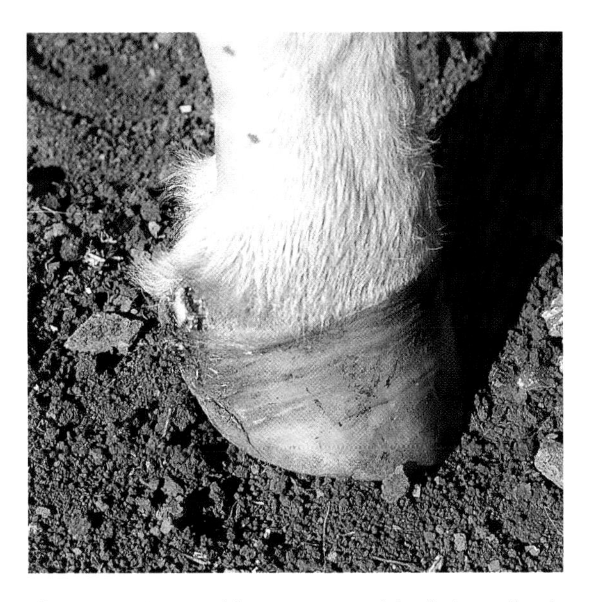

Figure 18.9 Heel haematoma with obvious discoloration over the heel bulb. In a pigmented foot it may be very difficult to see.

SOLE BRUISING AND HAEMATOMA

Profile

This is most often due to badly seated or too small shoes, or use of the horse on stony ground without conditioning or protection of the sole with leather or polypropylene protective pads. Other causes include fracture of the pedal bone, short or brittle broken back walls (which forces the horse to walk on the soles). Mild chronic laminitis with dropped soles will also contribute to solar bruising.

Clinical signs

The horse is usually lame and blood-streaked horn and, rarely, free blood under the sole of foot can be seen. Typical foot lameness with pain on percussion or pressure with hoof testers over the affected sole.

Diagnostic confirmation

- Visual appearance of the sole after paring away the outer layers of the sole. Pare away scaly layers of sole and blood-streaked horn will be found over areas of sole. In most cases it is confined to the toe.
- Widespread haemorrhage with a very lame horse could indicate pedal bone fracture. Radiography must be used at an early stage to eliminate this and other causes of bruising.

Treatment

Corrective farriery is vital using correctly fitted shoes and a protective pad of polypropylene under the shoe. Bar shoes with several opposing side clips to support the entire hoof wall are helpful. Specific causes of the bruising require specific treatment measures.

WALL BREAK-BACK

Profile

Repeated shoeing, brittle walls and incorrect shoe removal are contributing factors. Excessive dryness or wetting of the hoof wall and rough surfaces with unshod feet are relatively common aetiological aspects. Poor management is usually the principal cause although some horses have congenitally brittle hoof keratin. The role of biotin and methionine in the aetiology of hoof-wall defects is uncertain, but it does seem that deficiencies can cause obvious abnormalities of the periople (see Fig. 15.3) and histological evidence of keratin abnormalities.

Clinical signs

Portions of the hoof wall break out and expose the sensitive laminae (**Fig. 18.10**). The condition is not always painful, but reluctance to walk and pain on digital pressure over the damaged hoof can be encountered.

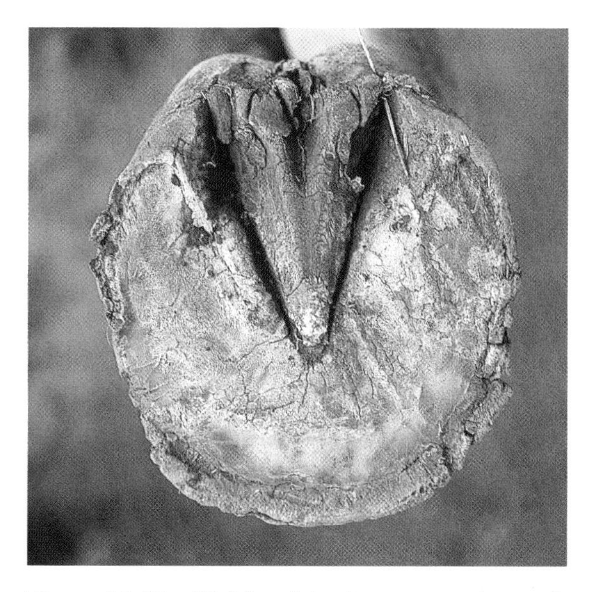

Figure 18.10 Wall break-back to expose the sensitive laminae.

Diagnostic confirmation

- Clinical appearance is typical.
- Radiographs may confirm underlying bone demineralization.

Treatment

A synthetic resin-bonded bandage is a useful supportive material. A protective leather undersole/pad should be fixed under the shoe; the pad may have to be glued over the sole and up the walls before applying the shoe if nail retention is difficult. Glue-on plastic shoes can be very useful as they minimize the damage to the horn. Resolution may take up to 3–6 months in an otherwise normal foot and much longer if there is underlying pathology. Addition of methionine and biotin to the diet can help restore hoof quality.

HOOF WALL RINGS/LAMINITIS

Profile

These are most often due to dramatic feed and

work changes, laminitic episodes or other causes of foot inflammation or prolonged periods of systemic illness. They can also follow 'therapeutic' or accidental blistering with strong iodine or even liquid mercurial blisters which are applied in an attempt to promote horn growth. Growth from such treatment is often wavy and irregular. Excessive stress or severe exercise can induce rings in the horn in endurance horses.

Laminitis produces the most marked changes and in the chronic form the hoof will have a series of rings plus a change in wall angle due to white line separation.

Chronic laminitis is characterized by lameness, 'laminitic' rings on the hoof, change in the hoof angle, and rotation of the third phalanx and presence of a laminar wedge – usually, bilateral lameness when due to metabolic changes, but a single weight-bearing foot can be affected where another foot or leg has been non-weight-bearing for a long period (**Fig. 18.11**). It also occurs in selenium poisoning (see p. 186) and Cushing's disease (see p. 269).

Clinical signs

Severe, often bilateral lameness with an exaggerated gait having an obvious, characteristic heel–toe foot placement pattern. Heavy 'ring-formation' of the hoof with excessive flaky horn growth. The hoof wall grows faster at the heels than the toe, which leads to dishing or slippering of the wall. Dramatic widening of the white line due to damage to the laminae is common.

A laminar wedge develops with a dropped sole where rotation of the third phalanx has occurred. Bruising of the sole just behind the white line on the anterior portion of the sole is common.

In severe cases, suppuration of dropped sole and prolapse of the pedal bone through the sole may occur.

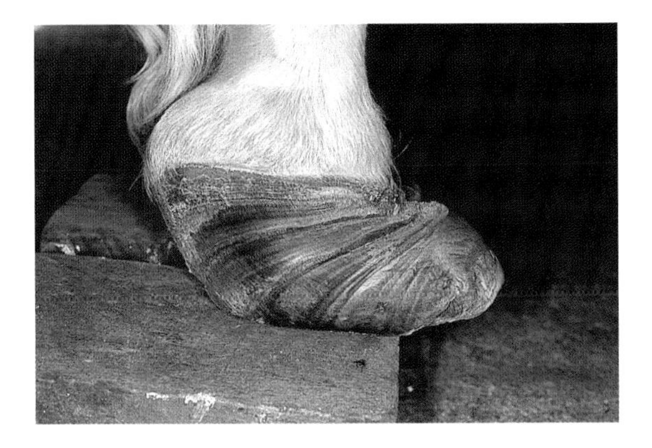

Figure 18.11 Typical rings and abnormal hoof growth of chronic laminitis which arises from abnormal and irregular horn growth.

Diagnostic confirmation

- Characteristic disease which has distinctive clinical and radiographic findings.

Treatment

Very careful farriery is required to correct the underlying disorder and the foot/hoof problems. Correction is a slow, costly procedure and the owner should be fully appraised of the likely prognosis. No specific treatment is applicable to the laminitic rings, although careful oiling and reshaping can help. Care must be taken not to damage the outer protective layers of the hoof as this may cause drying and cracking. Where reshaping of the hoof wall is required, hoof dressing on exposed keratin is advisable.

CANKER

Profile

Hypertrophic pododermatitis of the frog and adjacent structures seen predominantly in draught horses kept under unhygienic wet conditions. It has, however, been reported in all breeds and all ages of horse.

Clinical signs

Abnormal finger-like papillae of hypertrophic horn which bleeds easily, growing from frog and adjacent sole (**Fig. 18.12**). It can reach considerable proportions and can become infected and exudative.

Diagnostic confirmation

- Clinical appearance
- Characteristic histology showing chronic pododermatitis

Treatment

Surgical removal of all affected tissue is essential. Soaking and poulticing of the foot in a povidone–iodine soapy solution for 2–3 days before surgery is helpful. Surgical debridement should continue until healthy tissue is exposed over the whole area. After surgery the area should then be dressed with astringent or metacresolsulphonic acid or very diluted formalin solution (2%). Once

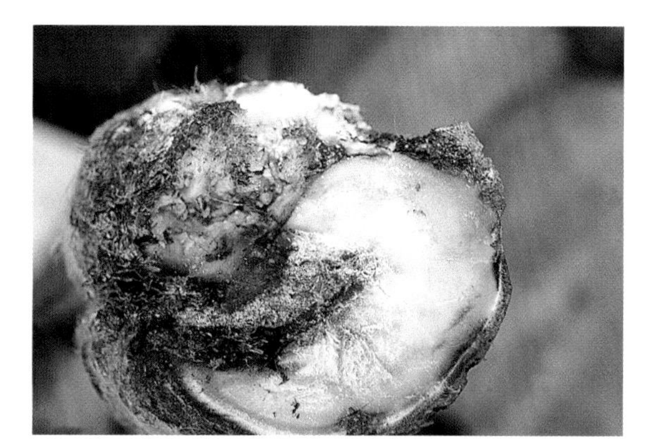

Figure 18.12 Canker showing abnormal finger-like papillae of hypertrophic horn which bleeds easily, growing from frog and adjacent sole.

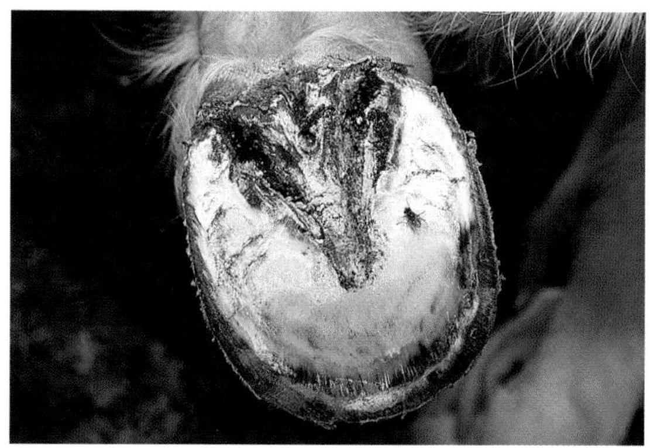

Figure 18.13 Thrush in the cleft of the frog – the clefts are filled with a foul-smelling black material.

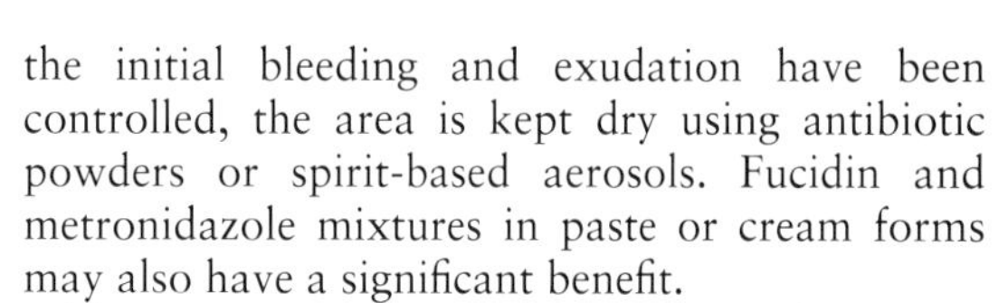

the initial bleeding and exudation have been controlled, the area is kept dry using antibiotic powders or spirit-based aerosols. Fucidin and metronidazole mixtures in paste or cream forms may also have a significant benefit.

Treatment is over many months and requires further debridement to control chronic hypertrophic growth. Benzoyl peroxide (2%) has been successfully used as a dressing, but the major requirement is to keep horse's feet clean and dry with daily dressings.

THRUSH

Profile

A degenerative exudative dermatitis of the central and collateral sulci of the frog characterized by a granular black discharge and a characteristic foul smell. Local factors such as deep cleft with narrow and occluding margins and general factors of lack of foot care, e.g. stabling of horses in wet, unhygienic conditions, are significant factors in the aetiology. Infection with a variety of microorganisms including *Fusobacterium necrophorus* is commonly present.

Clinical signs

Foul smelling, necrotic black discharge from the sulci of the frog (**Fig. 18.13**). Sometimes it is only detectable when a hoof pick or fine hoof knife is used deep in the clefts. There may be local or more extensive underrunning of sulci of the frog and in severe cases sepsis of the deeper structures of the foot. Swelling of leg and lameness occurs in some horses.

Diagnostic confirmation

- Typical appearance and features

Treatment

Debride all necrotic frog and underrun infected areas. Treat sparingly every day with 5% formalin solution worked into the cleft of the frog with a firm paint brush until all evidence of infection has cleared. Metronidazole paste applied twice daily for up to 3 weeks is often effective. Weekly foot bathing with 10% magnesium sulphate ($MgSO_4$) solution can be prophylactic. Ensure the horse is placed in clean, dry surroundings and eliminate contact with wet unsanitary conditions. Repeated debridement may be necessary.

Intravenous or oral potentiated sulphonamide compounds will assist in clearing the infection, particularly in cases with deep-seated infection.

LATERAL CARTILAGE NECROSIS (quittor)

Profile

Lameness associated with swelling and intermittent or persistent purulent discharge from a sinus tract over the area of the lateral cartilage. Usually associated with trauma (e.g. wire cuts or overreach injuries) to the lateral or medial heel areas with subsequent infection, inflammation and necrosis of the lateral cartilage.

Clinical signs

In the early stages a painful swelling over the area

of the lateral cartilage develops. A persistent or intermittent, usually scanty, purulent discharge develops, typically above the coronary band (**Fig. 18.14**). Periods of apparent healing are followed by repeated, though seldom increasingly severe, discharge. Local pain is not often marked during periods of discharge. In some cases the extent of the discharge can be minimal and show as a slight matting of the hair over the site. Lameness may or may not be obvious.

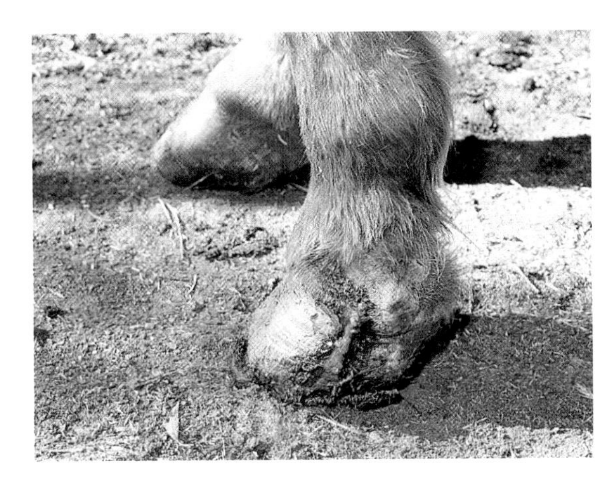

Figure 18.14 Quittor (necrosis of the lateral cartilages) resulting in a chronic purulent discharge from above the coronary band.

Diagnostic confirmation

- Characteristic history of injury to the coronary band over the lateral cartilage.
- Typical appearance of a chronic discharging sinus tract just above the coronary band.
- Plain and contrast radiography (using a catheter and contrast medium or a sterile blunt probe placed in the tract, will assist in assessing the extent of the problem and differentiate it from other causes of discharging coronary band sinus tracts such as 'seedy toe', white line disease, laminitis and solar sepsis.

Treatment

Surgical removal of all damaged cartilage under general anaesthetic is essential. Early lesions treated aggressively carry a good prognosis, while the outlook for extensive old lesions, especially when they involve the coronary band or coffin joint capsule, is much worse. Lameness often persists after surgery in the latter cases. Unilateral digital neurectomy can be considered as a palliative treatment if the surgical wound has healed satisfactorily.

SEEDY TOE/WHITE LINE DISEASE

Profile

Necrosis of the sensitive laminae, usually of the anterior wall of the hoof but it may affect all distal areas of the laminae, extending proximally towards the coronary band.

Cracks in the white line leading to infection and chronic laminitis with separation of the laminae in the area of the white line (usually at the toe), will cause this condition. Anaerobic fungi have been incriminated in some cases.

Clinical signs

Mild or sometimes moderate lameness is usual but not invariable. Examination of the foot will identify a chalky, crumbly white line region which can be easily gouged out with a foot knife. The adjacent hoof wall has a hollow behind it into which grit and other foreign matter is forced. Occasionally overt sepsis is present with a discharging tract at the coronary band above the region affected.

Diagnostic confirmation

- Characteristic clinical features.
- Lateral radiography clearly shows gas and foreign matter wedged into the area between the wall and the pedal bone.

Treatment

Small areas of seedy toe can be pared back to healthy tissue with a hoof knife. If the defect is spotlessly clean the defect can be packed with synthetic filler. If not clean the cavity should be packed tightly with a swab soaked in povidone–iodine or metronidazole and replaced daily. More severe cases will need to have the wall over the seedy portion completely removed and a small area of wall removed back to sound laminar tissue. The defect should not be filled permanently until all risk of haemorrhage is past and the area is certainly clean and infection free.

Extensive defects (some are very wide and as high as the coronet) should be extensively debrided after a shoe with supportive side clips has been applied to the foot to stabilize the distal margin.

The use of an electric burr allows a distal bridge of the hoof wall to be retained while removing all the damaged horn proximally and along the solar margin. Once all necrotic and infected tissue has been removed, the defect can be filled with synthetic acrylic filler. The shoe is then re-set and the horse rested in a stable with only light walking for 2 weeks. The shoe should be regularly re-set every 4 weeks at least and a close check kept on the repair patch to ensure that it remains firm and uninfected.

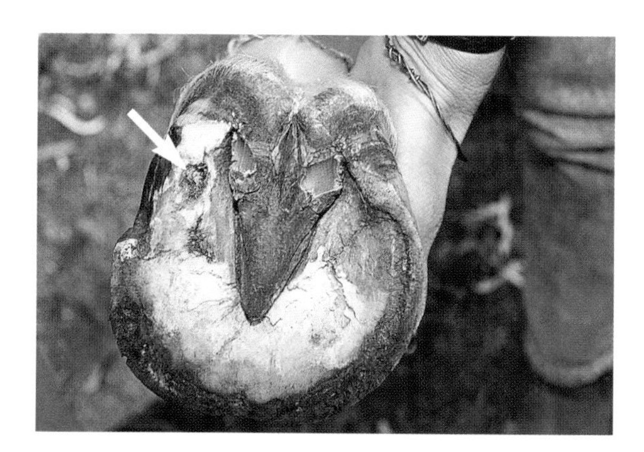

Figure 18.15 Corn (arrow). A foul-smelling purulent discharge (often but not always black in colour) can be released from many of these cases by careful paring and following of even the smallest black tract.

CORNS

Profile

Inflammation of the area between the wall and the bars of the foot known as the 'seat of corn'. This is caused through improper shoeing either because shoes are left on the foot too long or by use of poorly sized/undersized shoes. The heels of the shoe lie inside the wall and therefore cause excessive pressure on the seat of corn. However, it can also occur when the heels are allowed to drop by poor shoeing techniques causing tearing of the laminae and consequent bruising without direct shoe pressure. Pressure at this sensitive site causes bruising and necrosis of the horn, allowing infection to gain access to the bruised tissue.

Clinical signs

Acute lameness developing in a horse with poorly fitted shoes or overgrown feet. Warm or hot bulb of heel and a painful focus detectable at the seat of corn with hoof testers.

A focal red or black bruised area or blood-streaked horn or even pus and underrunning of the heel may be found when the shoe is removed and the foot is pared back (**Fig. 18.15**). A very small black focus may be all that can be seen on first glance.

Careful examination of the hoof wall at the heels may reveal a curled-under wall which causes pressure on the seat of corn and lamina problems with the urgent need for corrective farriery.

Diagnostic confirmation

- Clinical signs and examination of the seat of the corn.
- Palmar digital nerve block removes the lameness.

Treatment

Remove bruised solar tissue and, if infected, open and drain the region. Shoe with either a leather or polypropylene pad (possibly with a treatment plate) under the shoe. The defect should be packed with an antiseptic-soaked cotton wool plug. Antibiotics (such as penicillin) are often useful once the tract is draining freely, and the tetanus status is very important for infections of this type.

Where horses have thin-walled feet, leading to the heel wall turning under, heart-bar shoes can be used to prevent further bruising. It is essential to make sure shoes are fitted properly to prevent shoe pressure on the white line or the seat of corn. The heel is often cut down to sound tissue and the horse shod with raised, graduated heels to balance the foot and regain correct alignment. Plastic heel wedges are often used to retain foot level and balance **but** these frequently apply even more pressure to heels and may actually aggravate the problem. Alternatively, the heels can be reconstructed with synthetic acrylic filler and fibreglass mesh to restore normal conformation.

TUMOURS OF THE FOOT

Sarcoids are probably the commonest tumour located at the coronet and the treatment of these is extremely difficult. Such cases should be referred to a specialist centre where radiation or other means can be attempted. Nevertheless, there is still a high failure rate with the more aggressive types of fibroblastic tumours at this site. The more benign verrucose or occult lesions are far less common and can remain static for years (often until any insult, either accidental or iatrogenic is applied). They are probably best left alone unless full specialist facilities are available.

Squamous cell carcinoma and **melanoma** have also been reported at the coronary band. The prognosis for these is poor.

Two specific tumour types occur in and on the foot. These are the **sole fibroma** and the **keratoma** and are described in Chapter 19.

chapter 19

NEOPLASTIC CONDITIONS

Equine sarcoid	244
Basal cell carcinoma	252
Fibroma and fibrosarcoma	252
Haemangioma and haemangiosarcoma	253
Malignant fibrous histiocytoma (giant-cell tumour)	254
Leiomysosarcoma	254
Lipoma (liposarcoma)	254
Lymphangioma	255
Lymphoma	255
Lymphosarcoma (cutaneous histiocytic lymphosarcoma)	256
Mastocytoma (mast cell tumour) (equine cutaneous mastocytoma)	257
Melanoma and melanosarcoma	258
Neurofibroma	260
Ossifying fibroma (equine juvenile ossifying fibroma)	260
Squamous cell carcinoma	261
Sebaceous gland tumour	266
Sweat gland tumour	266
Fibroma of frog and sole	267
Keratoma	267
Equine Cushing's disease	269
Generalized lymphosarcoma	272

The incidence of skin tumours is relatively high in the horse and each tumour type has particular features which make early diagnosis important. By the time a solid tumour is clinically detectable it has already completed a major portion of its life cycle. The latent period before which a tumour becomes clinically detectable is highly unpredictable and will depend upon a number of characteristics such as the rate of replication versus cell death (the growth fraction), the inherent replication rate of the cells themselves (reflected crudely as the mitotic index or the proportion of cells undergoing mitosis at any one time) and the absolute number of tumour cells present. Some tumours are very slow growing while others are rapid. This means that equine tumours are usually only diagnosed when they are in a relatively advanced state. There is little which is predictable about cutaneous neoplasia.

The specific diagnosis of a tumour is very important, particularly with respect to the prognosis and possible treatment options. In some cases, such as the equine sarcoid, biopsy may be specifically contraindicated and a diagnosis may have to rely on other means. Some tumours are easily recognized clinically, e.g. melanoma, but others are much more difficult. Interference with a malignant tumour or incomplete surgical removal may result in a significant reduction in prognosis. Fortunately, the incidence of highly malignant tumours of equine skin is generally very low.

THE APPROACH TO A SUSPECTED SKIN TUMOUR

An instant diagnosis may sometimes be available through the definitive clinical character (such as melanoma). Where the mass is not so recognizable as to allow a definitive diagnosis to be made immediately, biopsy may be suggested: biopsy is usually definitive. However, the potential dangers of interference with any skin tumour must be considered carefully before performing any biopsy procedure. In many cases a reasoned judgement has to be made on the likely nature of the mass. Where biopsy is considered unavoidable, suitable therapeutic options should be available for treatment as soon as the results are known. Frozen sections examined immediately after removal may provide a rapid diagnosis, but this is often not feasible. In the case of very small tumours, total excisional biopsy (surgical removal) may be undertaken with some degree of safety.

Laboratory confirmation should always be undertaken and usually provides a positive diagnosis. Pathologists are usually highly skilled in recognizing the features of tumours. Where surgical removal is performed, all tissue removed should be submitted to the pathologist. Aspects of malignancy are clearly important (even if only retrospectively). Skilled pathologists are usually able to establish whether there is an adequate margin or whether excision has not been complete. A report of a 'safe margin of excision' is reassuring for the surgeon. Many tumours have local variations within the mass of tissue and examination of a relatively small piece may be misleading. For example, benign granulation tissue can be interspersed amongst a fibroblastic sarcoid; there may be an area of occult sarcoid around a smaller nodular or fibroblastic sarcoid; and there may be precancerous changes surrounding a squamous cell carcinoma lesion. A limited biopsy may provide the wrong information but extensive biopsy may be undesirable. The clinical examination and the experience of the clinician are therefore important.

Haematological responses including white cell and protein responses are generally not helpful in cutaneous neoplasia of any type. Cancer cachexia, characterized by weight loss, depression, anorexia, metabolic disturbances and general malaise which resolve after tumour treatment, is only rarely encountered in primary cutaneous neoplasia. However, where it does exist, it suggests that neoplastic lesions have significant secondary effects.

DIFFERENTIAL DIAGNOSIS OF SKIN NEOPLASIA

Common skin tumours
Fibroma/fibrosarcoma
Lymphoma
Lymphosarcoma
Melanoma/melanosarcoma
Neurofibroma (Schwannoma)
Ossifying fibroma
Sarcoid
Squamous cell carcinoma

Rare/unusual skin tumours
Basal cell carcinoma
Cutaneous mastocytoma
Giant cell tumours
Haemangioma/haemangiosarcoma
Histiocytoma (malignant/fibrous)
Lipoma/liposarcoma
Lymphangioma
Sebaceous gland tumour
Sweat gland tumour
Keratoma

Pituitary adenoma (adenoma of the pars intermedia) is an internal neoplastic tumour with skin manifestations recognized as Cushing's disease. The cutaneous manifestations (hirsutism, sweating, ectoparasitism and cutaneous abscessation) are not in themselves strongly suggestive of a tumour origin but are typical and easily recognized in most cases, especially when considered with other characteristic signs such as polydipsia/polyuria, supraorbital bulging, weight loss and laminitis.

DIAGNOSTIC PROCEDURES FOR NEOPLASIA

The majority of skin tumours fall into the nodular diseases category. There are some important features of diagnosis and treatment which should be appreciated before any interference is undertaken. These include aspects of malignancy and the tendency to recurrence.

Important diagnostic features include the following:

- Anatomical location(s) of the tumour(s)
- Elimination of other (non-neoplastic) (nodular) disease(s) such as allergy, infection, trauma and haematoma, preferably by clinical examination
- Number and similarity of tumours (multiple or single masses)
- Status of the draining local and regional lymph nodes
- Status of the surrounding tissue and any secondary effects (e.g. oedema, heat, pain, swelling)
- Presence of any systemic effects (weight loss, diarrhoea, physical deformities/abnormalities)

Physical examination

This must include:

1. A detailed, systematic clinical examination
2. Specific close examination of (all) the lesion(s) to establish individual extent and character
3. Examination of as much of the surrounding tissue and the appropriate draining lymph node(s) as possible.

All three of these have a strong influence on the prognosis.

The body condition of the horse and the health (or normality) of its system/organ functions may be seriously affected by some neoplastic disorders but much less so by others. Local invasion of tumour tissue may result in local distortions, physical alterations or functional problems, e.g. palpebral tumours may cause eyelid problems with secondary corneal ulceration or nasolacrimal obstructions with epiphora. Diffuse, ill-defined tumours may suggest malignancy or at least the prospect of treatment limitations. Few lymph nodes are readily palpable in the horse and further procedures such as endoscopy, radiography, ultrasonography and rectal examination may be required.

Cytological examination

All smears/aspirates obtained from tumours *must* be examined by an experienced pathologist. It is unacceptable to make a diagnosis without the help of such a specialist. The cell abnormalities are often subtle and difficult to interpret alongside artefactual alterations from sampling techniques. Malignant cells may be reported to exhibit some or all of the following:

- Irregular/bizarre cell size/shape with uneven/unusual staining
- Large obvious nucleoli within prominent/obvious nucleus with uneven staining and thickened nucleolar membranes
- High mitotic index (high proportion of cells in mitotic state)

Biopsy and histopathological examination (see The Approach to a Suspected Skin Tumour above and Chapter 3)

Biopsy of suspicious lesions is for the most part a sensible procedure. For the majority of skin lesions it is usually feasible under sedation and local analgesia alone. However, the equine sarcoid is probably best not subjected to biopsy unless an immediate therapeutic regimen can be applied (thus, a presumptive diagnosis is required). The interpretation of a biopsy relies heavily upon:

- Correct collection of a representative (diagnostic) specimen
- Correct processing (including fixation, section and staining)
- Careful examination by a qualified pathologist

Histopathology is compulsory for all excised tissues. There is little or no excuse for not submitting such specimens. These specimens will provide important information including the true (undistorted) characteristics of the tissue and the presence or absence of a clear line of demarcation to normal tissue. Unless every single tumour cell is removed, regrowth is likely and so, if only as an assessment of prognosis, surgical pathology is vital. If excision was not complete the owner can be warned that recurrence is likely; it is not then a disappointing surprise when the tumour recurs. Most owners will accept this more readily if communication is maintained.

Haematology and serum biochemistry

These are almost invariably very disappointing in skin neoplasia but may be significantly altered if:

- there is extensive organ involvement (either primary or secondary);
- there is significant secondary infection (either locally or systemically) as a result of impaired immune processes.

Radiology

This is sometimes useful in the horse but the anatomical difficulties make the benefit variable. Sinus and nasal involvement can be detected in some cases. Oblique and ventrodorsal projections are often required to establish the true extent but these are more difficult and in practice conditions may not be feasible. Thoracic radiography is sometimes indicated for highly malignant tumours but these are particularly unusual in equine skin apart from the lymphosarcoma complex.

Ultrasonography

A detailed ultrasonographic study of the region and the mass itself is often useful and is an underutilized aid. Space-occupying masses, fluid-filled cavities and displacements and distortions of the normal anatomy are easily recognized with experience.

EQUINE SARCOID

Profile

This is probably the most common cutaneous tumour found in horses worldwide. It is a locally aggressive fibroblastic tumour occurring in six clinically recognizable forms, all of which have a high propensity for recurrence. There is controversy over the aetiological role of papillomaviruses. A genome which closely resembles that of the bovine papillomavirus has been identified consistently in sarcoid tissue from donkeys and horses,[132] but no patent virus particle has yet been conclusively demonstrated. The distribution of the lesions and the epidemiology strongly suggest that flies are an important part of the pathogenesis.

Clinically and pathologically, sarcoids present most of the features of a true neoplasm. The predominant cell type is a malignant/transformed fibroblast with characteristic *in vitro* appearance and characteristics. Sarcoids generally have a high capacity for local tissue invasion into the dermis and subcutis. True metastatic dissemination does not occur, however. Tumours can appear in freshly healing wounds in previously normal horses, or re-occur at the same site following apparent complete surgical removal even up to 10 or more years later.

Individual horses may be genetically susceptible and a familial tendency to sarcoid has been identified. However, many horses may carry the genetic susceptibility to varying extent, possibly explaining the variations in numbers and types seen on individuals.

Sex (geldings more commonly) and age (1–6 years) predilections have been proposed, but no horse can be considered to be totally exempt from the condition on the grounds of sex, breed, colour or age. A familial tendency has also been identified, heavily supporting a genetic component.

The number of sarcoids affecting individual horses is very variable. Single lesions are frequently associated with wound sites. Sarcoids commonly multiply on the individual horse, sometimes very rapidly while some others remain relatively, or even completely, static for years. A few individuals show spontaneous full and permanent self-cure and a very few disappear spontaneously after being accidentally or intentionally (by biopsy) traumatized but these are exceptions rather than the rule. Interestingly, spontaneous remission usually means that the horse will not develop further lesions. However, the course of the condition is entirely unpredictable.

Clinical signs

Six distinct clinical entities which are noticeably different can be recognized.[86,133] Although each of these forms is commonly identifiable, it is important to recognize that the 'less severe' forms can rapidly progress to the more aggressive types, particularly if they are traumatized. Furthermore, the specific types may not be clearly identifiable in every case. It is, however, patently obvious that even the mildest forms are indeed sarcoid – *in vitro* cell cultures derived from these are typical and indistinguishable from those taken from the more aggressive lesions. These factors suggest that both cell and host factors are responsible in combination for the variety of forms.

Occult sarcoid

Predilection sites include the skin around the mouth and eyes, the neck and other relatively hairless areas of the body including the medial aspects of the forearm and thigh. Lesions show as hairless areas, often roughly circular. They usually contain one or more small cutaneous nodules (2–5 mm diameter) or roughened areas with a mild hyperkeratotic appearance (**Fig. 19.1**) but these may or may not be present or obvious in every case. An area of changed/altered, slightly thickened skin with thin hair coat and slight changes in hair pigment may be all that is seen (**Fig. 19.2**) and may be difficult to identify in winter-coated animals. The

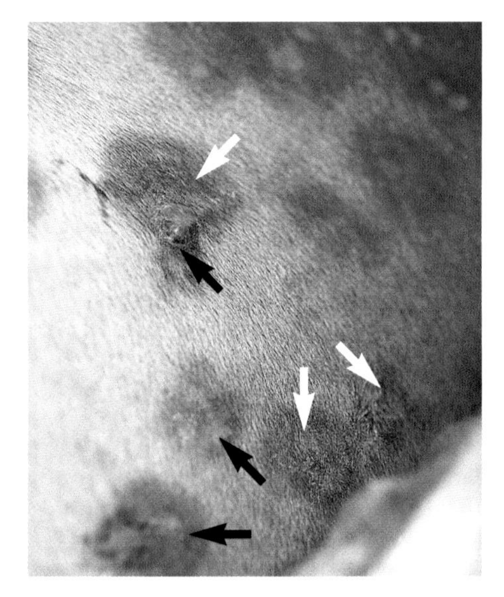

Figure 19.1 Occult sarcoid in the groin. Note that one or two of the lesions have a hyperkeratotic appearance (white arrows) with a few small nodules (black arrows).

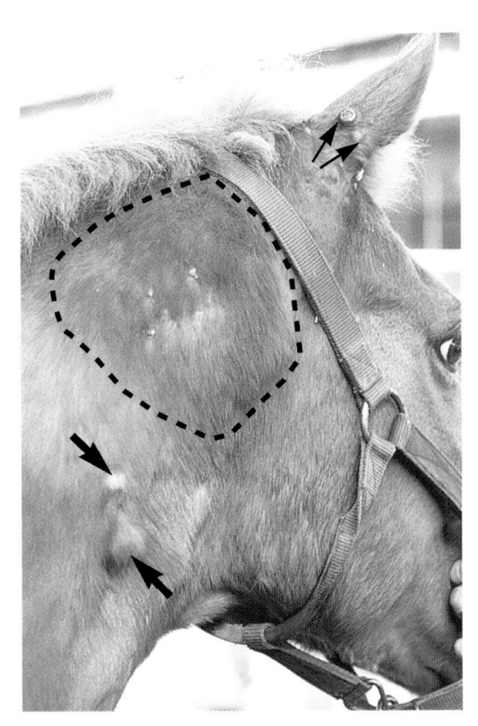

Figure 19.2 Occult sarcoid on the side of the neck, face and ear. Note the hair colour and density change. There are a few more obvious sarcoids of nodular and verrucose types present (arrows).

lesions are characteristically slow growing; they may progress to 'warty' verrucous growths (see Fig. 19.3) or if injured may develop rapidly into fibroblastic lesions (see Fig. 19.6). While the lesion remains as a static/quiescent hairless patch showing no evidence of growth in size or number of nodules, it may be wise not to interfere. Cases have existed for over 15 years without treatment or acceleration; however, extensive development of verrucose sarcoid or conversion into fibroblastic-type sarcoid usually demands immediate attention. This can occur at any time with or without apparent insult.

Differential diagnosis

- Dermatophytosis (ringworm)
- Blisters
- Burns
- Rub marks and chronic skin rubbing

Verrucous (warty) sarcoid

Predilection sites include the face, body and groin/sheath areas. The lesion has a characteristic wart-like growth in and on the skin (**Fig. 19.3**). Extensive areas can be affected and are often

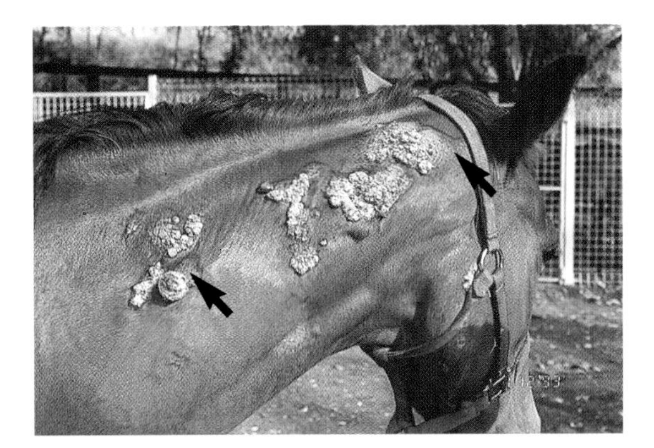

Figure 19.3 Verrucose sarcoid showing typical scaling and thickening. Note the occult area surrounding some of the more obvious tumour areas (arrows).

surrounded by an area of slightly thickened/changed skin (possibly reflecting a surrounding area of early occult sarcoid) with altered, thin hair-growth pattern.

Individual lesions may be sessile (flat-based) or pedunculated (with a narrow neck). The lesions are most often slow growing and not very aggressive until injured/insulted. However, small nodules may appear at any stage or over any area of the affected skin. These may develop a true fibroblastic character whether or not they are insulted or traumatized. Rubbing, biopsy, partial excision or minor or major trauma to the surface commonly result in a dramatic change to fibroblastic sarcoid over variable areas of the lesion.

Differential diagnosis

- Papillomatosis (warts)
- Chronic blistering
- Hyperkeratosis (e.g. chronic sweet itch)
- Equine sarcoidosis (chronic granulomatous disease)
- Squamous cell carcinoma (particularly of face)

Nodular sarcoid

Predilection sites include the groin, sheath or eyelid areas. The lesions are easily recognizable as firm, well-defined subcutaneous, spherical nodules of 5–20 mm diameter (**Fig. 19.4**) but can be much larger. The number of nodules varies widely – single, few, several or hundreds are common. The nodules usually lie under apparently normal skin (**Fig. 19.5**) and then may be freely movable. However, sometimes there are dermal and deep attachments which prevent independent movement

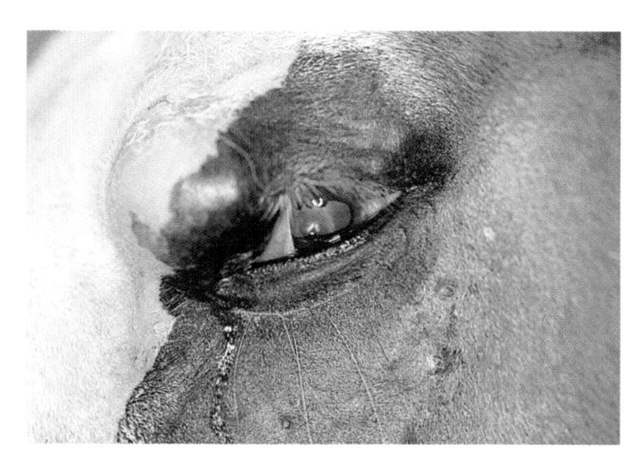

Figure 19.4 Nodular sarcoid in the eyelid with obstruction of the nasolacrimal duct causing epiphora. Note two smaller nodules on the face below the eye.

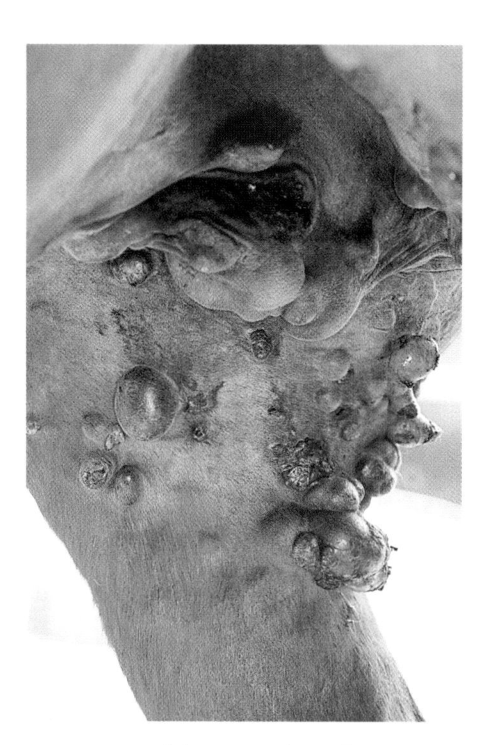

Figure 19.5 Nodular sarcoids in the groin. Some have ulcerated and become fibroblastic.

of the overlying skin and/or movement of the tumour mass relative to deeper tissue. The overlying skin may become thin over larger nodules and when these ulcerate they quickly take on a more aggressive fibroblastic character. A similar aggressive fibroblastic response commonly follows iatrogenic or accidental damage.

Differential diagnosis

- Fibroma
- Neurofibroma
- Equine eosinophilic granuloma
- Melanoma
- Collagen necrosis
- Dermoid cyst
- *Hypoderma* spp. (warble fly) cysts

Fibroblastic sarcoid

Predilection sites include the groin, eyelid, lower limbs and coronet, sites of skin wounds at any location and sites of any other types of sarcoid subjected to trauma or insult. The tumours have a characteristic aggressive, fleshy, ulcerated appearance and extensive local infiltration is common (**Fig. 19.6**). Both pedunculated and extensive sessile tumours with prominent ulceration and serum exudation are commonly encountered. The latter may reflect single or repeated insults to the 'lesser' forms but may develop spontaneously. They are common at sites of wounds (**Fig. 19.7**), and particularly on distal limb wounds, especially if other sarcoids are present elsewhere. Concurrent (excessive) granulation tissue growth serves to confuse the diagnosis. Accidental wounds which fail to heal may contain significant sarcoid components in the

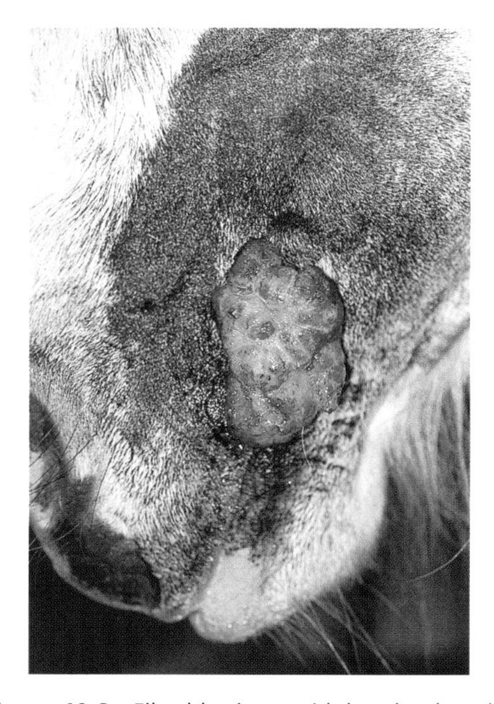

Figure 19.6 Fibroblastic sarcoid that developed at the site of a minor injury some 8 weeks previously.

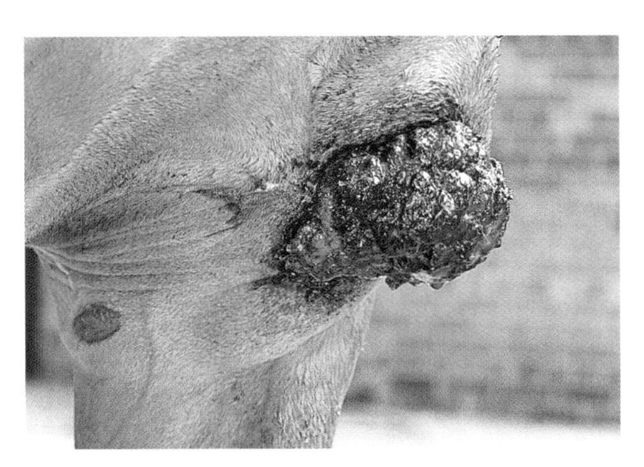

Figure 19.7 Fibroblastic sarcoid at the site of a previous wound which failed to heal. For several years prior to the injury the pony had had several verrucose sarcoids on the chest and extensive nodular lesions around one eye.

wound margins and irregularly and unpredictably mixed with granulation tissue.

Surgical wounds are also liable to sarcoid development. Dehiscence of the suture line within 2–7 days (or up to 5 years afterwards) for no apparent obvious reason may be suggestive of sarcoid development.

In spite of their aggressive appearance they do not metastasize but can spread locally in the dermis by local invasion/extension. Repeated insult (accidental or iatrogenic) appears to encourage local subdermal and dermal invasion. Therefore, tumours which have had previous unsuccessful treatment attempts can be extremely difficult to manage.

Differential diagnosis

- (Exuberant) granulation tissue
- Botryomycosis/fibrogranuloma
- Habronemiasis
- Neurofibroma/neurofibrosarcoma (ulcerated)
- Fibrosarcoma
- Squamous cell carcinoma
- Sweat gland tumour
- Pythiosis ('swamp cancer')

Mixed (verrucous, nodular and fibroblastic) sarcoid

Predilection sites include the face, eyelid, groin and medial thigh. This type of sarcoid probably represents a progressive/transient state between the verrucous/occult types and fibroblastic/nodular types (**Fig. 19.8**). Variations in proportion of the types is infinite and complex mixtures of any or all of the above types (containing both verrucous and fibroblastic elements) are common in long-standing lesions or those subjected to repeated minor trauma (such as rubbing by tack or harness). They become progressively more aggressive as more fibroblastic transformation takes place – a common consequence of biopsy or injury.

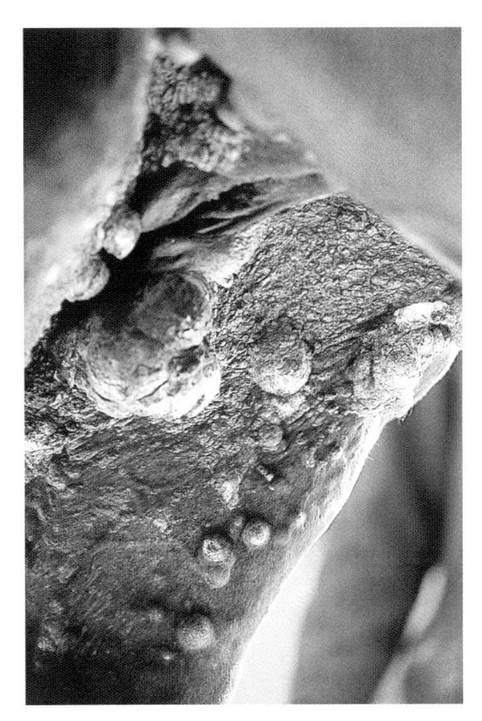

Figure 19.8 Extensive, ill-defined, mixed sarcoid in the groin showing elements of nodular, verrucose and occult types in particular with limited fibroblastic components arising from the other forms.

Differential diagnosis

- Little problem with recognition – the presence of more than one form of sarcoid in a single lesion is pathognomonic.
- Complex mixtures of granulation tissue in verrucose and/or fibroblastic sarcoid.
- Habronemiasis (particularly if affecting ulcerated verrucose sarcoid).

Malevolent sarcoid

This is a recently described variation[133] with predilection sites in the jaw, face, elbow and medial thigh areas in particular. A history of repeated trauma to other types of sarcoid, e.g. surgical interference, is commonly involved. However, some cases have no such history with spontaneous development of typical multiple, locally invasive sarcoids of nodular and fibroblastic character. Others show extensive infiltration of lymphatics (cords of tumour are commonly palpable) with numerous ulcerative nodules and surface involvement (**Fig. 19.9**). Although the local lymph nodes can be enlarged there are no reports of sarcoid tissue within them.

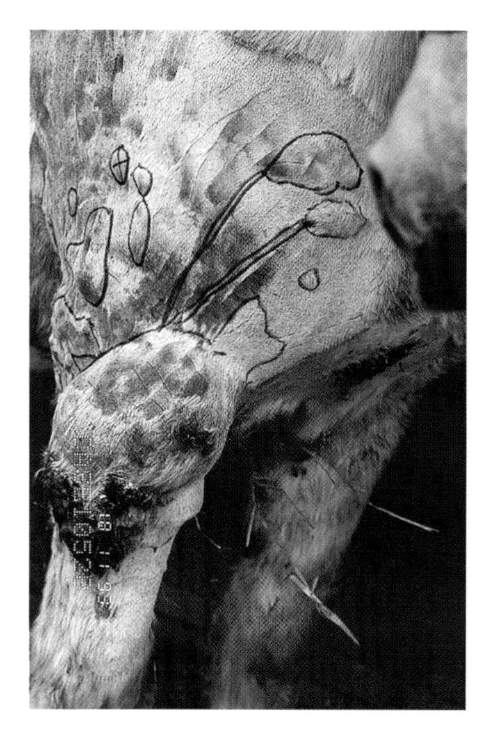

Figure 19.9 Malevolent sarcoid. The pen markings delineate the infiltrating cords of sarcoid which originated at a fibroblastic lesion on the elbow. Note the occult areas on the inside of the left leg.

Differential diagnosis

- Squamous cell carcinoma
- Subcutaneous mycosis
- Lymphangitis
- Glanders
- Enzootic lymphangitis
- Cutaneous histoplasmosis
- Lymphoma/lymphosarcoma (generalized or cutaneous histiocytic lymphosarcoma)

Diagnostic confirmation

- The clinical features are usually clearly recognizable but confirmation of the diagnosis is not always straightforward.
- Complications can arise when any of the differential diagnoses for the individual types is present simultaneously. Single lesions or single types on an individual horse are more difficult to diagnose definitively on clinical grounds alone. Multiple tumours with the characteristic features of more than one type of sarcoid on an individual horse make the diagnosis relatively simple – there is no other disease with the same range of clinical features and types.
- The tendency to progression of superficial (occult or verrucose) and nodular sarcoid to the more aggressive fibroblastic forms makes it important to obtain an early diagnosis and promptly consider appropriate treatment.
- Partial or excisional biopsy will almost always provide a definitive diagnosis but both carry attendant risks. A total excisional biopsy rather than a sample biopsy should be performed if this option is to be used and is feasible (see Chapter 3).
- A diagnosis may be made retrospectively when the tumour either becomes progressively more aggressive or the surgical site fails to heal normally. Wound breakdown and proliferation of fibroblastic tissue from the margins and depth of an excisional surgical site in a horse with other suspicious lesions are strong indicators that the lesion is a sarcoid. Early biopsy of this new tissue is indicated to confirm the presence of sarcoid and to eliminate other causes of wound breakdown (such as foreign body reactions, exuberant granulation tissue, etc.).
- Complications can arise particularly when sarcoid is diffusely mixed with granulation tissue. Biopsy may be very misleading if only one of the two distinctive tissue types is recognized in a particular specimen of the tissue.
- Hair pluckings and skin scrapings can be used to eliminate dermatophytosis (ringworm) and other ectoparasites in the case of occult and minor verrucose lesions. This procedure carries only minor risks of exacerbating a sarcoid.

Treatment

Treatment should follow as soon after diagnosis as possible. Suspicious lesions can justifiably be treated immediately after biopsy using an appropriate regimen (see below). In most cases diagnosis does not require a biopsy and so treatment can be instituted immediately.

▷ General treatment considerations

The prognosis for all cases is very guarded and owners must be made aware of the possible serious complications which can arise from this disease. Owners must be appraised of the limitations, cost and likely/possible outcome of the various treatment options. No case of sarcoid can be considered to be free of the disease, even following apparently successful treatment. There is a strong likelihood that prolonged or repeated treatments will be required. However, complete, spontaneous regression of tumours is occasionally seen and owners can then be reasonably assured that the condition is *unlikely* to recur.

Factors affecting choice of treatment methods

The value of the animal and the cost of treatment Many treatment methods are expensive and repeated treatments are commonly required both immediately and over the following years.

Previous treatments and history The prognosis for treatment is significantly worse if an unsuccessful attempt has been made previously.[19] Repeated failures make the prognosis very poor. Therefore, the best available option with the highest chance of success should always be used at the first attempt at treatment.[134]

Prognosis (likelihood of a successful outcome to the selected treatment method) Delays between biopsy and treatment may significantly alter the outlook.

Results of biopsy

- Delayed results may make treatment difficult or impossible or at least make the prognosis worse.
- Incorrect results, particularly when sarcoid is not diagnosed, are potentially disastrous. False positives are rare as the condition is easily recognized from biopsy specimens. There are, however, some occult or verrucose lesions and some mixtures of granulation tissue and sarcoid which are particularly difficult and require the opinion of an experienced pathologist.

Complication through co-existence of other factors such as granulation tissue, infection, myiasis, other neoplasia, etc., may alter both the histological and clinical appearance and may be misleading.

Facilities and practicality of the available treatment option. The best option may be economically or practically impossible. For example, radiation carries a generally good prognosis but is very restricted with respect to the size of tumour which can be treated and also requires special facilities. Extensive cryosurgery of multiple lesions may require prolonged general anaesthesia. Cisplatin is not currently widely available and AW4-LUDES cream is not available outside the United Kingdom (and is severely restricted even there).

The possibility of a contagious nature. The possibility of transmission to other horses in the group is important when considering treatment. Furthermore, there is little doubt that the condition can spread on the individual horse. The means for this are uncertain but flies are possibly involved in both aspects.

Treatment methods (see Table 19.1)

Many treatment methods including conventional and nonconventional approaches have been used with varying reported success. Only those which are documented and which are reported to have a benefit are considered here. Although isolated small lesions may respond well to surgical removal, incomplete excision (or even the use of biopsy punches) can precipitate rapid fibroblastic proliferation which can be difficult if not impossible to treat successfully. The general principles of the available treatment methods are described in Chapter 4. The various treatment methods described below may be more or less applicable to specific types of sarcoid. Currently there is no effective treatment regimen for the malevolent form of the disease.

Benign neglect is a realistic option in some cases where either the lesions are so extensive as to make any method impossible or so small as to make the cost of treatment seem unnecessary. For the latter cases this option should always be viewed with some caution as many cases become progressively worse.

Surgical methods

Ligation This is limited to small nodular lesions or fibroblastic lesions with a well-defined 'neck' (see Fig. 4.1). Occult and verrucose lesions and sessile fibroblastic and mixed sarcoids are not amenable to this treatment. Results with nodular lesions in the groin in particular are satisfactory.

Surgical excision There is a high rate of recurrence in all except the most confined and defined lesions following surgical excision.[135] Superficial (occult and verrucose) lesions can be effectively treated by wide excision provided that the wound can be closed and then protected during healing. Any delay in healing may be due to sarcoid

Table 19.1 Relative value[a] of treatment methods in the author's experience for the various forms of equine sarcoid.

	Treatment	Type of sarcoma				
		Occult	Verrucose	Nodular	Fibroblastic	Mixed
Surgical	Ligation	N/A[b]	N/A	***	#[c]	#
	Excision	***	*	***	*	*
	Cryosurgery	**	**	N/A	*	*
	Hyperthermia	**	*	N/A	*	N/A
	Electrocautery	**	**	***	*	*
	CO_2-YAG Laser	***	**	***	*	*
Cytotoxic/antimitotic	Topical (AW-4LUDES)	****	***	**	***	***
	Cisplatin	N/A	N/A	***	***	N/A
	Podophyllin	*	#	N/A	#	#
Immune methods	Autogenous vaccines	#	#	#	#	#
	BCG	N/A	N/A	****[d]	*** #	#
Radiation	Brachytherapy	N/A	N/A	*****	*****	***
	Teletherapy	*****	*****	*****	*****	*****

[a] *****, expected results over 80–90% success; ****, expected 60–80% success; ***, 40–60% success; **, 20–40% success; *, < 20% success.
[b] N/A, not appropriate modality.
[c] #, liable to be worse.
[d] BCG therapy has a good reputation in the treatment of nodular lesions around the eye but a poor one elsewhere. The results are particularly poor on limb or body lesions.

regrowth. This is usually a rapid development of fibroblastic sarcoid and complete or partial failure of the wound to heal.[136] Wound break-down within days of surgery is a common immediate indicator of failure to excise all the sarcoid tissue[137] but sarcoid regrowth can take up to 5 or more years to recur at the site.

Notwithstanding the limitations of surgery, excision of nodular lesions carries a somewhat better prognosis provided that the lesion is not attached to the skin and provided that the operative site is not contaminated with sarcoid tissue released by cutting into the lesion itself. Where these criteria can be met, the prognosis is usually quite good. Nodular lesions in the eyelids, however, are potentially very dangerous as they commonly have extensive ramifications through adjacent tissues and often extend into the muscles of the eyelids. Surgery almost always fails in these sooner or later.

Fibroblastic, mixed and malevolent sarcoids are not generally suitable for surgical excision alone. The prognosis following surgery can be improved somewhat by combining it with other modalities such as cryosurgery, topical cytotoxic compounds, intralesional cisplatin injections or radiation.

Cryosurgery Cryosurgery suffers from the same limitations as sharp excision. The margins of the lesion need to be defined and thermocouples placed so that the whole lesion is destroyed without damage to underlying or adjacent tissues. Cryosurgery is commonly employed[28] but on its own has a relatively poor success rate (except in the smallest and most defined lesions which carry a reasonable success rate). The reported benefit from cryoantigens released into the bloodstream which result in a resolution of lesions remote from the treated one[138] has not subsequently been substantiated. The selection of the site is also important as cryosurgery will inevitably result in extensive tissue destruction. Local scarring may have important effects on function. Furthermore, it is particularly difficult to apply in a controlled fashion to large areas and infiltrative lesions. It is not an appropriate method for tumours in and on the eyelid in particular.

Hyperthermia/radiofrequency hyperthermia Hyperthermia has produced some good results,[139] but repeated procedures are required and again the extent of the tumour has to be defined so that every sarcoid cell can be effectively destroyed. The method has not gained general acceptance.

Electrocautery Surgical electrocautery has advantages in that the margin of the lesion is effectively cauterized and so is extended beyond the incisional line. Furthermore, bleeding from the margins of the wound is minimal. However, its efficiency depends on the extent of the tumour and its locality. Scarring can be limited if primary closure of the wound is possible.

Laser surgery (CO_2-YAG laser excision) Laser excision is reported to have a high success rate, but again selection of the most appropriate lesions is very important. The major benefit appears to lie in the bloodless field of surgery and the low rate of recurrence may reflect the destruction of marginal cells which might be left viable by surgery or cryosurgery. The cosmetic results are, however, not often acceptable. Equipment is expensive and not readily available. It also requires very careful safety precautions.

Local/topical medication with cytotoxic or antimitotic compounds/chemotherapy

Topical chemotherapeutic agents including cytotoxic and antimitotic compounds such as 5-fluorouracil or cisplatin can be used effectively. They are limited, however, by their overall efficacy and the need to sustain medication over prolonged periods. However, when topically applied or injected into lesions they seem to have little or no untoward systemic effects.

Systemic cytotoxic or antimitotic compounds are probably irrelevant at this time.

Heavy-metal compounds (inorganic arsenic/antimony/mercury salts) These induce extensive tissue necrosis and scarring. Combinations of these compounds can limit the toxicity of each individual one but still maintain the efficacy. They are easy to apply and some complex mixtures of these with antimitotic, corticosteroid and cytotoxic drugs have a reasonable reputation (e.g. AW4-LUDES).[19]

Cisplatin (*cis*-diaminedichloroplatinum; DDP) (**Platinol**, Bristol Myers Oncology, USA; **Cisplatin Injection**, David Bull Laboratories, Warwick, UK and Mulgrave, Victoria, Australia) Good results are reported for small fibroblastic and nodular lesions in particular but it requires repeated injection into the site of the lesion.[140] In some cases it can be used in conjunction with surgical debulking. Emulsions made up from equal volumes of an aqueous solution of 1 mg cisplatin/ml and either sesame or almond oil may be used to provide a longer effect from each injection. A dose of 1 mg cisplatin per cubic centimetre of tumour is suggested but this can be very difficult to inject into the denser forms of sarcoid. This method is certainly worth exploring, although it is probably not applicable to verrucose or occult lesions. Furthermore, the material is not universally available and carries significant dangers for the operators.

Podophyllin Disappointing and unreliable results are common, with few good reports.

5-Fluorouracil Applied in ointment form under a bandage[141] or topically on a daily basis for some weeks. It can be successful on single, small occult or verrucose sarcoids and is also a useful material for controlling large areas of verrucose or occult sarcoid which cannot effectively be treated by any other means. Scarring is usually minimal, although the treated area can show marked reaction as cells are destroyed over a wide area of the surface of the skin.

Immunological methods

Treatment by means of vaccination has been undertaken by several research workers and is still performed by some practitioners. Bovine 'wart vaccine' has been used and was found valueless. It may indeed make the condition worse.[133] Pox vaccines administered intralesionally are also unsuccessful.

Vaccine (autogenous) Use of autogenous vaccines in treatment of the equine sarcoid is probably contraindicated. The method is based on the assumption that a viral aetiology is implicated and that the virus can then be used to induce a curative immune response. The results of this simple treatment suggest that this is not the case and if it worked it would surely have become universal practice. Many sarcoid cases which are treated with an autogenous vaccine are reported to be worse afterwards, with some cases developing several thousand lesions. The few cases which do resolve spontaneously suggest that there is some 'immunological' response available but autogenous vaccines do not appear to be the most appropriate way of inducing this.

Immunomodulation Immunomodulating proteins including various types of protein cell-wall fractions derived from Bacillus Calmette-Geurin (BCG) or other mycobacteria, or live, freeze-dried (lyophilized) BCG have been used widely.[142] The material is injected intralesionally at repeated intervals (see Chapter 4, p. 58). The technique carries a fair to good prognosis for treatment of nodular and some fibroblastic lesions in and around the eyelids in particular. The prognosis seems to be worse away from this area and some fibroblastic lesions on the limbs appear to be aggravated rather than treated and in fact become worse. The method is probably not appropriate for mixed, verrucose or occult lesions because the diffuse nature of the tumours precludes effective intralesional injection.

Radiation methods

Radiation (brachy- or tele-) therapy using gamma radiation carries a very good prognosis within the limits of the technology.[143] It is usually limited by cost and availability as well as the need to consider operator safety. It is therefore usually restricted to smaller lesions in areas for which no other method is suitable, such as the eyelids and over joints, etc. (see Fig. 4.6) The value of beta radiation delivered to superficial lesions is doubtful in view of its poor penetration through tissues (see Fig. 4.5). It is therefore not applicable to larger tumours with extensive tissue involvement. (See Chapter 4, p. 60.)

BASAL CELL CARCINOMA

Profile

A rare, slow-growing ulcerative tumour most often found on the face, neck, pectoral regions and trunk of older horses.

Clinical signs

Solitary, well-demarcated firm nodular dermal mass which frequently ulcerates. The margins of the lesion commonly develop a 'piled-up' raised appearance giving the impression of a crater (**Fig. 19.10**). Nonulcerating lesions are usually alopecic.

Differential diagnosis

- Granulation tissue
- Foreign body reaction
- Habronema
- Botryomycosis
- Fibroblastic sarcoid
- Fibroma (fibrosarcoma)
- Squamous cell carcinoma
- Other ulcerating tumours

Diagnostic confirmation

- Biopsy (excisional) is usually justified in small tumours.

Treatment

Surgical ablation is usually curative. Intralesional cisplatin or radiation can also be used effectively.

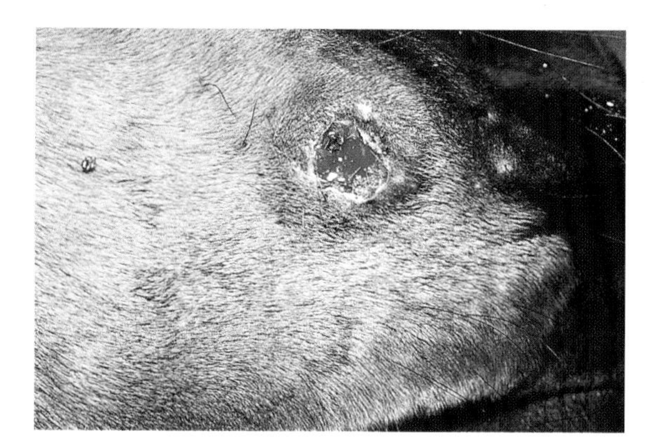

Figure 19.10 Basal cell carcinoma showing typical 'piled-up' margins and a central ulcerated area.

Prognosis

Good. Seldom if ever metastasizes or recurs at the site of full surgical excision.

FIBROMA AND FIBROSARCOMA

Profile

Uncommon tumour arising from dermal or subcutaneous fibroblasts. Older horses are more liable with predilection sites on the head, legs, neck and flanks. Fibroma is one of the commonest neoplasms encountered in the frog of the horse's foot. (See Fig. 19.26, p. 267.)

Clinical signs

Often single, firm or soft, well-circumscribed, dermal or subcutaneous nodules which may ulcerate or develop into a flattened, verrucous or fleshy, cauliflower-like lesion (**Fig. 19.11**). The surface may be hyperkeratotic in the early stages.

Differential diagnosis

- Sarcoid (nodular, verrucose, fibroblastic or mixed depending on type and stage)
- Exuberant granulation tissue
- Foreign body reaction
- Lymphoma/lymphosarcoma
- Other tumours (including keratoma of the foot)

Diagnostic confirmation

- Histological section of biopsy or whole tumour

Treatment

Total surgical excision or cryotherapy are often only partly successful. The best results are obtained

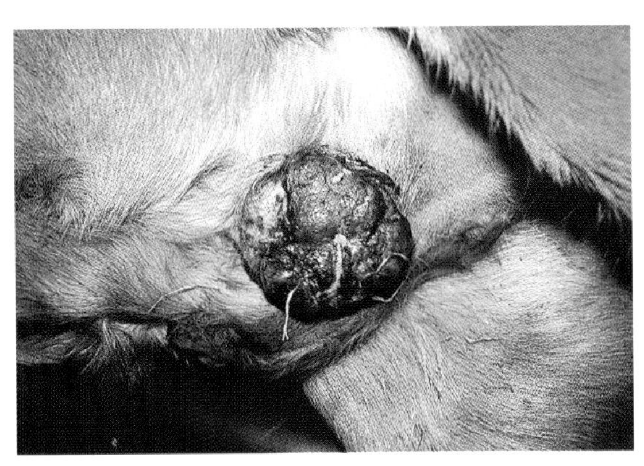

Figure 19.11 Fibrosarcoma in the girth region with a typically ulcerated, cauliflower appearance.

by radiation (teletherapy) but this is not widely available as an option.

Prognosis

Most fibromas are benign. Fibrosarcomas may be multiple and are locally invasive but normally have little or no tendency to metastasize.

HAEMANGIOMA AND HAEMANGIOSARCOMA

Profile

Uncommon cutaneous tumours of blood vessels. A congenital surface form (commonly referred to as a congenital vascular hamartoma) has been recorded in distal limbs of Arabian foals in particular. Affects elbow, groin, thorax and distal limbs (rarely eyelids/conjunctiva), associated with numerous tortuous, enlarged blood vessels. Many cases are regarded as vascular hamartoma. (A hamartoma is an abnormal accumulation of a normal tissue type and most often affects muscle (muscular hamartoma), blood vessels (vascular hamartoma) and dermal melanocytes.)

Clinical signs

The congenital form appears as a fleshy, proliferative, papilloma-like lesion restricted to skin surface which bleeds readily with minor trauma and which is very difficult to remove surgically without recurrence (**Fig. 19.12**).

Larger vascular hamartomas and haemangiomas can be found in the subcutaneous tissues (**Fig. 19.13**) and may involve the overlying skin.

Single lesions are commoner than multiple ones.

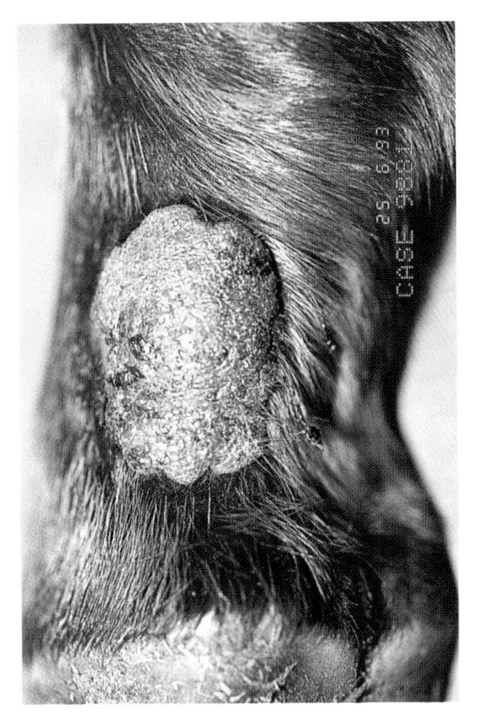

Figure 19.12 Congenital vascular haemangioma on the hind pastern of a 1-week-old Arabian foal.

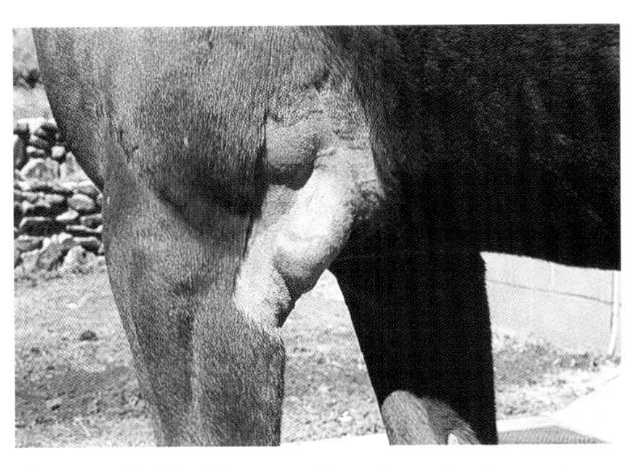

Figure 19.13 Haemangioma/vascular hamartoma in the elbow region.

Differential diagnosis

- Lymphoedema
- Viral papilloma (including the congenital form)
- Mixed, verrucose, fibroblastic, malevolent, sarcoid
- Exuberant granulation tissue

Diagnostic confirmation

- Biopsy (section or surgical removal) and histopathology

Treatment
Complete surgical ablation under general anesthesia followed by mesh, split- or full-thickness skin grafting of the resultant defect can be used but a high failure rate is common in the congenital form. They may sometimes respond to radiation teletherapy or brachytherapy.

Prognosis
Congenital forms are particularly difficult to resolve. Recurrences are common unless surgical excision is meticulous and the common sites make this problematical.

MALIGNANT FIBROUS HISTIOCYTOMA (GIANT-CELL TUMOUR)

Profile
Very rare tumours found in the neck and proximal regions of limbs.

Clinical signs
The lesions are characteristically solitary, firm and poorly circumscribed. They are locally invasive but very slow to metastasize.

Differential diagnosis
- Sarcoid (nodular, mixed and malevolent forms)
- Allergic collagen necrosis
- Insect bites and persistent urticaria
- Foreign body reactions

Diagnostic confirmation
- Biopsy shows characteristic histopathology

Treatment
Surgical excision can be difficult owing to invasive nature of tumour, but if performed meticulously can result in total resolution. Cryosurgery and laser excision are, theoretically at least, possible treatment methods.

Prognosis
Recurrence is common owing to the locally invasive nature of the tumour and the consequent difficulty in removal.

LEIOMYOSARCOMA

Profile
Rare muscle tumours often showing erosion of overlying skin.

Clinical signs
Clinically similar (identical) to squamous cell carcinoma. Early ulceration with minimal bleeding is common. The tumours grow moderately rapidly but have little local invasion. They commonly have a malodorous nature.

Differential diagnosis
- Squamous cell carcinoma
- Habronemiasis
- Deep dermal mycosis
- Bacterial infection of nonhealing wound/granulation tissue
- Botryomycosis

Diagnostic confirmation
- Surgical excision or biopsy and histopathology

Treatment
Total surgical removal or radiation are the only effective options.

Prognosis
Guarded. Some are very difficult to remove fully without damaging underlying tissues.

LIPOMA (LIPOSARCOMA)

Profile
Cutaneous lipomas are relatively uncommon when compared to other species and liposarcomas are very rare. Mesenteric lipomas are, however, very common in older horses where they can cause serious colic. The cutaneous tumours are formed from subcutaneous lipoid tissue primarily in aged horses. Fat/obese animals are most affected, but significant lipomas can also be found in some thin horses.

Clinical signs
Entirely subcutaneous, soft but well-defined, lobulated or smooth mass which may be mobile under the skin (**Fig. 19.14**). The tumours are slow to grow and may fluctuate in size with body condition.

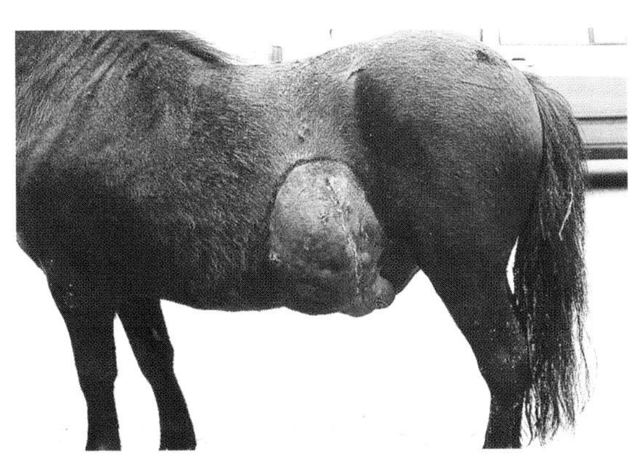

Figure 19.14 Subcutaneous lipoma in a Shetland pony mare. A surgical biopsy taken 2 weeks previously confirmed the nature of the multilobulated, soft, subcutaneous mass.

Differential diagnosis

- Sarcoid (nodular, mixed nodular and malevolent)
- Foreign body reactions
- Haematoma (organizing)
- Hernia
- Muscular, vascular or connective tissue hamartoma

Diagnostic confirmation

- Ultrasonographic examination is very useful (characteristic echo pattern).
- Histopathology (aspiration or biopsy).

Treatment

Surgical removal is effective and it may help to limit diet for some weeks before surgery. There is no recorded tendency to recurrence, but multiple tumours are possible.

Prognosis

Good, but other lipomas may develop locally or at other sites (internal and external).

LYMPHANGIOMA

Profile

A rare, benign tumour of lymphatic vessels located in axillary or inguinal regions of older horses.

Clinical signs

Multinodular or fluctuant subcutaneous masses occurring singly or in groups (**Fig. 19.15**). There is seldom any ulceration and tumours remain entirely subcutaneous.

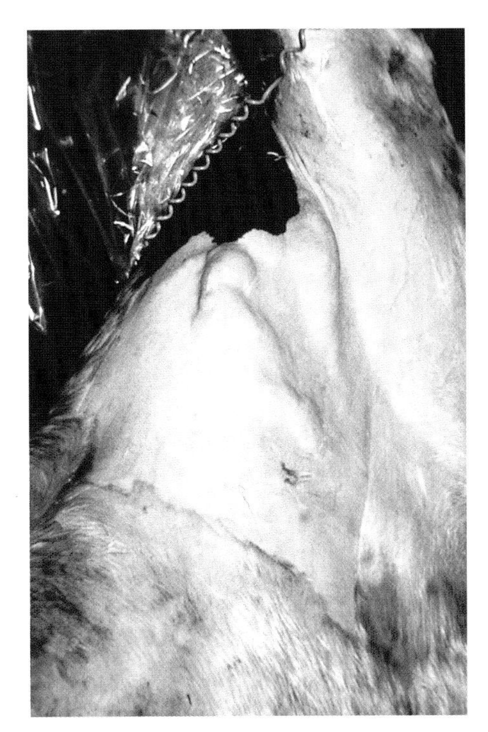

Figure 19.15 Lymphangioma on the sternum of an anaesthetized horse. Note the multinodular group of interconnected subcutaneous lesions.

Differential diagnosis

- Sarcoid (nodular and malevolent)
- Lymphoma
- Lymphosarcoma (generalized or cutaneous histiocytic type)

Diagnostic confirmation

- Surgical biopsy (or excision) and histopathology.
- Ultrasonography is useful.

Treatment

Surgical removal is usually feasible and effective. Radiation by teletherapy may be used in cases where the site precludes surgery.

Prognosis

Guarded; some will recur and multiple tumours can be present.

LYMPHOMA

Profile

Any tumour involving the lymphoid tissue can be termed a lymphoma. They are commoner in older

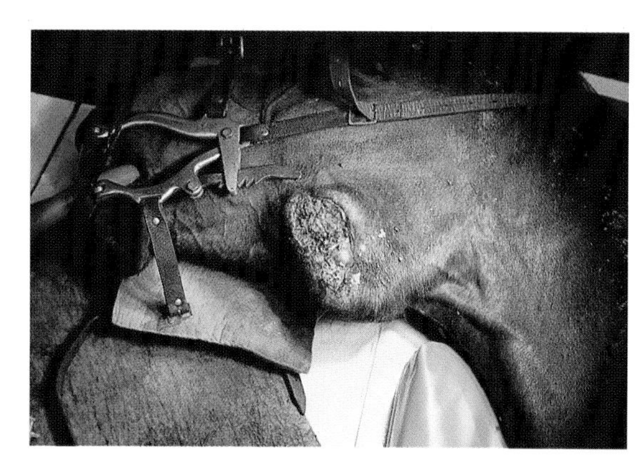

Figure 19.16 Ulcerated lymphoma on the skin of the face.

horses in the region of the jaw and distal limb but can occur at any site. A significant number of cases are tentatively linked to the presence of ovarian granulosa cell tumour in mares.

Clinical signs

Depressed, ulcerated lesion involving subcutaneous infiltration giving a diffuse, ill-defined character. A slight discharge with some scab formation over nonhealing ulcerated skin is usual (**Fig. 19.16**).

Differential diagnosis

- Fibroma, fibrosarcoma
- Sarcoid (multiple or single nodular or malevolent)
- Foreign body reaction/fibrosis
- Scarring/cicatrization of skin (particularly after a wound which has been very slow to heal)

Diagnostic confirmation

- Clinical features.
- Biopsy or surgical ablation and histopathology.
- Ultrasonography and radiography may help.
- Careful rectal and ultrasonographic (or assay of hormones) should establish the presence of a primary granulosa cell tumour in mares.

Treatment

Surgical removal or radiation teletherapy (or brachytherapy) are the only options likely to be effective. The possible value of cisplatin is uncertain at this time. Removal of a primary granulosa cell tumour may resolve secondary lymphoma-like cutaneous masses.

Prognosis

Very guarded; the prognosis depends heavily on treatment efficiency. The prognosis is significantly worse for lymphomas not associated with operable granulosa cell tumours.

LYMPHOSARCOMA (CUTANEOUS HISTIOCYTIC LYMPHOSARCOMA)

Profile

Infrequent tumour affecting the skin only. Middle-aged to old horses are most often affected and present with generalized lesions (trunk, limbs and neck). Some cases are possibly related to a primary ovarian granulosa cell tumour. A very similar appearance with a very much worse prognosis is presented by the cutaneous lesions of generalized lymphosarcoma.

Clinical signs

Multiple, subcutaneous nodules (1–35 mm diameter) are typical (**Fig. 19.17**). The lesions may appear suddenly and then may regress slightly and reappear at irregular intervals. Later the nodules become persistent and slowly enlarge. Lesions are also found in nasal and oral mucosa and the pharynx. There may be an associated dyspnoea or possible dysphagia. Cutaneous lesions may ulcerate and become infected, producing a thin, purulent or seropurulent discharge (**Fig. 19.18**).

Concurrent systemic signs include depression, weight loss, generalized lymphadenopathy, ventral oedema, undulating fever, respiratory distress,

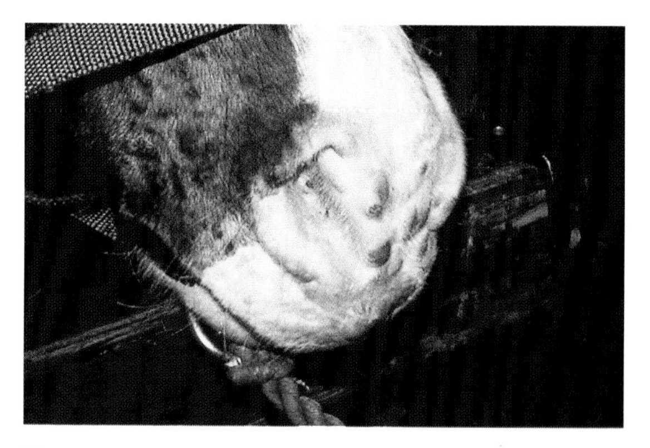

Figure 19.17 Cutaneous histiocytic lymphosarcoma nodules over the muzzle and face. There were many others over the body, nasal cavity and pharynx. Many of the cutaneous ones were ulcerated.

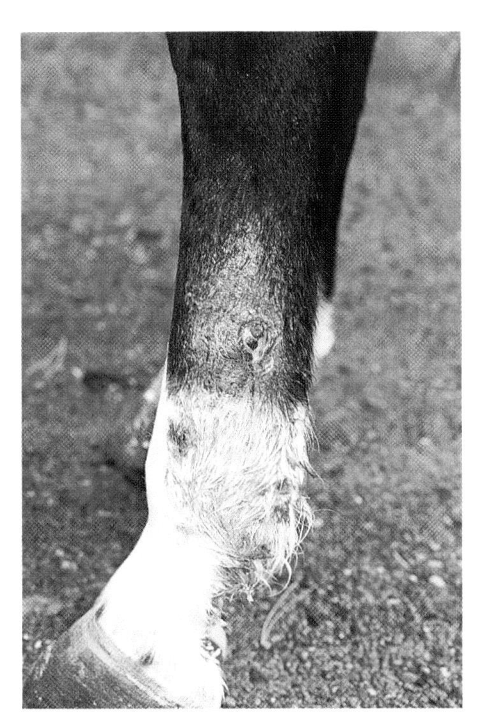

Figure 19.18 Cutaneous histiocytic lymphosarcoma lesions which have ulcerated and produce a thin plasma-like discharge. This mare had a concurrent ovarian granulosa cell tumour.

reduced exercise tolerance, colic and intestinal malabsorption with or without diarrhoea. Anaemia and intermittent hypercalcaemia are also present in some cases but all these signs are far more prominent in the more rapid course characteristic of generalized lymphosarcoma with cutaneous involvement.

Differential diagnosis

- Intestinal, thoracic or generalized lymphosarcoma with cutaneous metastases
- Cutaneous or subcutaneous lymphoma/lymphangioma
- Sarcoid (malevolent or nodular forms)
- Cutaneous histoplasmosis
- Ulcerative lymphangitis (*Corynebacterium pseudotuberculosis*)
- Farcy (equine cutaneous glanders)
- Multiple insect bite reactions
- Idiopathic collagen necrosis/nodular paniculitis/eosinophilic collagen necrosis
- Urticaria

Diagnostic confirmation

- Biopsy of nodules and/or enlarged lymph nodes
- Fine needle aspiration and direct cytology (impression smears of ulcerated lesions is often disappointing with heavy inflammatory infiltration and infection)
- Endoscopy of nasal cavities and pharynx
- Serum chemistry and haematology
  - elevation of liver enzymes indicates liver involvement
  - intermittent elevation of serum calcium
  - elevated serum globulin and plasma fibrinogen with reduced serum albumin concentration
  - occasionally lymphopenia or leukaemia
  - paracentesis of thorax or peritoneal cavity for cytological examination of exfoliating cells. Note, however, that many lymphosarcoma lesions occurring in the body cavities are not exfoliative and so cytology of fluid aspirates may be disappointing.
- Evaluation of bone marrow (requires skilled pathologist)

Treatment

Surgical removal of ulcerating masses is palliative only. Single ulcerating lesions can be effectively removed if the horse is only affected by the cutaneous form of the condition.

Removal of a concurrent ovarian granulosa cell tumour may be curative. In all cases of confirmed histiocytic lymphosarcoma in mares, a detailed clinical examination must be directed to establish the presence or otherwise of a granulosa cell tumour.

Supportive therapy is very important. Iron deficiency anaemia and recurrent infections and infestations with ectoparasites and gastrointestinal parasites are common due to impaired immune status.

Prognosis

True histiocytic cutaneous forms carry a reasonable prognosis with some cases living for up to 5 or more years following diagnosis. The prognosis will depend heavily on the extent of involvement and any secondary complications such as intractable limb oedema, weight loss and parasitism. Primary granulosa cell tumours should be investigated thoroughly in all cases. Generalized (internal) lymphosarcoma cases seldom live for more than a few months from diagnosis and the progression is so rapid that differentiation from the cutaneous disease is relatively simple.

MASTOCYTOMA (MAST CELL TUMOUR) (EQUINE CUTANEOUS MASTOCYTOMA)

Profile

A rare tumour occurring more frequently in young or middle-aged male horses than in females or older horses.

Clinical signs

Usually single, cutaneous nodule (2–20 mm diameter) with a focal aggregation of mast cells, eosinophils, fibrinoid necrosis of collagen and, occasionally, mineralization of contents. The surface may be normal, hairless or ulcerated. Multiple lesions can occur and appear to be less responsive to treatment.

Differential diagnosis

- Sarcoid (nodular form especially if centre is necrotic – when it may be softer)
- Eosinophilic/allergic collagenolytic granuloma complex
- Insect bite/sting
- Cutaneous amyloidosis

Diagnostic confirmation

- Fine needle aspirate/biopsy or impression smears
  - Giemsa stain reveals heavy eosinophil and mast cell infiltration with metachromic granules
- Biopsy, histopathology

Treatment

Surgical ablation is often effective. Intralesional injection of distilled water (may require 2–4 treatments at 4–6 day intervals) or triamcinolone or methylprednisolone acetate can also be useful. Oral cimetidine (5 mg/kg q 24 h for 3–6 weeks) has been suggested as a treatment. This has still to be substantiated. The value of cisplatin is uncertain. The low numbers of cases make the treatments difficult to compare clinically.

Prognosis

A good prognosis is usual. Some lesions undergo spontaneous resolution without apparent reason. The theoretical dangers associated with surgery are poorly quantified in the horse.

MELANOMA AND MELANOSARCOMA

Profile

Melanotic hamartomas are 'depots' of melanin pigment and are commonly found in the linings of the guttural pouches (particularly overlying major blood vessels) and on oral and other mucosae. These may vary from time to time in location and size.

Melanomas are benign tumours of melanocytes. They are noninvasive and cause disruption by space-occupying bulk.

All the common variations are largely (but not exclusively) limited to grey horses. Other colours can be affected with typical melanomas. Almost all grey horses over 6–8 years of age will have one or more melanomas at some location. Some families of grey horses have a higher incidence (possible genetic predisposition).

They are commonly found around anus, vulva, tail and prepuce (and also in guttural pouch), less commonly in parotid salivary and lymph nodes, eyelids, lips, and occur sporadically anywhere on or in the body (iris, internal organs or foot[144]).

Melanosarcomas are rapidly invasive and metastasize early and widely but are rare. Their effects in tissues are dependent on their relative number and size, the extent of space-occupying size and the extent of tissue interference.

Clinical signs

Small (or larger), hard spherical nodules in skin or subcutis (**Fig. 19.19**). Some lesions may ulcerate and discharge a thick, black, tarry discharge. Single discrete nodules may have pedicle or may be coalescent with many lesions (often hundreds or more of variable sizes). Growth is characteristically slow.

Melanomas can occur at almost any site and can reach considerable size. Those developing in the parotid lymph nodes and salivary glands and subcutaneous lesions are most obvious. Secondary signs are possible, including interference with any other organ such as the spinal cord (ataxia and weakness), trachea (dyspnoea/stertor), jugular groove and guttural pouch (Horner's syndrome), heart muscle (arrhythymias), etc.

Differential diagnosis

- Habronemiasis
- Parotid salivary gland pathology
- Warble fly (*Hypoderma bovis*)
- Cutaneous collagen necrosis/allergic collagenolytic granuloma
- Sarcoid (nodular form)
- Lymphoma/lymphosarcoma
- Mast cell tumours
- Fibroma/fibrosarcoma

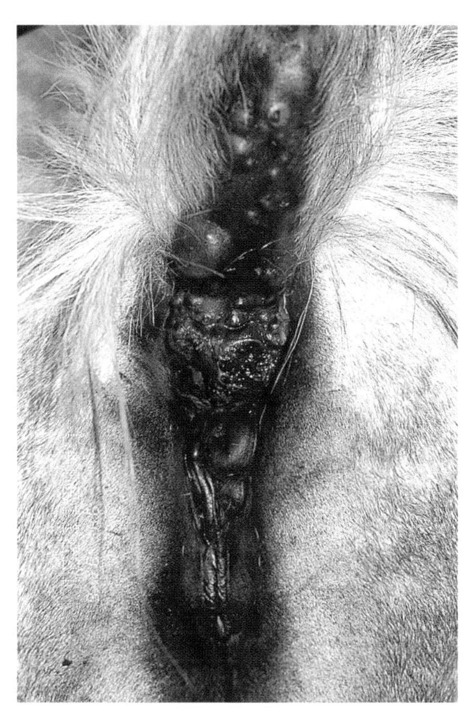

Figure 19.19 Melanomas in the perineum. Nodular and ulcerated forms are common at this site and can reach alarming size without affecting the well-being of the horse.

Diagnostic confirmation

- Appearance and location are characteristic.
- Biopsy by fine needle aspirate is a very simple and very positive test – the back pigmented material is obvious and pathological examination is usually not required except to establish the true character of the cells themselves.
- Complete removal and histopathology.
- It is possibly unwise to partially excise a melanoma.

Treatment

Surgical removal Single small tumours (<3 cm diameter) are usually more successfully treated by wide surgical excision or cryonecrosis therapy. Surgical removal of troublesome lesions is possible and even ligation of pedunculated lesions may be effective in isolated lesions where this is feasible. (**Note:** Surgical excision alone can in some horses stimulate rapid tumour regrowth caused by stimulation to abnormal melanoblasts in proximity to the surgical site.[22])

Cryosurgery Cryonecrosis using a double freeze–thaw cycle is effective in treating ulcerated and discharging lesions and is useful for tumours which are inaccessible to total surgical excision, e.g. in the anal sphincter area. The tumour is surgically debulked as far as possible and the remaining inaccessible area is treated by cryotherapy. However, this rarely 'cures' the problem but it allows a further useful life span for the treated horse.

Cisplatin by intralesional injection Tumours less than 3 cm diameter should be debulked first and a vegetable oil-based emulsion of cisplatin injected into the base of the tumour at the rate of 1 mg/cm^3 of tissue every second week for 4 treatments. The drug is irritant and the use of 22–25G needles is advisable to stop leakage following injection. Injection is continued as the needle is withdrawn to deposit the drug along the needle track. Injections should be spaced 5–8 mm apart.[140] Treatment is limited to small tumours but such melanomas will resolve. The relative risks of tumour and treatment will not support the method in most cases. Recurrence may occur around 7–8 months following therapy. Repeat treatments may follow the same procedure.

(**Note:** Cisplatin powder has to be freshly prepared and when reconstituted is only stable at room temperature for approximately 15 hours. It is difficult to obtain in many parts of the world. Systemic toxicity may be a problem but the treatment has been used on stallions and pregnant brood mares without ill effects. Post-treatment therapy with penicillin or potentiated sulphur drugs, plus an anti-inflammatory such as phenylbutazone is advisable to minimize post-injection swelling and discomfort.)

Cimetidine The role of histamine (H_2) and growth of tumours may be related to activation of T suppresser cells. As cimetidine is a potent H_2-blocker, it has been used experimentally on melanomas. Its successful use appears to be related to tumours which are showing active growth. Where growth has been minimal or even static, the response is reportedly poor. Cimetidine administered orally at 2.5 mg/kg three times daily or (less satisfactorily) 7.5 mg/kg given once or twice daily for 6–12 weeks may have some benefit but reported results are mixed. Some report excellent resolution,[21] others describe no noticeable changes. If the drug is seen to have a beneficial effect then it should continue daily until there is no further improvement. A response is indicated by a slow decline to 50% of pre-treatment size and occurs during the first 6 weeks of treatment. The progression of the tumours may be halted for months to years following cessation of treatment.

If no significant effect is seen by 3 weeks, it is probably not worth continuing. Regrowth on cessation of treatment is also reported.

Prognosis

Individual tumours on other than grey horses can be surgically removed with little risk but slightly more caution should be exercised with grey horses. Although the majority of 'black' lumps are benign and almost every grey horse will eventually develop them, no melanoma should be belittled. Severe aggressive melanosarcomas may be very dangerous with widespread dissemination.

NEUROFIBROMA

Profile

Fibrous tumour of nerve endings which can occur anywhere associated with nerve tissue but is predominantly recorded in the upper and lower eyelids of middle-aged to older horses. The relationship between these masses and nodular sarcoids is debatable, but it seems likely that although the two tumours are similar in many respects they are pathologically distinct.

Clinical signs

Small 1–10 mm hard *subcutaneous* nodules and subsequently very much larger multiloculated masses(> 25 mm diameter) (**Fig. 19.20**). Multiple and cording lesions may be seen and larger lesions in particular cause erosion through overlying skin and develop into granulomatous-type lesions very similar in appearance and behaviour to fibroblastic sarcoid. However, they rarely show overlying hair loss until ulceration occurs.

Differential diagnosis

- Sarcoid (nodular and malevolent). Some pathologists consider the neurofibroma to be a variant of nodular sarcoid found in the eyelids.
- Mastocytoma (mast cell tumour).
- Cutaneous histiocytic and generalized lymphosarcoma.
- Cutaneous nodules caused by insect bites and allergic collagen necrosis but these seldom conflict with the location of neurofibromas.

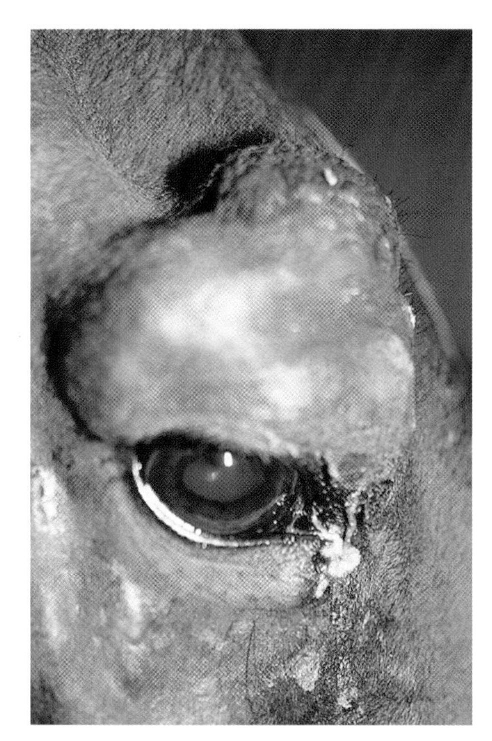

Figure 19.20 Neurofibroma in the upper eyelid with multiple nodules of varying size. Eyelid distortion resulted in a purulent ocular discharge.

Diagnostic confirmation

- Biopsy or excision and histopathology.
- Fine needle aspirates are usually impossible to obtain owing to the extreme density of the tissues and the paucity of intercellular matrix.

Treatment

Complete surgical removal carries a good prognosis but is extremely hard to achieve. Seeding nodules are easily overlooked and tumours recur in a different site on the eyelid in approximately 25–50% of cases where surgical excision is attempted.

Intralesional injection of BCG (or similar immunomodulating proteins, see Chapter 4) over an extended period can be effective but is far less effective than against nodular sarcoid in the same site.

Intralesional cisplatin may be effective.

Gamma radiation brachytherapy using iridium-192 linear array sources (or teletherapy) is highly effective but very limited in availability.

Prognosis

A very guarded prognosis is justified because complete resolution is almost impossible to achieve with a single surgical intervention.

BCG therapy carries about 40% success for periorbital lesions.

Radiation is very effective (brachytherapy using iridium-192 linear sources). Gold-198 is less effective because of the slow rate of replication of the cells involved and the short half-life of the isotope.

OSSIFYING FIBROMA (EQUINE JUVENILE OSSIFYING FIBROMA)

Profile

Fibro-osseous tumour mass growing from mandible, maxilla or premaxilla characteristically occurring in young horses between birth and 12 months of age. Many horses are born with the mass, which grows slowly over the following months to create a physical disability and visible abnormality. It is often only observed when the mass distorts the mouth or protrudes between the lips or interferes with eating or respiration.

Clinical signs

Smooth, mucosa-covered, hard bony mass extruding from maxilla, mandible or premaxilla. There may be displacement or destruction of the roots of the incisor teeth. Rapid growth and locally aggressive nature may create early ulceration (**Fig. 19.21**). The ulcerated mass rapidly becomes impacted with food material and infected. A malodorous smell is often present.

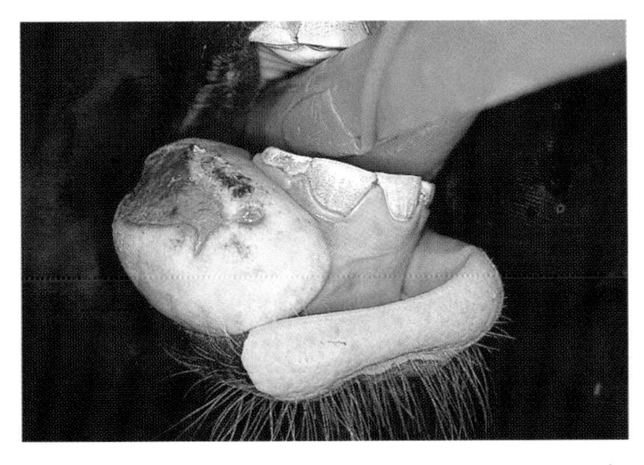

Figure 19.21 Ossifying fibroma (equine juvenile ossifying fibroma).

Differential diagnosis

- Adamantinoma
- Odontoma
- Intra-osseous carcinoma
- Soft-tissue carcinoma
- Squamous cell and undifferentiated oral carcinoma
- Dental maleruption/malformations
- Sarcoid

Diagnostic confirmation

- Biopsy
- Ultrasonography
- Radiography (lateral and occlusal projections)
  - bony proliferation of bone usually with teeth displacement; may shows dense bone or as highly invasive destructive bone lesion

Treatment

Wide surgical excision is the only practical option for the most part. Recurrences are common unless the mass is excised effectively and the resultant defect in dentition of structure of the bony components makes the outlook poorer. Radiation therapy is effective but very limited in availability and application.

Prognosis

A guarded prognosis is warranted – many recur in spite of aggressive surgical excision involving extensive mandibular or maxillary bone removal.

SQUAMOUS CELL CARCINOMA

Profile

This is an invasive tumour of squamous cells of the skin, respiratory mucosa and paranasal sinuses and of the gastrointestinal and reproductive tracts (see Table 19.2). Chronic high UV light challenge is suggested as being a significant aetiological factor in the skin and eye forms while in penile forms smegma may be responsible. In one study[145] squamous cell carcinoma in the horse predominantly affected the external genitalia but these results are possibly unusual. Squamous cell carcinomas of the third eyelid, corneo–scleral junction and eyelids are probably equally important, particularly in selective breeds; for example, Clydesdale horses in Australia more frequently have tumours of the lips and eyes than of the prepuce and penis while in the United Kingdom it is somewhat the reverse.

Penile forms in younger horses tend to be much more aggressive and commonly metastasize to

Table 19.2 Squamous cell carcinoma.

Form/location	Features	Assumed carcinogen	Type of horse affected	Nature
Ocular				
Palpebral	Proliferative	UV light/pale skin	All ages/sex Pale skin	Slow, benign
	Ulcerative	UV light/pale skin	All ages /sex Pale skin	Rapid, destructive
Nictitans	Proliferative	UV light/pale skin	All ages/sex Pale skin	Slow, benign
	Ulcerative	UV light/pale skin	All ages/sex Pale skin	Slow, destructive
Conjunctival	Proliferative	UV light/pale skin	All ages/sex Pale skin	Slow, benign
Cornea[a]	Invasive	UV light/pale skin	Any	Slow, corneal opacity
Penile				
Penile shaft	Proliferative/ benign	Smegma	Aged geldings	Benign, local infiltration
Penile shaft	Ulcerative/invasive	Smegma	Geldings (> 6 y)	Highly malignant
Prepuce	Ulcerative/invasive	Smegma	> 5 y	Highly malignant
Vulval				
Labial	Proliferative	UV/smegma	Pale skin	Slow, benign
	Ulcerative	UV/smegma	Pale skin	Local invasion
Clitoral	Proliferative	Smegma	> 10 y	Slow benign
	Ulcerative	Smegma	> 6 y	Local invasion, possibly malignant
Cutaneous				
Face	Ulcerative/proliferative	UV light	Clydesdale Pale skin	Highly invasive, low malignancy
Perineal	Ulcerative	UV light	Pale skin (> 6 y)	Slow, destructive
Respiratory tract				
Sinus/nasal cavity/pharynx	Proliferative, invasive	Not known	> 6 y	Slow, space-occupying mass
Alimentary tract				
Gastric	Aggressive	Not known, possible bacteria/parasites	> 12 y	Highly malignant, invasive.

[a]Carcinoma *in situ*.

regional lymph nodes. Extension to involve preputial ring or primary preputial lesions is a serious complication. Most of the other cutaneous/superficial forms have little tendency to metastasize.

In mares, clitoral proliferative forms are commoner than ulcerative labial forms.

The skin of the perianal region can develop an ulcerative form in horses with nonpigmented skin. The facial forms are probably commonest in Clydesdale breed, especially where these are kept in tropical and subtropical areas.

Ocular forms include benign, proliferative and aggressive ulcerative palpebral and nictitans forms. The benign types at all sites in the eye are usually slow-growing and proliferative. The ulcerative forms which are the preserve of the eyelids and the nictitans are faster and locally destructive. Proliferative conjunctival squamous cell carcinoma is relatively common at the lateral limbus (corneoscleral junction). The corneal form ('carcinoma *in situ*') is slowly invasive but usually remains very superficial. All types may be slow-growing or highly invasive but remain largely restricted to superficial tissues of the palpebral skin, conjunctival/corneal epithelium. In contrast to the bovine condition, ocular squamous cell carcinoma in the horse is only rarely malignant. The nictitans (third eyelid) form is usually slow-growing and proliferative but sometimes aggressive and ulcerative.

Nasal, paranasal sinus and pharyngeal forms are less common. They are usually fast-growing and exert their main effects by occupying space within the respiratory tract with nasal, facial and pharyngeal distortions, dyspnoea and dysphagia. They are

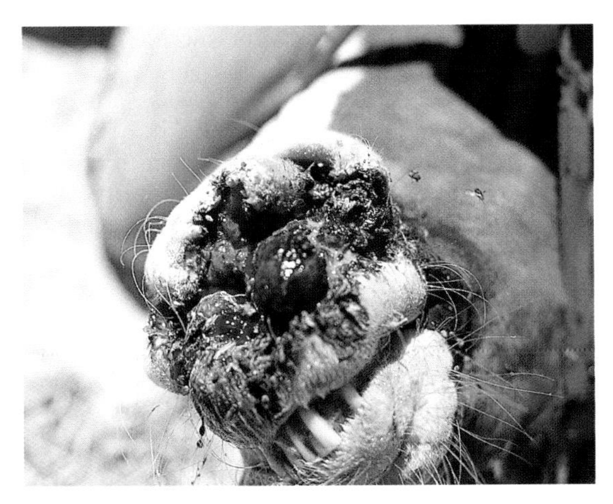

Figure 19.22 Squamous cell carcinoma with extensive tissue destruction on the face. The affected area was white skinned.

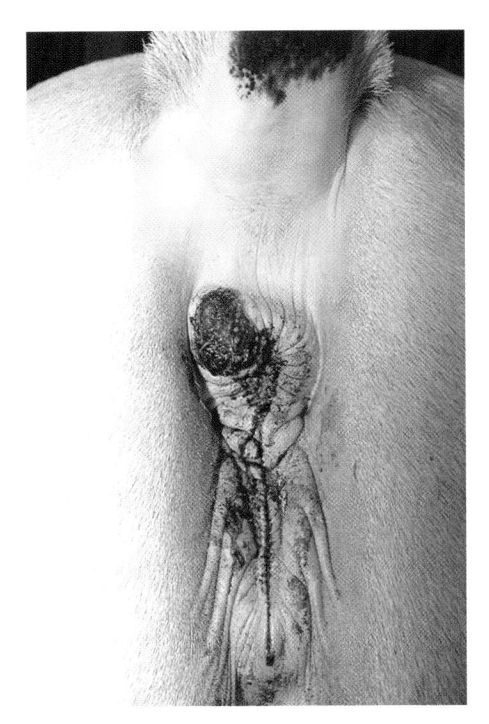

Figure 19.23 Squamous cell carcinoma of the perianal skin. Note the tissue destruction and shallow ulcer developing on the nonpigmented skin.

occasionally highly malignant. The gastric form is restricted to older horses with a possible connection to recurrent gastric ulceration (however caused) and *Habronema musca* or *Draschia* spp. lesions in the stomach. The tumour is extremely malignant, with direct transperitoneal spread and metastatic dissemination to liver, lungs and other organs.

Clinical signs

Precancerous changes which may be detected include thickening and mild exfoliation and ulceration of the skin; these are usually very obvious on the preputial skin of older geldings. Changes will present different signs at the relevant sites. Initially, however, early signs are not usually detected and a small, granulating 'sore' on the skin which may be depressed below skin level is often the first report.

Invasive forms are aggressively ulcerative and erode into normal tissue. All types have varying degrees of malodour, even with early lesions. The skin at any site can be affected but nonpigmented nasal and facial skin (**Fig. 19.22**) and perineal skin (**Fig. 19.23**) are probably commonest.

Nasal and oral lesions are often missed in the early stages and malodorous breath and blood

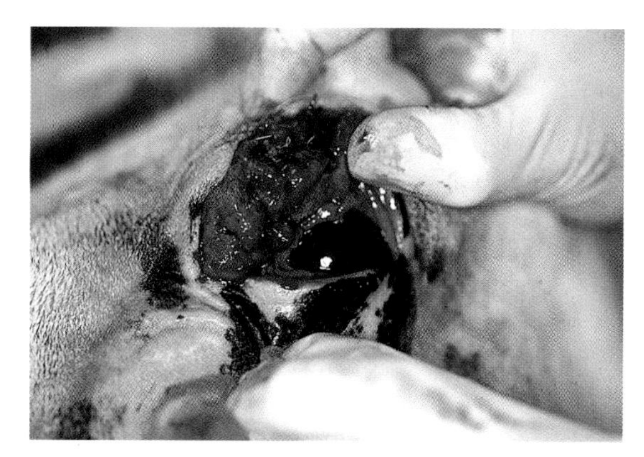

Figure 19.24 Squamous cell carcinoma. Destructive, proliferative palpebral form in a Clydesdale gelding.

staining of the saliva and nasal mucus may be reported first. Lesions affecting the pharynx may pass unnoticed until dysphagia and stertor develop. Secondary infection is common within the respiratory and alimentary tracts.

Eyelid lesions often start as white, raised plaques at the edge of the eyelid and proceed to extensive ulceration and destruction of the eyelid, rapidly and progressively invading the peri-orbital tissues (**Fig. 19.24**). Nictitans and conjunctival forms are very common and here the earliest stages may be noted as blood staining of the tears. They may progress rapidly as appearance changes to a granulomatous and ulcerated lesion.

The penile forms may vary from single or multiple pedunculated or sessile 'cauliflower' type to smooth or ulcerated and highly invasive masses giving a wooden feel to the free end of the penis.

Vulval tumours are often slow-growing and proliferative in the clitoral form but are more often ulcerative in labial forms.

Systemic signs may be relatively minor unless secondary metastatic spread has occurred. Weight loss, colic and chronic intestinal bleeding are signs of the gastric form, which carries a very poor prognosis and a short fulminating course. Secondary tumours can develop at any site (including the spinal cord, vertebral bodies, lungs, liver and spleen) from any form but, apart from the severe, malignant penile form and gastric squamous cell carcinoma, most are not malignant and even local lymph node involvement is unusual.

Differential diagnosis

- Sarcoids (fibroblastic and verrucose/mixed lesions)
- Melanoma
- Papilloma (especially nictitans and vulval proliferative forms)
- Mast cell tumour
- Spindle cell sarcoma
- Lymphosarcoma (cutaneous and generalized)
- Exuberant granulation tissue
- Botryomycosis
- Habronemiasis
- Phycomycosis and other fungal tumours
- Other causes of colic/weight loss/anaemia and protein-losing enteropathy

Diagnostic confirmation

- Surgical biopsy or scrape biopsy
- Impression smears possible for eye lesions
- Total excisional biopsy for histopathological examination

Treatment

Wide surgical excision, cryotherapy, irradiation, immunomodulation and chemotherapy are used with degrees of success related to the invasiveness and accessibility of the tumour.

Early tumours are more successfully removed surgically with complete remission in most cases. Intralesional injection of cisplatin has been found to be useful in some cases and this is simple and relatively noninvasive.

Immunomodulation with BCG derivatives (see Chapter 4) has disappointing effects in the horse (compared to the bovine).

Prior to the application of any treatment method, a full clinical appraisal must be performed to assess the extent of local and generalized spread of carcinoma. Attention must be paid to the likely secondary effects of treatment such as scarring, failure to remove all the tumour tissue, etc. Carcinomas are usually highly susceptible to gamma or beta radiation and where this is practical it can be applied effectively. Penile forms are often resolved completely by penile amputation but in younger horses with a 'wooden' penile shaft the prognosis is poor or hopeless. In all cases secondary spread to regional lymph nodes (including the iliac nodes which can be palpated per rectum) supports a hopeless prognosis and there is little point in subjecting the animal to surgery.

Systemic chemotherapy is not feasible in the horse and in any case carcinoma is probably less responsive than other tumours.

Specific treatment methods (see Table 19.3)

Surgical ablation Where wide excision can be

Table 19.3 Relative value[a] of treatment modalities for treatment of common forms of cutaneous squamous cell carcinoma from the authors' experience

	Surgical ablation	Cryosurgery	Immunomodulation	Cytotoxic/ antimitotic	Radiation
Cutaneous	**	**	*	**	**** (β) (γ)
Labial	*	**	N/A[b]	***	**** (γ)
Clitoral	***	**	N/A	**	**** (γ)
Penile					
< 8 y	*	N/A	N/A	N/A	N/A
> 10 y	****	N/A	N/A	N/A	N/A
Palpebral	N/A	**	*	*	**** (γ)
Nictitans	****	***	*	N/A	N/A
Corneolimbal	**	**	N/A	N/A	**** (β)
Carcinoma *in situ*	**	*	N/A	N/A	**** (β)

[a] * = unlikely to be effective; ** = effective in some cases or partially effective; *** effective or partially effective in most cases; **** likely to be effective in almost all cases (the best approach).
[b] N/A, not applicable or invariably fails to help.

performed, results are usually good, e.g. amputation of tail, enucleation/exenteration of eye with complete removal of eyelids, amputation of penis. Very good results can usually be predicted on proliferative lesions on the third eyelid. Less successful results are obtained with long-standing invasive tumours on eyelids, prepuce, mouth and, to a lesser extent, the vulva in the mare. Due consideration should be given to the secondary effects of the surgery including scarring and skin/tissue deficits.

Cryotherapy (See Chapter 4 for general principles.) This can be performed on squamous cell carcinoma lesions either directly (facial, anal, nictitans, eyelid and conjunctival forms) or after surgical debulking. It is more likely to be successful in very early cases and is unsuccessful in rapidly or widely invasive tumours. The use of 2 or 3 freeze–thaw cycles is recommended. Cryosurgery gives only moderate results and is particularly poor around the eyes and mouth; while it can be very effective on limbal conjunctival and corneal lesions,[146] in these circumstances the control of the freezing process has to be meticulous.

Cytotoxic chemicals and antimitotic drugs (See Chapter 4.) Topical application of antimitotic drugs, e.g. 5-fluorouracil and prednisolone (or other corticosteroids), may help but have a poor reputation in most cases. The intralesional injection of cisplatin has been found to be effective in some cases.[147]

Immunomodulation (See Chapter 4.) BCG cell wall extracts (or live BCG bacillus) has been used successfully in some forms of bovine ocular squamous cell carcinoma. The equine condition (at all sites) does not seem to be nearly as responsive, with very disappointing results.

Radiation therapy (See Chapter 4.) This is probably the most reliably effective of all treatments, with good results expected in all cutaneous forms of the condition. Radioactive implants with gold-198 and iridium-192 isotopes offer increased chances of resolution.[148] Interstitial implants of cobalt-60, caesium-137, iridium-192 or gold-198 have all been successfully applied. Where the tumour mass is thin, e.g. corneal carcinoma *in situ*, or where debulking can be employed to reduce the mass of tumour tissue to <3 mm, strontium-90 probes/plaques (which are potent beta radiation emitters) can also be successfully used. Corneal squamous cell carcinoma presents a serious challenge. Such tumours can be treated by means of sharp-excision lamellar keratectomy to clear the cornea and conjunctivectomy if the conjunctiva is also invaded, followed by 8000–10 000 rads of beta radiation fractionated over 5 days. Over 80% of such lesions may respond[149] with little recurrence.

The results of radiation brachytherapy are usually very satisfactory with a good cosmetic effect and a low recurrence rate, although the full effects may not be obvious for some months. Teletherapy is a very effective treatment for most forms of the disease which have no systemic dissemination but is unlikely to be available except under very particular and specialized circumstances.

As with all tumours, the radiation dose should be accurately calculated and careful placement of the implants can maximize the effect. Nevertheless, some tumours will recur in time. These irradiation procedures usually require referral to specialist centres with qualified radiologists and specialized facilities for radiation protection.

Prognosis

Fortunately most (but by no means all) cutaneous forms of the condition tend to remain fairly local. Extensive local spread is rare in any case but is much more common than wide metastatic dissemination. The major exception to this is the penile form which occurs in younger geldings (< 8 years of age). In these, the presence of a hard, wooden feel to the free end of the penis is a bad prognostic sign.

Gastric squamous cell carcinoma and to a lesser extent nasal and pharyngeal forms are often highly malignant.

Any secondary involvement of the local lymph nodes should be viewed with suspicion and it may be justifiable to biopsy this to check for metastatic tumour. If this is present then the prognosis is very poor and it is not justifiable to subject the animal to surgery or other treatments.

Prevention

Penile forms can be prevented by regular sheath inspections and washing of suspected cases showing precancerous changes or abnormal accumulations of smegma. The greater incidence of squamous cell carcinoma of the penis occurs in older geldings, usually ponies or work horses which are less likely to receive regular cleaning of the prepuce and penis.[150] Consequently, therapy should also be aimed at the regular cleansing of the prepuce and penis of this group of horses. This also particularly applies to the 'colour' type horses (Appaloosas, Piebald and Skewbald, Palominos, and to a lesser extent, grey horses). Regular washing of the clitoral region of mares may help to prevent occurrence. Avoidance of other predisposing factors can be helpful but is usually difficult (avoidance of UV light in pale-skinned horses). Regular anthelmintic worming regimens and minimization of gastric ulceration may be useful but the gastric condition is very rare and so these measures directed at prevention are probably disproportionate to the value.

SEBACEOUS GLAND TUMOUR

Profile

These are rare tumours arising from sebaceous gland cells in adult to aged horses. They may occur at any cutaneous site and the causative factors are unknown.

Clinical signs

Solitary masses which vary from nodules to alopecic lobulated growths. They are usually slow-growing and benign in nature.

Differential diagnosis

- Dermoid cyst
- Sarcoid (nodular or fibroblastic)
- Neurofibroma
- Nodular collagenolytic granuloma/eosinophilic collagen granuloma
- Insect and insect bite reactions
- Foreign body reactions

Diagnostic confirmation

- Biopsy or surgical excision and histopathology

Treatment

Surgical excision or cryotherapy are effective with little chance of recurrence.

SWEAT GLAND TUMOUR

Profile

Uncommon tumour of apocrine sweat glands occurring in older horses, most commonly around ears and vulva. It is usually very benign in character.

Clinical signs

Single firm or cystic dermal nodules which are nonpainful, slow-growing and nonalopecic (**Fig. 19.25**). The lesions have a striking clinical resemblance to nodular sarcoids and neurofibromas but are histologically distinctive.

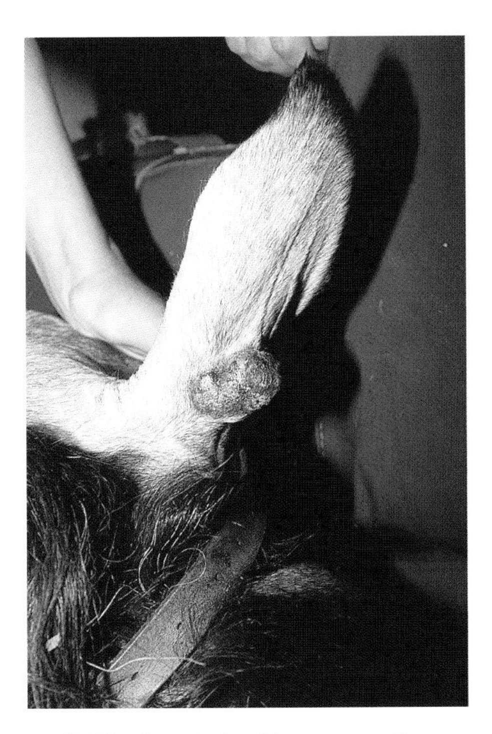

Figure 19.25 Sweat gland tumour on the ear.

Differential diagnosis
- Nodular sarcoid
- Neurofibroma
- Fibroma
- Foreign body reaction
- Insect bites/stings and migrations (e.g. *Hypoderma bovis*, warble fly)
- Allergic/eosinophilic collagen necrosis

Diagnostic confirmation
- Biopsy/surgical excision and histopathology

Treatment
Complete surgical ablation is curative.

Prognosis
A good prognosis can be given.

FIBROMA OF FROG AND SOLE

Profile
A soft, fleshy tumour, usually in the frog region, affecting horses of all breeds. It rarely causes lameness and is most often found incidentally during dressing of the foot.

Clinical signs
A well-circumscribed, moist tumour resembling granulation tissue often in the frog region. The margins of the tumour are well defined (**Fig. 19.26**).

Differential diagnosis
- Canker of the foot
- Thrush
- Keratoma
- Granulation tissue
- Foot sepsis

Diagnostic confirmation
- Clinical appearance
- Characteristic histology from biopsy

Treatment
Complete surgical removal is usually very effective. Very careful deep incision may be required to ensure complete removal but the defined margins of the mass make this relatively simple.

- Cut down to base of tumour:
  - if on the sole, curette down to pedal bone;
  - if in the frog dissect down very carefully to avoid opening into the deep flexor tendon sheath;

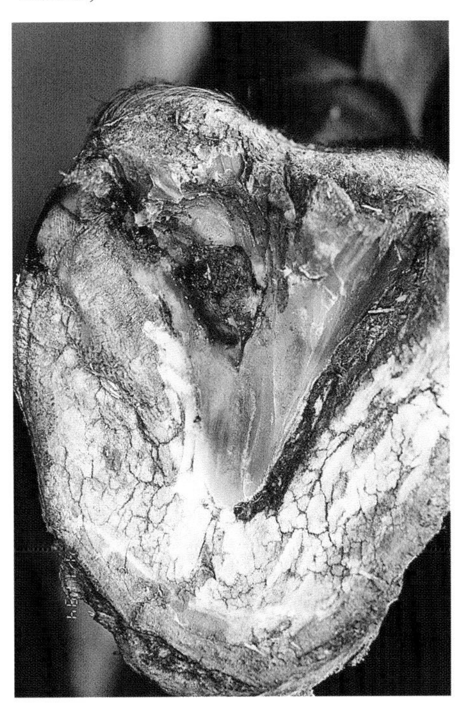

Figure 19.26 Fibroma of the frog/sole. Note the well defined appearance.

- pack wound and keep dry.

The resultant wound is packed with antiseptic swabs and is kept scrupulously clean during healing with the help of a plastic boot or treatment plate. Recovery is slow, but repeat surgery is not usually required.

KERATOMA

Profile

A tumour of keratin-producing cells in the inner surface of the hoof wall or sole resulting in a keratin-containing core between the wall and the pedal bone. Most commonly lesions are found at the toe or quarter.[151] It may result from injury or chronic irritation[152] so that it may not be true neoplasm, or may occur spontaneously. Lameness is a consequence of pressure on adjacent sensitive tissue. If the tumour impinges on the pedal bone itself, lysis can occur.

Clinical signs

Insidious onset of mild and intermittent but progressive lameness,[153] which probably arises from intracapsular pressure, is often the first presenting sign. Later some change in the outline of the wall and sole contour can occur. Sometimes they are identified incidentally during foot paring and shoeing, having shown no evidence of any problems. Sole keratomas are usually circular 0.5–2 cm diameter. The wall keratoma may cause considerable distortion on bulging of the toe region of the hoof (**Fig. 19.27**). The tumour often extends from the coronary band to the distal margin of the hoof (**Fig. 19.28**). The white line is patently abnormal with a circular distortion of dense, rubbery white tissue. A few cases are patently infected with submural abscess.

Diagnostic confirmation

- Characteristic changes in contour of the wall and sole.
- Radiological examination will often identify the mass and any underlying destruction or distortion of the pedal bone.

Differential diagnosis

- Cysts in the pedal bone usually have no concurrent wall or sole distortion.

Treatment

Surgical removal of overlying wall with careful and

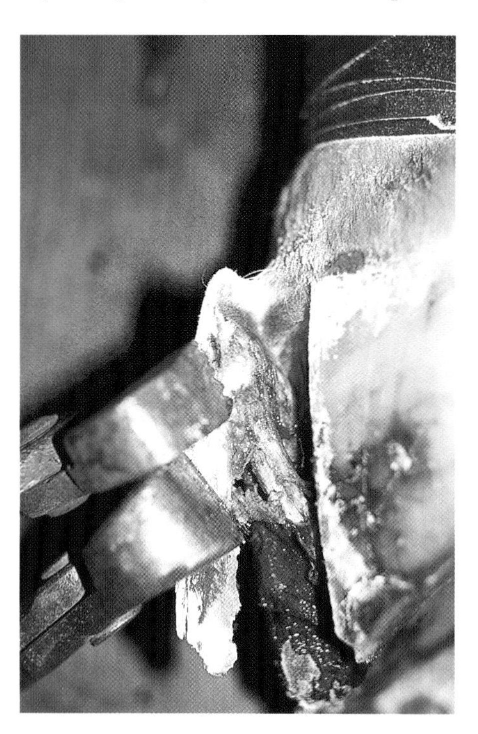

Figure 19.27 Keratoma of the foot extending from the solar margin to the coronet.

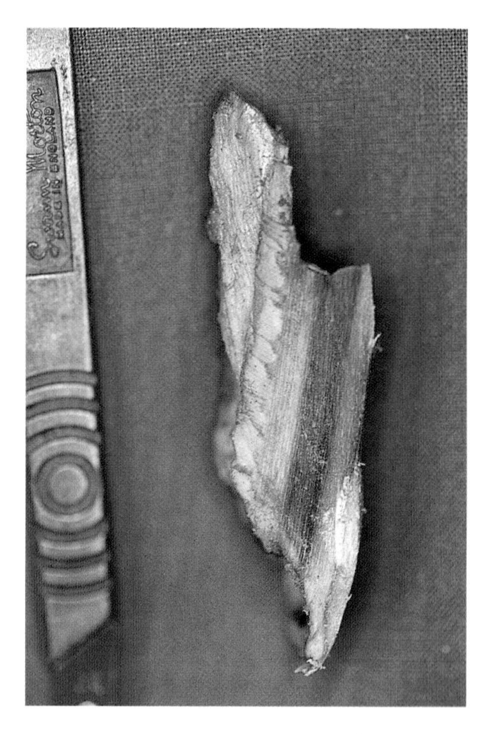

Figure 19.28 Keratoma of the foot – surgical specimen.

complete resection and curettage of tumour from underlying bone is necessary.[154] Complete removal of a hoof-wall keratoma usually results in an extensive wall defect at the toe. It is particularly important to dissect out the proximal limit of the mass, which may be at or just below the coronary band. It is helpful to leave a bridge of wall at the distal margin of the hoof to provide support. Alternatively, a plate can be screwed to the wall of the hoof to provide a stable hoof capsule. A shoe can be applied before surgery to ensure that the defect is not subjected to excessive movement after surgery and to provide additional support for the hoof bridge. The defect can be packed until healing is underway and then filled with acrylic resin filler for a more permanent repair which will often allow the horse to be used earlier in the course of recovery.

The tumour has a relatively high rate of recurrence, but it is not certain whether recurrences are the result of failure to remove the entire mass or genuine recurrence. Most authors report an excellent overall prognosis provided that the whole lesion is removed and any possible causative factors are eliminated.[155]

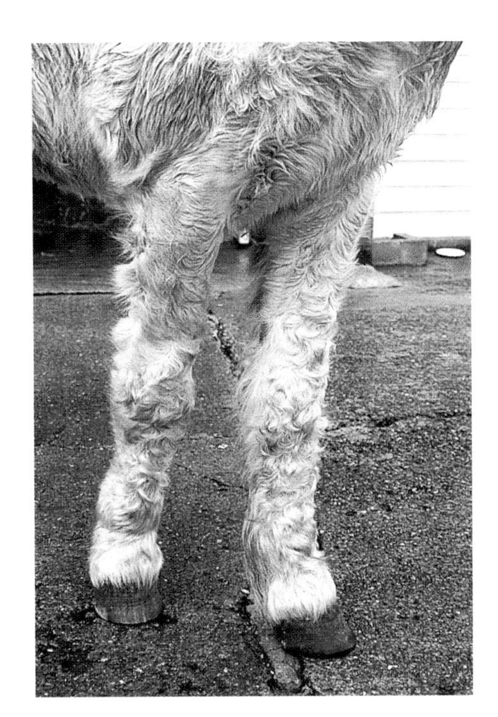

Figure 19.29 Pituitary hirsutism. Pituitary adenoma/Cushing's disease is the only cause of significant hirsutism in the horse.

INTERNAL NEOPLASTIC TUMOURS WITH SKIN MANIFESTATIONS

EQUINE CUSHING'S DISEASE

Profile

Equine Cushing's disease is almost always due to the very common tumour of pars intermedia of the neurohypophysis occurring in horses and ponies over 12–15 years of age. The condition is very rare in animals under 7–10 years of age. No breed, sex or colour predisposition has been established, but ponies and geldings may be over-represented (possibly because they are commonly kept to older ages than larger horses). Tumours may be very small (almost invisible) but functional while others may be large enough to cause physical effects but have little physiological effect.[156]

Clinical signs

The early signs of polyuria and polydipsia may be difficult to detect. Often the earliest evidence is a failure of hair coat shedding which is commonly ascribed to 'old age'. One or more episodes of laminitis which has characteristic features which are somewhat different from the 'normal' pony laminitis are also commonly reported in the early stages. The laminitis is characterized by a failure to respond to nonsteroidal drugs and may have a lesser digital pulse than might be expected from the severity of the condition.

Cutaneous signs include:

- Hirsutism (failure to shed hair, rapid regrowth of curly, longer than normal hair (8–10 cm long)) with a greatly increased density and patchy areas of longer hair (**Fig. 19.29**). The mane and tail are almost never affected.
- Sweating (hyperhidrosis) giving the coat a clammy feel and soaked appearance (**Fig. 19.30**)
- Secondary bacterial cutaneous infections with *Staphylococcus* spp. and *Dermatophilus congolensis* are common.
- Parasitism (including ectoparasites such as lice or mites) is common.
- Oral ulceration which shows no evidence of healing (**Fig. 19.31**) and oral and cutaneous abscessation.

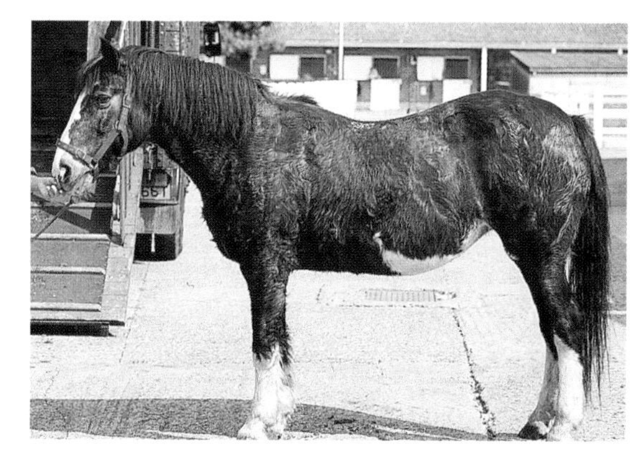

Figure 19.30 Pituitary adenoma/Cushing's disease showing hirsutism and sweating giving the coat a soaked appearance. Secondary skin infections and infestations are common.

Other body system signs include:

- Periodontal disease/loose teeth.
- Laminitis (recurrent, mild to severe) with lesser digital inflammatory response than might be expected from the severity of signs.
- Intestinal parasitism (even ascarids can be present in large numbers).

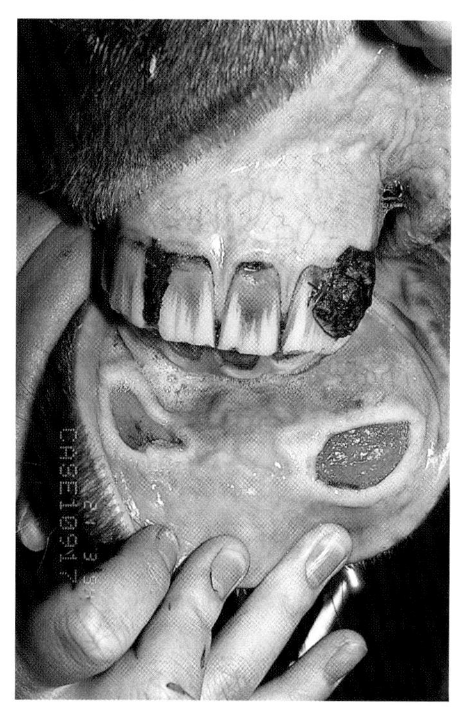

Figure 19.31 Pituitary adenoma/Cushing's disease. Oral ulceration showing a singular lack of healing is a common sign. Other dental and oral lesions may be present also.

- Cataract and/or central blindness (amaurosis) (resulting from direct pressure on the optic nerves).
- Supraorbital swellings and a pendulous abdomen (possibly the result of fat redistribution).

Systemic signs include:

- Polydipsia and polyuria (PD/PU) associated with glycosuria/hyperglycaemia.
- Weight loss and loss of muscle tone ('sway back' appearance).
- Immunosuppression with recurrent internal and external bacterial, fungal and parasitic infections.
- Intermittent or persistent pyrexia.

Differential diagnosis

- Seborrhoea
- Diabetes mellitus
- Diabetes insipidus
- Chronic arsenical poisoning
- Renal failure
- Other causes of laminitis
- Other causes of hyperhidrosis (including phaeochromocytoma – functional tumour of the adrenal medulla)
- Other causes of immunosuppression (lymphosarcoma complex usually)

Note: True pancreatic islet-related diabetes mellitus is extremely rare, most cases showing significant hyperglycaemia/glycosuria and polyuria/polydipsia can safely be assumed to be suffering from Cushing's disease, and particularly when at least one other characteristic sign is present.

Table 19.4 The relative frequencies of the major clinical signs described in one study involving animals with a confirmed diagnosis of equine Cushing's syndrome[156]

Clinical sign	Frequency (%)
Hair-coat changes	94
Weight loss	88
Lethargy	82
Laminitis	82
Polydipsia/polyuria	76
Sweating	59
Tachypnoea	41
Tachycardia	29
Skin infections	24
Sinusitis	18
Oral ulceration	18
Bulging supraorbital fat	18
Neurological signs	6

Table 19.5 Clinicopathological findings in horses with Cushing's syndrome due to pituitary adenoma[156]

Parameter	Values in Cushing's cases	Reference range	Percentage of cases showing this sign
Blood glucose (mmol/l)	>5.6	3.5–4.5	94
Basal cortisol (nmol/l)	> 155	25–155	53
Serum insulin (μIU/l)	> 50	5–36	Uncertain
Eosinophil count (10^9/l)	0	0.5–1.2	69
Neutrophil count (10^9/l)	> 6.5	2.5–5.5	75

Diagnostic confirmation

- Classical clinical signs.
  - pituitary adenoma is the only clinical condition known to cause hirsutism in the horse.
- Hyperglycaemia (fasting level 8–16.75 mmol/l is consistent with presence of tumour).[157]
- Diagnosis can be confirmed by
  - adrenocorticotrophic hormone (ACTH) stimulation test (see Chapter 3);
  - dexamethasone suppression test[158] (or a combination of this with ACTH stimulation test[156,159]);
  - thyroid releasing hormone response;[160]
  - blood cortisol concentrations;*
  - blood/urinary cortisol excretion ratios;†
  - insulin assay.‡

* Normal blood cortisol concentrations will vary from 55 nmol/l to 125 nmol/l with a strong diurnal rhythm. Cushingoid horses will often have gross elevations of resting levels and a significant loss of diurnal rhythm.

† Urinary excretion ratio is calculated from the concentrations of cortisol in the blood and urine obtained at the same time. Cushingoid horses commonly show an inordinately high excretion ratio, i.e. they are excreting significant amounts of cortisol in the urine (this should be minimal in normal horses).

‡ Normal insulin concentrations around 5–36 μIU/ml. Cushingoid horses show around 5–120 μIU/ml.

Note: The technicalities of the diagnostic tests are to be found in laboratory and other medical texts.

Currently there is no practical method of imaging the pituitary gland in a live horse and so definitive confirmation relies on diagnostic tests.

A diagnosis can be made based on the presence of one or more of the major clinical signs with glycosuria/hyperglycaemia.

Treatment[161]

Bromocriptine mesylate (*Parlodel*, Sandoz Pharmaceuticals, UK) has antiserotonin and antihistamine effects. At a daily oral dose of 10 mg total dose daily for 3–12 weeks a significant number of mildly affected horses will show an improvement. Daily oral dosing of 0.04 mg/kg in the morning and 0.02 mg/kg in the evening has been advocated.[162] The dose can be gradually reduced once a significant therapeutic benefit is achieved but it may take some weeks, with hair loss being the first sign of a beneficial effect. If no improvement is detected after 2 weeks an alternative drug should be used. The injectable formulations of bromocriptine can cause painful swellings and this approach is probably not necessary anyway.

Cyproheptadine hydrochloride (*Periactin*, MSD, UK) suppresses the pituitary–adrenal axis. It is administered orally at 0.6 mg/kg q 12 h for the first week. The dose is increased to 0.8, 1.0, 1.2 mg/kg each succeeding week. Initial doses of 0.25 mg/kg twice daily can be used with progressive increases to effect. Early improvement is reflected in reducing thirst. Hair normalization may be seen within 1–3 weeks. Serum cortisol concentrations may take longer to fall (and may never reach normal concentrations), therefore laminitis may not improve in the earliest stages. Horses which fail to respond to this drug will often benefit from pergolide treatment (see below).

Pergolide (*Celance*, Ciba Ltd, UK) is a dopamine antagonist drug which can safely be administered orally at 1 mg daily for a horse of any size. Alternatively, an exact dose can be calculated at 0.014 mg/kg orally. It has been reported to be very effective in some cases but others do not respond.

Horses with significant hirsutism will often benefit from regular clipping. Management of intercurrent infections (using appropriate antibiotics and anthelmintics), weight loss (through careful feeding management) and control of laminitis (through routine foot care, possibly supplemented by use of corrective farriery) is very important. Most cases will also benefit from sustained ectoparasite and endoparasite control measures.

Prognosis

Therapy can prolong life by 2–3 years or more but is expensive and needs to be sustained or at least administered intermittently. Effective treatment results in a dramatic change in hair quality and quantity, a reduction in blood glucose and a reduction in the polyuria/polydipsia. Changes in plasma cortisol are often slow or disappointing.

Complications such as extreme weight loss and weakness, severe recurrent laminitis, central blindness and serious buccal and intestinal infections and infestations are indicators of a poor/reduced prognosis.

GENERALIZED LYMPHOSARCOMA

Profile

Widespread malignant proliferation of lymphoid cells in multiple organs occurs in generalized forms of lymphosarcoma. Although the disease affects internal organs in an aggressive way, skin is not often involved.

Clinical signs

Cutaneous nodules of variable size and number which may ulcerate represent the cutaneous manifestation. There are no predictable features of the disease apart from its rapidly progressive course and highly fatal prognosis.

Skin bruising or an unexpected degree of surface damage and haemorrhage from relatively trivial surface trauma to mucous membranes (such as nasal or tracheal endoscopy) can be significant signs of high capillary fragility. This is sometimes encountered in generalized or splenic forms of lymphosarcoma in particular.

Most cases show vague clinical signs of weight loss, inappetance and intermittent or fluctuating pyrexia. The course of the disease is rapid with death (or euthanasia) usually occurring within 6 months. Significant generalized lymphadenopathy is commonly encountered but may be absent. Significant signs of internal organ involvement such as diarrhoea, renal failure, hepatic failure and cardiorespiratory signs (including forelimb oedema, often one limb at first, ventral oedema, jugular engorgement and pulsation, pleural or abdominal fluid accumulations) are related to the organs affected by the disease and are very variable. Undulant fever is reported.

Differential diagnosis

- Other nodular diseases
- Cutaneous histiocytic lymphosarcoma
- Nodular and malevolent sarcoid
- Cutaneous collagen necrosis
- Eosinophillic granuloma

Diagnostic confirmation

- Clinical signs.
- Haematological findings (including hypercalcaemia and low globulin and albumin concentrations). A very low proportion of affected horses are overtly leukaemic but lymphocyte counts of over 100×10^9/l are recorded.
- Biopsy of cutaneous nodules for enlarged lymph nodes may be diagnostic.

Treatment

No treatment is effective for generalized lymphosarcoma. The course is usually rapid with most cases being destroyed within 6 months of diagnosis. Noncutaneous signs may be much more significant with respect to the prognosis. Cutaneous histiocytic lymphosarcoma has a much slower course with individuals surviving for up to 4–6 years or more in some cases. It is therefore very important to establish the diagnosis at an early stage. Usually a skilled pathologist is required. However, if the course is rapid and inexorable then a diagnosis of generalized lymphosarcoma is probably justified.

Note: Cutaneous lumps showing histopathological evidence of cutaneous lymphoma may develop in mares secondary to an ovarian granulosa cell tumour. Typical stallion-like behaviour (or benign anestrus) accompanied by skin nodules having the histopathological features of (T cell-rich) B cell lymphoma is a characteristic history. The cutaneous nodules may regress when an oral progestogen (such as allyltrenbolone) is administered for the infertility, but usually recur when therapy is stopped. Removal of the granulosa cell tumour may cause full regression of the skin problem. The role of oestrogen receptors is uncertain.

REFERENCES

1. Cotran RS, Kumar V and Robbins SL (1989) Inflammations and repair. In: Cotran RS, Kumar V and Robbins SL, eds. *Robbin's Pathological Basis of Disease*, 4th edn. WB Saunders, Philadelphia, pp. 39–86.
2. Grant DI (1991) Fungal skin disease. In: *Skin Diseases in the Dog and Cat*. Blackwell Scientific, London, p. 54.
3. Evans AG and Stannard AA (1986) Diagnostic approach to equine skin disease. *Compendium of Continuing Education for Veterinary Practitioners* **8**; 652–660.
4. McGavin MD and Fadok VA (1984) Factors limiting the usefullness of histopathological examination of skin biopsies in the diagnosis of large animal dermatoses. *Veterinary Clinics of North America, Large Animal Practice* **6**; 203–213.
5. Evans AG (1992) Dermatophilosis – Diagnostic approach to non-pruritic, crusting dermatitis in horses. *Compendium of Continuing Education for Veterinary Practitioners* **14**; 1618–1623.
6. Swiderski CE and McLure JJ (1995) Immunodiagnostic assays. *Veterinary Clinics of North America, Equine Practice* **11**; 455–489.
7. Fadok VA and Greiner EC (1990) Equine insect hypersensitivity: Skin test and biopsy results correlated with clinical data. *Equine Veterinary Journal* **22**; 236–240.
8. Littlewood JD (1997) Diagnostic procedures in equine skin disease. *Equine Veterinary Education* **9**; 174–176.
9. Fadok VA (1995) Overview of equine pruritus. *Veterinary Clinics of North America, Equine Practice* **11**; 1–9.
10. Spurlock SL and Hanie EA (1989) Antibiotics in the treatment of wounds. *Veterinary Clinics of North America, Large Animal Practice* **5**; 465.
11. Magdesian KG, Hogan PM, Brumbaugh G, Bernard WW, Chaffin MK and Cohen ND (1994) Pharmocodynamics of gentamicin administered once daily by the intravenous and intramuscular routes. *Proceedings of the 40th Annual Convention of the American Association of Equine Practitioners*, pp. 115–116.
12. Geor R (1997) Aminoglycoside dosing. In: Robinson NE, ed. *Current Therapy in Equine Medicine* 4. WB Saunders, Philadelphia, pp. 476–478.

13. Paterson S (1997) Dermatophytosis in 25 horses – a protocol of treatment using topical therapy. *Equine Veterinary Education* **9**; 171–173.
14. Robinson NE (1987) Table of common drugs: approximate doses. In: Robinson NE, ed. *Current Therapy in Equine Medicine 2*. WB Saunders, Philadelphia, p. 761.
15. Paterson S and Orrell S (1995) Treatment of biting lice (*Damalinea equi*) in 25 horses using 1% selenium sulphide. *Equine Veterinary Education* **7**; 304–306.
16. Barth D and Sutherland IH (1983) *Proceedings of the 12th World Veterinary Congress, Perth, Australia*, p. 14.
17. Stannard AA (1994) Corticosteroid therapy. *Proceedings of Workshop on Equine Dermatology, European Society of Veterinary Dermatologists, Newmarket, UK*.
18. Theon AP (1997) Cisplatin treatment for cutaneous tumours. In: Robinson NE, ed. *Current Therapy in Equine Medicine 4*. WB Saunders, Philadelphia, pp. 372–377.
19. Knottenbelt DC and Walker JA (1994) Topical treatment of the equine sarcoid. *Equine Veterinary Education* **6**; 72–75.
20. Bill R (1997) Anti-inflammatories. In: *Pharmacology for Veterinary Technicians*, chapter 12. Mosby, London, p. 277.
21. Goetz TE, Ogilvie GK, Keegan KG, Johnson PJ (1990) Cimetidine for the treatment of melanoma in 3 horses. *Journal of the American Veterinary Medical Association* **196**; 449–452.
22. Goetz TE and Long MT (1993) Treatment of melanoma in horses. *Compendium of Continuing Education* **15**(4); 608–610.
23. Manning TO (1983) Pemphigus foliaceus. In: Robinson NE, ed. *Current Therapy in Equine Medicine 1*. WB Saunders, Philadelphia, pp. 541–542.
24. Latimer CA (1987) Diseases of the adnexa and conjunctiva. In: Robinson NE, ed. *Current Therapy in Equine Medicine* 2nd ed. WB Saunders, Philadelphia, p. 442.
25. Grier RL, Brewer WG, Paul SR *et al.* (1980) Treatment of bovine and equine ocular squamous cell tumours by radio frequency hyperthermia. *Journal of the American Veterinary Medical Association* **177**; 55–58.
26. Hoffman KD, Kainer RA and Schideler RK (1983) Radio-frequency, current-induced hyperthermia for the treatment of equine sarcoid. *Equine Practice* **5**; 24–32.
27. Joyce JR (1975) Cryosurgery for removal of equine sarcoids. *Veterinary Medicine for Small Animal Clinicians* **70**; 200–203.
28. Fretz PB and Barber SM (1987) Prospective analysis of cryosurgery as the sole treatment for equine sarcoids. *Veterinary Clinics of North America* **10**; 847–850.
29. Lane JG (1977) The treatment of equine sarcoids by cryosurgery. *Equine Veterinary Journal* **9**; 127–128.
30. Wheat JD (1964) Therapy for equine sarcoids. *Modern Veterinary Practice* **45**; 62.
31. Page EH and Tiffany LW (1967) Use of autogenous equine fibrosarcoma vaccine. *Journal of the American Veterinary Medical Association* **150**; 177.
32. Rebhun WC (1987) Immunotherapy for sarcoids. In: Robinson NE, ed. *Current Therapy in Equine Medicine 2*. WB Saunders, Philadelphia, pp. 627–638.
33. Wyman M, Rings MD, Tarr MJ and Aldin CL (1977) Immunotherapy in equine sarcoid: a report of two cases. *Journal of the American Veterinary Medical Association* **171**; 449–451.
34. Vaneslow BA, Abetz I and Jackson ARB (1988) BCG emulsion immunotherapy of equine sarcoid. *Equine Veterinary Journal* **20**; 444–447.
35. Hepler DI and Lueker DC (1980) Letter to the Editor. *Journal of the American Veterinary Medical Association* **176**; 390.
36. Coombe KA (1994) Primary parotid lymphoma in a 10 year old Hanovarian gelding. *Equine Veterinary Education* **6**; 91–94.
37. Turrel JM and Koblik PD (1983) Techniques of after-loading iridium-192 interstitial brachytherapy in veterinary medicine. *Veterinary Radiology* **24**; 278–279.
38. Frauenfelder HC, Blevins WE and Page EH (1982) Sr^{90} for the treatment of periocular squamous cell carcinoma in the horse. *Journal of the American Veterinary Medical Association* **180**; 307–309.
39. Blood DC and Studdert VP (1988) *Baillière's Comprehensive Veterinary Dictionary*. Baillière Tindall, London.
40. Moens Y and Kombe AH (1988) Molluscum contagiosum in a horse. *Equine Veterinary Journal* **20**; 143–145.
41. Atwell RB and Summers PM (1977) Congenital papilloma in a foal. *Australian Veterinary Journal* **53**; 229.
42. Williams AM (1997) Papillomatosis: warts

and aural plaques. In: Robinson NE, ed. *Current Therapy in Equine Medicine 4*. WB Saunders, Philadelphia, pp. 398–390.
43. Pascoe RR, Spradbrow PB and Bagust TJ (1969) An equine genital infection resembling coital exanthema associated with a virus. *Australian Veterinary Journal* **45**; 166–170.
44. Welsh RD (1990) Corynebacterium pseudotuberculosis in the horse. *Equine Practice* **12**; 7–18.
45. White SD (1988) Corynebacterial folliculitis in a horse. *Journal of the American Veterinary Medical Association* **193**; 89–90.
46. Pascoe RR (1983) Dermatophilosis. In: Robinson NE, ed. *Current Therapy in Equine Medicine 1*. WB Saunders, Philadelphia, pp. 553–554.
47. Pascoe RR (1989) *Equine Dermatoses*, 3rd edn. University of Sydney Post Graduate Foundation in Veterinary Science No. 30. University of Sydney, Australia.
48. Rose RJ and Hodgson DR (1993) Hemolymphatic diseases. In: *Manual of Equine Practice*. WB Saunders, Philadelphia, p. 335.
49. Scott DW (1988) Immunologic diseases. In: *Large Animal Dermatology*. WB Saunders, Philadelphia, p. 321.
50. Pascoe RR (1979) The epidemiology of ringworm in racehorses caused by *Trichophyton equinum* var. *autotrophicum*. *Australian Veterinary Journal* **55**; 403–407.
51. Pascoe RR (1984) Infectious skin diseases of horses. *Veterinary Clinics of North America, Large Animal Practice* **6**(1); 27–46.
52. Pascoe RR (1973) Dermatophyte infection in the horse. Fellowship Thesis, Royal College of Veterinary Surgeons, London, UK.
53. Hiddleston WA (1970) The use of griseofulvin mycelium in equine animals. *Veterinary Record* **87**; 119.
54. Desplenter L (1989) Dermatophytosis in animals: Topical treatment and environmental control with enilconazole. Advances in Veterinary Dermatology. In: *Proceedings of the First World Congress of Veterinary Dermatology, Dijon*, pp. 453–454.
55. Pascoe RR and Connole MD (1974) Dermatomycosis due to *Microsporum gypseum* in horses. *Australian Veterinary Journal* **50**; 380–383.
56. Boomker J (1977) Black grain mycetoma (maduromycosis) in horses. *Ondesterpoort Journal of Veterinary Research* **44**; 249.
57. Miller RI (1980) Black grained mycetoma in two horses. *Australian Veterinary Journal* **56**; 347.
58. McEntee M (1987) Eumycotic mycetoma. Review and report of a cutaneous lesion caused by *Pseudallescheria boydii* in a horse. *Journal of the American Veterinary Medical Association* **191**(11); 1459–1461.
59. Kaplan W (1975) Equine phaeohypomycosis caused by *Drechslera apicifera*, cited by Scott DW (1988) *Large Animal Dermatology*, WB Saunders, Philadelphia.
60. Evans AG (1990) Alterations in skin. In: Smith BP, ed. *Large Animal Internal Medicine*. Mosby, St Louis, pp. 209–238.
61. Scott DW (1988) Dermatohistopathology. In: *Large Animal Dermatology*. WB Saunders, Philadelphia, pp. 29–49.
62. Bridges CH and Emmons CW (1961) A phycomycosis of horses caused by *Hypomyces destruens*. *Journal of the American Veterinary Medical Association* **138**; 579.
63. Moriello KA, DeBoer DJ and Semrad SD (1998) Diseases of the skin. In: Reed SM and Bayly WM, eds *Equine Internal Medicine*. WB Saunders, Philadelphia, pp. 534–536.
64. Restrepo LF, Morales LF, Robledo M, Restrepo A, Tenica C and Correa de I (1973) *Antioquia Medica* **23**; 13–25; cited by RI Miller (1980) Treatment of equine phycomycosis by immunotherapy and surgery. *Australian Veterinary Journal* **57**; 377–382.
65. Pascoe RR (1973) The nature and treatment of skin conditions observed in horses in Queensland. *Australian Veterinary Journal* **49**; 35–40.
66. McMullan WC, Joyce JR, Henselka DV and Heitmann JM (1977) Amphotericin B for the treatment of localised subcutaneous phycomycosis in the horse. *Journal of the American Veterinary Medical Association* **170**; 1293–1298.
67. Eaton SA (1993) Osseous involvement by *Pythium insidiosum*. *Compendium of Continuing Education for Practising Veterinarians* **15**(3); 485–488.
68. Miller RI (1981) Treatment of equine phycomycosis by immunotherapy and surgery. *Australian Veterinary Journal* **57**; 377–382.
69. Newton JC and Ross PS (1993) Case notes and commentary: Equine pythiosis – an

overview of immunity. *Compendium of Continuing Education for Practising Veterinarians* **15**; 491–493.
70. Alfaro AA and Mendoza L (1990) Four cases of equine bone lesions caused by *Pythium insidiosum*. *Equine Veterinary Journal* **22**(4): 295–297.
71. Terrel TG and Stookey JL (1973) *Besnoitia bennetii* in two Mexican burros. *Veterinary Pathology* **10**; 177–184.
72. Davis WP, Peters DF and Dunstan RW (1997) Besnoitiosis in a miniature donkey. *Veterinary Dermatology* **8**; 139–143.
73. Van Heerden J, Els HJ, Raubenheimer EJ and Williams JH (1993) Besnoitiosis in a horse. *Journal of the South African Veterinary Medical Association* **64**; 92–95.
74. Robertson A (1976) *Handbook on Animal Diseases in the Tropics*. British Veterinary Association, London.
75. Littlewood JD, Rose JF and Paterson S (1995) Oral ivermectin paste for the treatment of chorioptic mange in horses. *Veterinary Record* **137**; 661–663.
76. Barbet JL, Baxter GM and McMullen WC (1991) Diseases of the skin. In: Colahan PT, Mayhew IG, Merritt AM and Moore JN, eds. *Equine Medicine and Surgery*, 4th edn, American Veterinary Publications, Goleta CA, pp. 1569–1736.
77. Schumacher MJ, Schmidt JO, Egan NB and Dillon KA (1992) Biochemical variability of venoms from individual European and Africanized honey bees (*Apis mellifera*). *Journal of Allergy and Clinical Immunology* **90**; 59–65.
78. Staempfli HR and Kaushik A (1993) Clinical reactions of horses to venoms from winged stinging insects. *Equine Veterinary Education* **5**; 259–261.
79. Arundel JH (1978) Parasites of the horse. *Veterinary Review*, no. 18. Post Graduate Foundation for Veterinary Science, Sydney, Australia.
80. Dewes HF and Townsend KG (1990) Further observations on *Strongyloides westeri* dermatitis. Recovery of larvae from soil and bedding and survival in treated sites. *New Zealand Veterinary Journal* **38**; 34–37.
81. Scott DW (1988) Dermatohistopathology. In: *Large Animal Dermatology*. WB Saunders, Philadelphia, p. 49.
82. Scott DW (1988) *Large Animal Dermatology*. WB Saunders, Philadelphia.
83. Herd RP and Donham JC (1983) Efficacy of ivermectin against *Onchocerca cervicalis* microfilarila dermatitis in horses. *American Journal of Veterinary Research* **44**; 1102.
84. Stannard AA (1994) Erosive and ulcerative diseases. In: *Proceedings of Workshop on Equine Dermatology, European Society of Veterinary Dermatology, Newmarket, UK*, pp. 77–83.
85. Kohn CW, Johnson GC, Garry F, Johnson CW, Martin S and Scott DW (1989) Mechanobullous disease in a 2 month-old Belgian foal. *Equine Veterinary Journal* **21**; 297–301.
86. Knottenbelt DC and Pascoe RR (1994) *A Colour Atlas of Diseases and Disorders of the Horse*. Mosby-Wolfe, London.
87. Wellington JR and Scott DW (1991) Equine keratinizing cutaneous cysts. *Equine Practice* **13**; 8–17.
88. Stone WC (1990) The pathologic mineralization of soft tissue calcinosis circumscripta in horses. *Compendium of Continuing Education for Practising Veterinarians* **12**; 1643–1648.
89. Gell PGH and Coombs RRA (1964) *Clinical Aspects of Immunology*. FA Davis, Philadelphia.
90. Stannard AA (1994) Urticaria. *Proceedings of Workshop on Equine Dermatology, European Society of Veterinary Dermatologists, Newmarket, UK*.
91. Evans AG (1987) Recurrent urticaria due to inhaled allergens. In: Robinson NE, ed. *Current Therapy in Equine Medicine 2*. WB Saunders, Philadelphia, p. 619.
92. Degler JM (1997) Pruritic dermatoses. In: Robinson NE, ed. *Current Therapy in Equine Medicine 4*. WB Saunders, Philadelphia, pp. 377–381.
93. Evans AG (1990) Diseases of skin. In: Smith B, ed. *Large Animal Medicine*. CV Mosby, Philadelphia, pp. 1258–1260.
94. Rosser EJ, Ihrke PJ, White SD, *et al.* (1983) Equine pemphigus foliaceus. *Equine Veterinary Science* **3**(1); 14.
95. Schlipf JW (1997) Dermatologic conditions associated with crusts and scales. In: Robinson NE, ed. *Current Therapy in Equine Medicine 4*. WB Saunders, Philadelphia, pp. 381–386.
96. George LW and White SL (1984) Autoimmune skin diseases of large animals.

Veterinary Clinics of North America, Large Animal Practice **6**; 79–86.

97. Stannard AA (1994) Pastern and cannon leukoclastic vasculitis. In: *Proceedings of Workshop on Equine Dermatology, European Society of Veterinary Dermatologists, Newmarket, UK.*
98. Stannard AA (1994) Systemic lupus erythematosus. In: *Proceedings of Workshop on Equine Dermatology, European Society of Veterinary Dermatologists, Newmarket, UK.*
99. Stannard AA (1994) Alopecia areata. In: *Proceedings of Workshop on Equine Dermatology, European Society of Veterinary Dermatologists, Newmarket, UK.*
100. Stannard AA (1994) Linear keratosis. In: *Proceedings of Workshop on Equine Dermatology, European Society of Veterinary Dermatologists, Newmarket, UK.*
101. Stannard AA (1994) Sarcoidosis. In: *Proceedings of Workshop on Equine Dermatology, European Society of Veterinary Dermatologists, Newmarket, UK.*
102. Cotran RS, Kumar V and Robbins SL (eds) (1994) *Robbin's Pathological Basis of Disease*, 5th edn. WB Saunders, Philadelphia.
103. Scott DW (1997) Erythema multiforme in dogs, cats and horses: Literature review and case material from Cornell. *Proceedings of the British Veterinary Dermatology Study Group, Stratford upon Avon, 1997.*
104. Marshall C (1991) Erythema multiforme in two horses. *Journal of the South African Veterinary Association* **62**; 133.
105. Scott DW, Walton DK, Slater MR, *et al.* (1987) Immune-mediated dermatoses in domestic animals. *Compendium of Continuing Education* **9**; 539.
106. Dunham RJ (1979) *The Evaluation of 'Sumifly' for the Control of Queensland Itch (Culicoides brevitarsus) on Horses.* Shell Research Report, Melbourne, Australia.
107. Karcher LF, Scott DW, Paradis M and Anderson WI (1990) Sterile nodular panni culitis in five horses. *Journal of the American Veterinary Medical Association* **196**; 1823–1826.
108. Hawthorne T (1988) Equine amyloidosis. *Proceedings of the Veterinary Medical Forum of the American College of Veterinary Internal Medicine* **6**; 332.
109. van Andel ACJ, Gruys E and Kroneman J (1988) Amyloid in the horse; a report of nine cases. *Equine Veterinary Journal* **20**; 277.
110. Allen D, Clark ES and Murray MJ (1990) Disorders of the small intestine. In: Smith BP, ed. *Large Animal Internal Medicine.* CV Mosby, St Louis, pp. 654–659.
111. Thomsett LR (1984) Non-infectious skin diseases of horses. *Veterinary Clinics of North America, Large Animal Practice* **6**; 59–78.
112. Mattocks AR and Jukes R (1992) Detection of sulphur-conjugated pyrrolic metabolites in blood and fresh or fixed liver tissue from rats given a variety of toxic pyrrolizidine alkaloids. *Toxicology Letters* **63**; 47–55.
113. Mattocks AR and Jukes R (1991) The identification of hepatotoxic pyrrolizidine alkaloid exposure in horses by the demonstration of sulphur-bound pyrrolic metabolites on their haemoglobin. *Veterinary and Human Toxicology* **33**; 286–287.
114. McKenzie RA (1994) Plant poisoning in horses in Australia. *Proceedings of the 16th Bain Fallon Memorial Lectures.* Australian Veterinary Association, pp. 24–29.
115. Hillyer HM and Taylor FGR (1997) Cutaneous manifestations of suspected hypothyroidism in a horse. *Equine Veterinary Education* **4**; 116–118.
116. Irvine CHG and Evans MJ (1977) Hypothyroidism in foals. *New Zealand Veterinary Journal* **25**; 354.
117. Fadok VA and Wild S (1983) Suspected cutaneous iodism in a horse. *Journal of the American Veterinary Medical Association* **183**; 1104–1106.
118. Hintz HF (1993) Nutrition and skin disease. In: Robinson NE, ed. *Current Therapy in Equine Medicine 3.* WB Saunders, Philadelphia.
119. Harrington DD, Walsh J and White V (1973) Clinical and pathological findings on horses fed zinc deficient diets. In: *Proceedings of the Third Equine Nutrition and Physiology Symposium, USA.*
120. McLean J and Jones WE (1983) Depigmentation: copper supplement therapy, a case report. *Equine Veterinary Science* **3**; 208.
121. Meijer WCP (1962) Vitiligo in seven horses and five cattle. *Tidescrift voor geeneskunde* **87**; 411–425.
122. Pascoe RR (1973) The nature and treatment of skin conditions observed in horses in

Queensland. *Australian Veterinary Journal* **49**; 35–40.

123. Yu AA (1997) Dermatologic conditions associated with abnormal pigment. In: Robinson NE, ed. *Current Therapy in Equine Medicine 4*. WB Saunders, Philadelphia, pp. 391–393.
124. Stannard AA (1987) Hyperesthetic leukotrichia. In: Robinson NE, ed. *Current Therapy in Equine Medicine 1*. WB Saunders, Philadelphia, p. 647.
125. Scott DW (1988) Unilateral papular dermatosis. In: *Large Animal Dermatology*. WB Saunders, Philadelphia.
126. Rothwell TL and Birch CB (1991) Unilateral papular dermatitis in a horse. *Australian Veterinary Journal* **68**; 122–123.
127. Hackett RP, Dimock BA and Bentnick-Smith J (1983) Quantitative bacteriology of experimentally incised skin wounds of horses. *Equine Veterinary Journal* **15**; 37.
128. Knottenbelt DC (1997) Equine wound management; are there significant differences in healing at different sites on the body? *Veterinary Dermatology* **8**(4); 273–290.
129. Britton JW (1970) Wound management in horses. *Journal of the American Veterinary Medical Association* **157**; 1585–1589.
130. Bertone AL (1989) Management of exuberant granulation tissue. *Veterinary Clinics of North America, Equine Practice* **5**; 551–562.
131. Trotter GE (1989) Technique of wound closure. *Veterinary Clinics of North America, Large Animal Practice* **5**; 499–505.
132. Reid SW and Smith KT (1992) The equine sarcoid: Detection of papillomaviral DNA in sarcoid tumours by use of consensus primers and the polymerase chain reaction. *Proceedings of the Sixth International Conference on Equine Infectious Diseases, Cambridge, UK*, pp. 297–300.
133. Knottenbelt DC, Edwards SER and Daniel EA (1995) The diagnosis and treatment of the equine sarcoid. *In Practice* (supplement to *Veterinary Record*) **17**: 123–129.
134. Genetsky RM, Biwer RD and Myers RK (1983) Equine sarcoid: causes, diagnosis and treatment. *Compendium of Continuing Education* **5**; 416–420.
135. Jackson C (1936) The incidence and pathology of tumours of domestic animals in South Africa. *Ondesterpoort Journal of Veterinary Science and Animal Industry* **6**; 378–385.
136. Brostrom H (1995) *Equine Sarcoids: A clinical, epidemiological and immunological study*. Department of Medicine and Surgery, Faculty of Veterinary Medicine, Swedish University of Agricultural Sciences, Uppsala, Sweden, pp. 37–39.
137. Ragland WL, Keown GH and Spencer GR (1970) Equine sarcoid. *Equine Veterinary Journal* **2**; 2–11.
138. Lane JG (1977) The treatment of equine sarcoids by cryosurgery. *Equine Veterinary Journal* **9**; 127–133.
139. Hoffman KD, Kainer RA and Schideler RK (1983) Radio-frequency current induced hyperthermia for the treatment of equine sarcoid. *Equine Practice* **5**; 24–31.
140. Theon AP, Pascoe JR, Carlson GP and Krag DN (1993) Intratumoral chemotherapy with cisplatin in oily emulsions in horses. *Journal of the American Veterinary Association* **202**; 261–267.
141. Roberts D (1970) Experimental treatment of equine sarcoid. *Veterinary Medicine for the Small Animal Clinician* **65**; 67–73.
142. Rebhun WC (1987) Immunotherapy for sarcoids. In: Robinson NE, ed. *Current Therapy in Equine Medicine 2*. WB Saunders, Philadelphia, pp. 637–639.
143. Turrel JM, Stover SM and Gyorgyfalvy J (1985) Iridium-192 interstitial brachytherapy of equine sarcoid. *Veterinary Radiology* **26**; 20–24.
144. Honnas CM, Liskey CC, Meagher DM, Brown D and Luck EE (1990) Malignant melanoma in the foot of a horse. *Journal of the American Veterinary Medical Association* **197**; 756–758.
145. Silvassy IP, Brown JW and Dalgreen RR (1972) Prepucial carcinoma in a horse. *Veterinary Medicine for the Small Animal Clinician* **67**; 1329–1330.
146. Lavach D (1989) *Large Animal Ophthalmology*. Lea and Febiger, Philadelphia, p. 273.
147. Theon AP, Pascoe JR, Madigan JE, Carlson G and Metzer MS (1997) Comparison of intratumoral administration of cisplatin versus bleomycin for treatment of periocular squamous cell carcinoma in horses. *American Journal of Veterinary Research* **58**; 431–436.
148. Wyn-Jones G (1983) Treatment of equine cutaneous neoplasia by radiotherapy using iridium-192 linear sources. *Equine Veterinary Journal* **15**; 361–365.

149. Rebhun WC (1990) Treatment of advanced squamous cell carcinoma involving the equine cornea. *Veterinary Surgery* **19**; 297–302.
150. Howarth S, Lucke VM and Pearson H (1991) Squamous cell carcinoma of the equine external genitalia: a review and assessment of penile amputation and urethrostomy as a surgical treatment. *Equine Veterinary Journal* **23**; 53–58.
151. Honnas CM (1997) Keratomas of the equine digit. *Equine Veterinary Education* **9**; 203–207.
152. Lloyd KCK, Peterson PR, Wheat JD, Ryan AE and Clark JH (1988) Keratomas in horses: seven cases (1975–1986). *Journal of the American Veterinary Medical Association* **193**; 967–970.
153. Chaffin MK, Carter GK and Sustaire D (1989) Management of a keratoma in a horse; a case report. *Equine Veterinary Science* **9**; 323.
154. Honnas CM, Pelsos JG, Carter GK and Moyer W (1994) Surgical management of incomplete avulsion of the coronary band and keratomas in horses. *Veterinary Medicine* **89**; 984–988.
155. Wagner PC, Balch-Burnett O and Merrit F (1986) Surgical management of keratomas in the foot of the horse. *Equine Practice* **8**; 11.
156. Hillyer MH, Taylor FGR, Mair TS, Murphy D, Watson TGD and Love S (1992) Diagnosis of hyperadrenocorticism in the horse. *Equine Veterinary Education* **4**; 131–134.
157. Beech J and Garcia MC (1991) Disease of the endocrine system. In: Colohan PT, Mayhew IG, Merritt AM, Moore JN, eds. *Equine Medicine and Surgery*, 4th edn, vol. II. American Veterinary Publications, Goleta, CA, 1737–1751.
158. Beech J (1987) Evaluation of thyroid, adrenal and pituitary function. *Veterinary Clinics of North America* **3**; 649–660.
159. Knottenbelt DC (1997) *Formulary of Equine Medicine*. Liverpool University Press, p. 43.
160. Beech J and Garcia M (1985) Tumors of the pituitary gland (pars intermedia). In: Robinson NE, ed. *Current Therapy in Equine Medicine 2*. WB Saunders, Philadelphia, pp. 182–185.
161. Murphy DJ and Love S (1996) Diagnosis and treatment of equine pituitary adenoma (Cushing's disease). In: *Veterinary Annual*, vol. 36. Blackwell Scientific, Oxford, pp. 302–308.
162. Kolk JH van de (1997) Equine Cushing's disease. *Equine Veterinary Education* **9**; 209–214.

INDEX

Page numbers in **bold** refer to figures.

abscesses, 72, 97–9, **98**
  cheek, 98–9, **99**
  in streptococcal dermatitis, 107
acetate tape skin sampling, 26–7
acetic acid
  as antiseptic, 36
  as lavage fluid, 213
actinic dermatoses, 183–5, **184**
actinomycotic mycetomas, 115
acyclovir, 37
adhesive tape skin sampling, 26–7
adrenocorticotrophic hormone, for anhidrosis, 199
aesthenia, 146–7, **146**, **147**
albinism, 148–9, **149**
allergic/autoimmune diseases, 155–81
  alopecia areata, 168–9, **168**
  amyloidosis, 176–7, **176**
  atopy, 160–1, **161**
  axillary nodular necrosis, 177, **177**
  contact hypersensitivity, 173–4, **174**
  diagnosis, 155–6
  drug eruption, 174–5, **174**
  eosinophilic collagen necrosis, 177–8, **178**
  erythema multiforme, 170–1, **171**
  food hypersensitivity, 161
  granulomatous disease, 178–9, **179**
  insect hypersensitivity, 171–3, **172**
  leukocytoclastic vasculitis, pastern/cannon, 165–6, **165**
  linear keratosis, 169, **169**
  lymphoedema, 175–6, **175**
  panniculitis, 176
  pemphigus foliaceus, 162–3, **162**, **163**
  pemphigus vulgaris, 163–4, **163**
  purpura haemorrhagica, 180–1, **181**
  sarcoidosis, 169–70, **170**
  seborrhoea, 179–80, **180**
  systemic lupus erythematosus-like syndrome, 166–8, **166**, **167**
  urticaria, 156–60, **157**, **158**, **159**
  vasculitis, 164–5, **164**
allergy testing, 32–4, **33**
aloe vera, 53
alopecia, 68
  areata, 168–9, **168**
  classification of causes, **69**, **70**
  definition, 9, 18, 68
  linear, 169, **169**
  in nodular syndromes
    nonpruritic, 75
    pruritic, 74
  see also hypotrichosis
Altenaria, in mycetoma, 115
aminoglycosides, 41, 43
amphotericin B, 44, 47
  for phaeohyphomycosis, 116
  for pythiosis, intravenous, 119
amphoterics, 43
amyloidosis, cutaneous, 176–7, **176**
anaesthesia, for wound management, 209
  see also tranquillization
anagen defluxion, 199–200, **200**
anamnesis *see* history
anaphylactic response, **6**
  after BCG immunotherapy, 58
anatomy of skin, 3–4
angio-oedema, 158–9, **159**
anhidrosis, 199, **199**
antibiotics, 38–42
  for abscess, 98
  appropriateness checklist, 38
  for dermatophilosis, 105
  duration, 40, 42
  for folliculitis, 100
  lavage fluids, 213
  prophylactic, 38, 42
  route of administration, 40, 41–2
  selection, 39, 40–1
    sensitivity testing, 26
  side-effects, 38
  spectrum of activity, 41
  summary table, 43
antifungal agents, 42, 44–5
  appropriateness checklist, 38
  fungicides, for ringworm, 113
  summary table, 46–7
antigen-antibody complexes, in hypersensitivity reaction, **8**
antihistamines, 52
  for insect hypersensitivity, 173
  for urticaria, 160
antinuclear antibody testing, 32
antiseptics, 36
antiviral agents, 37–8
Appaloosa breed, congenital disorders
  mane/tail dystrophy, 147–8, **148**
  parentage syndrome, 149–50
Arabian fading syndrome, 150, **150**
arsenic
  poisoning, 187
  topical
    paste, 51
    for sarcoid, 251

arteritis, viral, 93
arthritis, septic, wound complication, 210
Aspergillus, antifungal treatment, 44
Astragulus, selenium accumulation, 186
atheroma, 152–3, **152**
atopy, 160–1, **161**
aural plaque, 95, **95**
aurothioglucose, 52
autoimmune diseases *see* allergic/autoimmune diseases
avermectin, 48
  for chorioptic mange, 124
AW(3)4–LUDES, 51
axillary nodular necrosis, 177, **177**

Bacillus Calmette–Guerin (BCG), 57–60
  in tumour treatment
    neurofibroma, 260
    sarcoid, 251
    squamous cell carcinoma, 265
bacterial diseases, 97–109
  abscess, 97–9, **98**
    cheek, 98–9, **99**
  dermatophilosis, 102–6, **102**, **103**, **104**, **105**
  folliculitis/furunculosis, 99–100, **99**
    pastern, 100–1, **100**
    streptococcal, 107–8, **107**
  glanders, 108–9, **108**
  granuloma, 101–2, **101**
  staphylococcal, 106–7, **106**
  ulcerative lymphangitis, 109, **109**
bacterial infections
  alopecia in, 69, 70
  nodular syndromes in, 74, 75
  pastern dermatitis in, 83
  pruritus in, 67
  scaling/crusting, 77
  weeping/seeping, 79
  and wound healing, 207
bandaging
  hoof support, 228
  injuries, 220–1, **220**, **221**
  of wounds, 216
    compression, 215
basal cell carcinoma, 252, **252**
basidiobolomycosis, 117, 118, **118**
basophils, in inflammatory response, 5
bastard strangles, 97, 107
bee stings, 133, 134, **135**
gamma-benzene hexachloride, for psoroptic mange, 126
besnoitiosis, 121–2, **121**
betamethasone, 48, 49
biopsy, 27–32
  fixatives, 28
  indications, 27
  limitations, 27
  methods, 28–30, **28**, **29**, **30**
  for *Onchocerca* detection, 31
  in phaeohyphomycosis, 115–16
  recommendations for quality, 31–2
  specimen handling, 30, **30**, **31**
  of tumours, diagnostic, 241, 243
  types, 27–8
biotin, and hoof quality, 193, *193*
bites, insect, 133–6, **133**, **134**, **135**
black-flies, bites, 133–4, **134**
blood supply, and wound healing, 207–8
blood vessels, wounding damage, exploration, 212
blow-fly strike, 136
boil, 99
bot parasites, avermectin against, 48
botryomycosis, 101–2, **101**
brachytherapy, 60–1, **61**
  of sarcoid, 251–2
  of squamous cell carcinoma, 265
branding
  freeze, 218, 222
  hot, 219, 222
bromocryptine mesylate, for Cushing's disease, 271
bruising
  sole, 234
  in traumatic injury, 216
buffalo fly, 131, 133, **133**
burns
  chemical, 223–4, **223**, **224**
  rope/wire, 220–1
  thermal, 218–20, **219**
  see also traumatic injury
bursae, 73
bursatti, 117–19, **118**
bursitis, 225–6, **226**

calcinosis circumscripta, 153, **153**
Calliphora infestation, 136
Callitroga, 136
cancer *see* neoplasms
canker, 235–6, **236**
cannon leukocytoclastic vasculitis, 165–6, **165**
'capped hock', **226**
carbuncle, 99
carcinomas
  antimitotic therapy, 51
  basal cell, 252, **252**
  immunotherapy, BCG, 58
  squamous cell *see* squamous cell carcinomas
casts, for coronary band injuries, 231
cautery, 54–5
  see also electrocautery
cellulitis, 73
  in traumatic injury, 216
cephalosporins, 43
cheek abscess, 98–9, **99**
cheloid, 222, **223**
  definition, 9–10
chemical alopecia, 69
chemical burns, 223–4, **223**, **224**
chemical pruritus, 69
chemical/toxic dermatoses, 183–8
  actinic, 183–5, **184**
  plant poisoning, 185–6, **186**
  poisoning
    arsenic, 187
    mercury, 187–8, **187**
    selenium, 186–7, **186**
chemotherapy, of sarcoid, 252
chigger mite, 127–8, **128**
chloramphenicol, 43
chlorhexidine, 36, 37
  for folliculitis control, 100
  lavage fluid, 212
  shampoo, for ringworm, 113
chlorinated hydrocarbon parasiticides, 45
Chorioptes equi, 123, **124**
  identification, 24
chorioptic mange, 123–4, **123**, **124**
  and pruritus, 66
Chrysomyia bezziana, 136
cimetidine
  antineoplastic action, 52
  for melanoma/melanosarcoma, 259
cisplatin
  intralesional, for melanoma/melanosarcoma, 259
  topical, 51
    for sarcoids, 251
clostridial abscess, 97–8

coital exanthema, 95–6, **96**
collagen necrosis/granuloma, eosinophilic, 177–8, **178**
compression bandaging, 215
conchal cyst, 150, **151**
congenital/developmental diseases, 145–53
  albinism, 148–9, **149**
  Appaloosa parentage syndrome, 149–50
  calcinosis circumscripta, 153, **153**
  conchal cyst, 150, **151**
  dentigerous cyst, 151, **151**
  dermoid cyst, 151–2, **152**
  epidermoid cysts, 152–3, **152**
  epidermolysis bullosa, 146, **146**
  epitheliogenesis imperfecta, 145, **145**
  fading syndrome, 150, **150**
  hyperelastosis cutis, 146–7, **146**, **147**
  hypotrichosis, 147–8, **148**
  mane/tail dystrophy, 147–8, **148**
  vascular hamartoma, 253, **253**
  see also genetic disorders
contact hypersensitivity, 173–4, **174**
Coombs' sensitivity reactions, 6, 7–8, 7, 8, 9
copper
  deficiency, 192
  and melanin production, 80
corns, 238, **238**
coronary band
  disorders, **88**
  dystrophy, 200–1, **200**
  injuries, 230–2, **231**
coronet dermatitis syndrome, 82
corticosteroids, 48–50
  anti-inflammatory action, 6
  for insect hypersensitivity, 173
  and laminitis, 35
  for leukocytoclastic vasculitis, 166
  topical, as antimitotics, 51–2
  see also prednisolone
Corynebacterium paratuberculosis, in ulcerative lymphangitis, 109
Corynebacterium pseudotuberculosis, abscess, 97
cracks, hoof, 228–30, **228**, **229**
crust, definition, 9
  see also scaling/crusting syndrome
cryosurgery/cryonecrosis, 55–7, **56**
  of melanoma/melanosarcoma, 259
  of sarcoids, 250
  of squamous cell carcinoma, 264, 265
cryptococcosis, equine, 117, **117**
Culicoides
  bites, 133
  control measures, 173
  hypersensitivity, 171–3, **172**
  irritation, 130–1, **130**
  repellants, 48
  in ventral midline dermatitis, 131, **131**
Curvularia geniculata, in mycetoma, 114
Cushing's disease, 269–71, **269**, **270**
cutaneous aesthenia, 146–7, **146**, **147**
cypermethrin, 48
cyproheptadine hydrochloride, for Cushing's disease, 271
cysts, 75
  conchal, 150, **151**
  definition, 9
  dentigerous, 151, **151**
  dermoid, 151–2, **152**
  epidermoid, 152–3, **152**
cytokines, in post-inflammatory repair, 6
cytology, in tumour diagnosis, 243
cytotoxic response, 7
cytotoxic therapy, 51

Damalinia equi infestation, 137–9, **137**, **138**, **139**
debridement of wounds, 213–14
decubitus ulcers, 220–1, **220**, **221**
Demodex species, 126, **127**
  identification
    D. caballi, 25
    D. equi, 24, 25
demodicosis, 126–7, **127**
dentigerous cyst, 151, **151**
depigmentation, idiopathic, 195–6, **195**, **196**
Dermanyssus gallinae infestation, 128–9, **129**
dermatitis
  coronet dermatitis syndrome, 82
  pastern, **83**, 201–2, **201**
  photodermatitis, in dermatophilosis, 102, 105, 106
  staphylococcal, 106–7, **106**
  streptococcal, 107–8, **107**
  ventral midline, 131–2
  viral papular, 93–4, **93**
dermatographism, in urticaria, 157, **157**, 159
dermatophilosis, 102–6, **102**, **103**, **104**, **105**
Dermatophilus congolensis
  in dermatophilosis, 102, **105**, 106
  identification, 23, 26
dermatophytosis
  and alopecia, 69
  and pruritus, 67
  see also antifungal agents; fungal diseases; fungal infections
dermatosparaxis, 146–7, **146**, **147**
dermoid cyst, 151–2, **152**
derris, 45
developmental diseases *see* congenital/developmental diseases
dexamethasone, 48, 49
diagnosis
  approach, 11
  basis, 3
  confirmation, 19–20
  differential, 19
  examination
    clinical, 17–18
    form, 11, **12–16**
  history taking, 17
  problem list, 18–19
  tests *see* tests, diagnostic/investigative
diarrhoea scalding, 224, **224**
dietary restriction/provocation tests, 32
diets
  fat/oil supplementation, 191
  hypoallergenic, in food allergy, 160
  see also nutritional disorders
disinfectants, 36–7
dourine, 122, **122**
Drachia megastoma infestation, 139–41, **139**, **140**
Drechslera spicifera, in phaeohyphomycosis, 115
dressings *see* bandaging; casts
drug eruption, 174–5, **174**
drugs *see by particular drug*
dry dermatoses *see* scaling/crusting syndrome

ear drops, for psoroptic mange, 126
Echidnophaga gallinacea infestation, 129–30
ectoparasites, and pruritus, 66
ectoparasiticides, 45, 48
Ehlers-Danlos syndrome, 146–7, **146**, **147**
electrocautery, 54
of sarcoids, 250–1
endocrine disorders
hypothyroidism, 189
iodism, 189–90, **190**
energy deficit, 191
enilkonazole, 44, 47
enteritis, chronic eosinophilic, 178–9, **179**
enzyme-linked immunosorbent assay (ELISA) allergy testing, 33–4
in urticaria, 160
eosinophilic collagen necrosis, 177–8, **178**
eosinophilic enteritis, chronic, 178–9, **179**
eosinophils, in inflammatory response, 5
epidermoid cysts, 152–3, **152**
epidermolysis bullosa, 146, **146**
epitheliogenesis imperfecta, 145, **145**
epizootic lymphangitis, 117, **117**
equine viral arteritis (EVA), 93
equine viral papular dermatitis, 93–4, **93**
erosion, definition, 10
erythema multiforme, 170–1, **171**
erythromycin, 43
etisazole, for phaeohyphomycosis, 116
exanthema, coital, 95–6, **96**
exclusion tests, 32
exuberant granulation tissue, 214–15, **214**, 217–18, **217**
eye disorders, habronemiasis, 139–41, **139**, **140**
see also ocular squamous cell carcinoma

fading syndrome, 150, **150**
farcy, 108
African, 117, **117**
fat (dietary), supplementation, 191
fenbendazole, for onchocerciasis, 142
fenvalerate fly repellent, 173
fibroblastic sarcoid, 246–7, **246**, **247**
mixed, 247, **247**
fibroma/fibrosarcoma, 252–3, **253**
of frog/sole, 267, **267**
ossifying fibroma, 261, **261**
fine needle aspirate, 28
method, 29, **30**
fissure, definition, 10
'fistulous withers', 226, **226**
fixatives, for biopsies, 28
fleas
and pruritus, 67
stickfast, 129–30
Florida leaches, 117–19, **118**
5–fluorouracil, topical, 51
for sarcoids, 251
for squamous cell carcinoma, 265
fly control, 173
repellents, 48, 173
fly strike, 136–7, **137**
folliculitis, 99–100, **99**
pastern, 100–1, **100**
streptococcal, 107–8, **107**
food hypersensitivity, 161
foot *see* hoof disorders
foreign bodies, and wound healing, 207
formaldehyde fumigation, 37
freeze brands, 218
frog disorders, **86**
fibroma, 267, **267**
fumigation
formaldehyde, 37
fungal diseases, 111–19
granuloma, 72
granuloma/pythiosis, 117–19, **118**
histoplasmosis, 117, **117**
microsporosis, 113–14, **114**
mycetoma, 114–15, **115**
phaeohyphomycosis, 115–16, **116**
sporotrichosis, 116–17, **116**
trichopytosis, 111–13, **111**, **112**
fungal infections
alopecia in, 69, 70
nodular syndromes in, 74, 75
pastern dermatitis in, 83
pruritus in, 67
scaling/crusting, 77
weeping/seeping, 79
fungi, culture, 26
fungicides, for ringworm, 113
see also antifungal agents
furunculosis, 99–100, **99**
Fusobacterium necrophorus, in canker, 236

genetic disorders, hoof defects, 228
see also congenital/ developmental diseases
giant-cell tumour, 254
glanders, 108–9, **108**
and differential diagnosis, 19
see also pseudoglanders
gnats *see Culicoides*
gold therapy, 52, 60–1, **61**
granulation tissue, exuberant, 214–15, **214**, 217–18, **217**
granulocytes, in inflammatory response, 5
granuloma
bacterial, 101–2, **101**
eosinophilic collagen, 177–8, **178**
fungal, 117–19, **118**
granulomatous disease, generalized, 178–9, **179**
'grass warts', 94–5, **94**, **95**
vaccination, 57
'greasy heel' syndrome, 83, 88, 202–3, **202**
pastern folliculitis in, 100
griseofulvin, 44, 46
oral, for ringworm, 113
growth factors, in post-inflammatory repair, 6
gyrate urticaria, 158, **159**

habronemiasis, 139–41, **139**, **140**
haemangioma/haemangiosarcoma , 253–4, **253**
Haematobia irritans, 131
bites, 133, **133**
haematology, 18
in tumour diagnosis, 243
haematoma, 73
heel, 233, **233**
sole, 234
in traumatic injury, 216
Haematopinus asini infestation, 137–9, **137**, **138**, **139**
hair
pigmentation changes, 80
sampling, 23–4
see also alopecia
hamartoma, vascular, 253, **253**
harvest mite
identification, 24
infestation, 127–8, **128**

heavy metals, for sarcoid topical treatment, 251
heel cracks, 229, **229**
  treatment, 230
helminths
  avermectin for, 48
  and pruritus, 67
hernia, nodules, 73
herpesvirus infections
  acyclovir for, 37
  coital exanthema, 95–6, **96**
hexachlorophene, 36, 37
Hippobosca, bites, 133, 134, **134**
hirsutism, in Cushing's disease, 269, **269**
histiocytic lymphosarcoma, 256–7, **256**, **257**
histiocytoma, malignant fibrous, 254
histoplasmosis, 117, **117**
history
  taking, 17
  in wound management, 208–9
homeopathic therapy, 53
hoof disorders, 84, 227–39
  canker, 235–6, **236**
  clinical examination, 227
  corns, 238, **238**
  coronary band, **88**
    injuries, 230–2, **231**
  cracks, 228–30, **228**, **229**
  frog, **86**
    fibroma, 267, **267**
  genetic defects, 228
  heel haematoma, 233, **233**
  lateral cartilage necrosis, 236–7, **237**
  neoplastic
    fibroma, 238–9, 267, **267**
    keratoma, 267–9, **268**
    sarcoids, 238–9
  seedy toe, 237–8
  sole, **86**
    bruising/haematoma, 234
    fibroma, 267, **267**
    wounds, 232–3, **232**
  thrush, 236, **236**
  wall, **87**
    break-back, 234, **234**
    rings/laminitis, 234–5, **235**
hoof quality, and biotin/methionine, 193, *193*
horn fly *see Haematobia*
horse fly, 131, 133
horse pox, 91–2, **91**
hydrogen peroxide, 36
  lavage fluid, 212–13
hydroxyzine hydrochloride, 52
hyperaesthetic leuko(melano)trichia, 198, **198**
hyperelastosis cutis, 146–7, **146**, **147**
hyperpigmentation, definition, 10
hypersensitivity
  contact, 173–4, **174**
  food, 161
  insect, 171–3, **172**
    and pruritus, 67
  responses, 4, **6**, 7–8, **7**, **8**, **9**, 155
hyperthermia, surgical
  radiofrequency, 55, 250
  of sarcoids, 250
hypertrophic scar, 222, **222**
hypodermiasis, 132, **132**
hypopigmentation, 10
hypopyon, in SLE-like syndrome, 167, **167**
hypothyroidism, 189
hypotrichosis, 147–8, **148**

iatrogenic/idiopathic disorders
  anagen defluxion, 199–200, **200**
  anhidrosis, 199, **199**
  burns, firing/branding, 218, 219, **219**
  coronary band dystrophy, 200–1, **200**
  'greasy heel' syndrome, 83, 88, 100, 202–3, **202**
  hyperaesthetic leuko(melano)trichia, 198, **198**
  leukoderma, 196–7, **196**
  leukotrichia, **196**, 197, **197**
  pastern dermatitis, **83**, 201–2, **201**
  unilateral papular dermatosis, 198–9, **199**
  vitiligo, 195–6, **195**, **196**
idiopathic disorders *see* iatrogenic/idiopathic disorders
imidazoles, 44, 47
immune responses, 155
immune-mediated diseases *see* allergic/autoimmune diseases
immunofluorescence tests, 32
immunotherapy, 57–60
  immune stimulants, 52–3
  immunomodulation, 57–60
  of sarcoid, 251
  of squamous cell carcinoma, 265
  vaccination, 57
impression smears, 28
  method, 29–30, **30**
inflammation, 4–7
  acute response, 4–5
  chronic, 5–7
  Coombs' sensitivity reactions, 4, **6**, 7–8, **7**, **8**, **9**
inflammatory nodules, 72
injuries *see* traumatic injury
  see also wounds
insect bites/stings, 133–6, **133**, **134**, **135**
insect hypersensitivity, 171–3, **172**
insecticides, 45, 48
iodide therapy
  agents, 44, 46
  for phaeohyphomycosis, 116
  for sporotrichosis, 116
  see also povidone-iodine
iodine
  deficiency, 191–2
  topical, for sporotrichosis, 116–17
iodism, 189–90, **190**
  see also hypothyroidism
iridium-192 therapy, 60–1, **61**
irrigation of wounds, 209, **209**
itraconazole, 44
ivermectin, 48
  for habronemiasis, 141
  for louse infestation, 139
  for mange
    chorioptic, 124
    sarcoptic, 126
  for onchocerciasis, 142–3
Ixeuticus robusta, bites, 135, **135**

keratoma, 268–9, **268**
keratosis, linear, 169, **169**
ketoconazole, 44, 47
  for phaeohyphomycosis, 116
'kunkers'
  of mycetoma, 114
  of pythiosis, 117

laceration, 216
lameness, in foot disorder syndrome, 86, 87
  see also hoof disorders
laminitis, 234–5, **235**
  and corticosteroids, 35, 48–9, 50
  in foot disorder syndrome, 86
  see also hoof disorders

Lampona cylindrata, bites, 135, **135**
laser surgery, of sarcoids, 250, 251
lateral cartilage necrosis, 236–7, **237**
lavage, of wounds, 212–13
lavender foal syndrome, 148–9
lethal-white foal syndrome, 148–9
Leucaena leucocephala, poisoning, 185–6, **186**
leukocytoclastic vasculitis, pastern/cannon, 165–6, **165**
leukoderma, 196–7, **196**
leukotrichia, **196**, 197, **197**
 hyperaesthetic, 198
leukotrienes, 6
levamisole, as immunomodulator, 53
lice
 and alopecia, 69
 infestation, 137–9, **137**, **138**, **139**
 ivermectin against, 48
 and pruritus, 66, 67
lichenification, definition, 10
ligation, surgical, 54, **54**
 of sarcoids, 249
lime sulphur, 45
Lindane, for psoroptic mange, 126
'line firing', 218, 219, **219**
linear keratosis, 169, **169**
lipoma, 254–5, **255**
 surgical excision, 53
liver failure, photosensitization in, 184, **184**, 185
louse *see* lice
louse fly, bites, 133, 134, **134**
lupus erythematosus, diagnosis, antinuclear antibody, 32
 see also systemic lupus erythematosus-like syndrome
lymphangioma, 255, **255**
lymphangitis
 epizootic, 117, **117**
 ulcerative, 109, **109**
lymphocytes, in inflammatory response, 5
lymphoedema, 175–6, **175**
lymphoma, 255–6, **256**
lymphosarcoma, 256–7, **256**, **257**
 generalized, 272
macrolides, 43
macrophages, in inflammatory response, 5
macule, definition, 8
malevolent sarcoid, 247–8, **248**
malic acid
 as antiseptic, 36
 as lavage fluid, 213
malignancy *see* neoplasms
malignant fibrous histiocytoma, 254
Malleomyces mallei, in glanders, 108
mane dystrophy, 147–8
mange
 chorioptic, 66, 123–4, **123**, **124**
 demodectic, 126–7, **127**
 and pruritus, 66
 psoroptic, 124–6, **125**
 sarcoptic, 126, **126**
 see also mites
mast cell tumour *see* mastocytoma
mast cells, in inflammatory response, 5
mastocytoma, 258
 surgical excision, 53
mebendazole, for onchocerciasis, 142
melanin, 80
melanocytes, and pigmentation, 80
melanoma/melanosarcoma, 258–60, **259**
 antimitotic therapy
  systemic, 52
  topical, 51
melanotrichia, hyperaesthetic, 198
mercury poisoning, 187–8, **187**
mercury, for sarcoid topical treatment, 251
metalloproteinases, in inflammatory response, 6–7
metazoan diseases *see* parasitic diseases
methionine, and hoof quality, 193, *193*
methylprednisolone, 48, 49
 for urticaria, 160
 see also corticosteroids; prednisolone
metronidazole, 41, 43
Michel's medium for biopsy preservation, 28
miconazole, 44, 47
 shampoo, 113
microfilariasis, 141–3, **142**
microsporosis, 113–14, **114**
 see also ringworm
Microsporum, antifungal therapy, 44–5
midge *see Culicoides*
Mills wound irrigator, 209, **209**
mimosa poisoning, 185–6, **186**
mites
 and alopecia, 69
 avermectin compounds against, 48
 identification, 24
 infestations
  Dermanyssus gallinae, 128–9, **129**
  trombiculidiasis, 127–8, **128**
 and pruritus, 66, 67
 see also mange
molluscum contagiosum, 92, **92**
mosquitoes, bites, 134, **134**
'mud rash', **104**
mycetoma, 114–15, **115**
mycosis
 and alopecia, 69
 and pruritus, 67
 see also fungal diseases; fungal infections
myiasis, 136–7, **137**

natamycin, 44–5, 47
necrotic disorders
 axillary necrosis, 177, **177**
 eosinophilic collagen, 177–8, **178**
 lateral cartilage, 236–7, **237**
 pressure necrosis, 220–1, **220**, **221**
 seedy toe, 237–8
needle aspirate *see* fine needle aspirate
nematodes
 infestation, 139–41, **139**, **140**
 larvae, identification, 24
neonatal wart, 94, **94**
neoplasms, 241–72
 basal cell carcinoma, 252, **252**
 diagnosis, 241–3
 fibroma/fibrosarcoma, 252–3, **253**
  of frog/sole, 267, **267**
 foot, 238–9
 in foot disorder syndrome, 87, 86, 88
 haemangioma/haemangiosarcoma, 253–4, **253**
 in hair disorders, 69, 70

histiocytoma, malignant fibrous, 254
internal, with skin manifestations, 269–72
Cushing's disease, 269–71, **269, 270**
lymphosarcoma, generalized, 272
keratoma, 267–9, **268**
lipoma, 254–5, **255**
lymphangioma, 255, **255**
lymphoma, 255–6, **256**
lymphosarcoma, 256–7, **256, 257**
mastocytoma, 257–8
melanoma/melanosarcoma, 258–9, **258**
neurofibroma, 260, **260**
nodular, 72, 75
ossifying fibroma, 260–1, **261**
sarcoid *see* sarcoid
scaling/crusting, 77
sebaceous gland tumour, 266
squamous cell carcinoma *see* squamous cell carcinoma
surgical excision, 53
sweat gland tumour, 266–7, **267**
treatment
antimitotic, 51
radiotherapy, 60–2, **61**
surgical, 53, 54–6
see also by individual disease
tumour growth rate, 241
weeping/seeping, 79
see also tumour, definition
nerves, damage in wounding, exploration, 212
neurofibroma, 260, **260**
neutrophils, in inflammatory response, 5
nitroimidazoles, 43
Nocardia, in mycetoma, 115
nodular disorders
axillary necrosis, 177, **177**
eosinophilic collagen necrosis, 177–8, **178**
sarcoid, 245–6, **246**
mixed, 247, **247**
nodules, 72
classifications
clinical, **74–5**
physical, **73**
definition, 9, 19
nonsteroidal anti-inflammatory drugs, action, 6
nutritional disorders, 191–3
alopecia, 69
foot disorder syndrome, 87, 88
pigmentary changes, 81
nystatin, 44, 46

ocular squamous cell carcinoma, 261, 262
clinical signs, 263, **264**
treatment, 264–5
oil (dietary), supplementation, 191
Onchocerca, biopsy technique, 31
onchocerciasis, 141–3, **142**
opsonins, 5
organophosphates, 45
ossifying fibroma, 261, **261**
oxygenation, and wound healing, 208
oxyuriasis, 143, **143**
Oxyuris equi, detection, 26–7

panniculitis, 176
papillomata, grass wart, vaccination, 57
papillomatosis, 94–5, **94, 95**
congenital, 94, **94**
see also warts
papillomavirus, in sarcoid, 244
papular disorders
unilateral dermatosis, 198–9, **199**
viral dermatitis, 93–4, **93**
papule, definition, 8
parasites, identification in groomings, 22
parasitic diseases, 123–43
chorioptic mange, 123–4, **123, 124**
Culicoides see Culicoides
demodicosis, 126–7, **127**
habronemiasis, 139–41, **139, 140**
hypodermiasis, 132, **132**
insect bites/stings, 133–6, **133, 134, 135**
myiasis, 136–7, **137**
onchocerciasis, 141–3, **142**
oxyuriasis, 143, **143**
pediculosis, 137–9, **137, 138, 139**
poultry red mite, 128–9, **129**
protozoal, 121–2, **121, 122**
psoroptic mange, 124–6, **125**
sarcoptic mange, 126, **126**
stickfast fleas, 129–30
tromiculidiasis, 127–8, **128**
ventral midline dermatitis, 131–2
parasitic infections
alopecia in, 70
nodular syndromes in, 74, 75
pastern dermatitis in, 83
pruritus in, 67
scaling/crusting in, 77
weeping/seeping in, 79
parasiticides, 45, 48
pastern, disorders of
dermatitis, **83**, 201–2, **201**
folliculitis, 100–1, **100**
leukocytoclastic vasculitis, 165–6, **165**
pediculosis, 137–9, **137, 138, 139**
see also lice
Pelodera, identification, 24
pemphigus
foliaceus, 162–3, **162, 163**
vulgaris, 163–4, **163**
penicillins, 41, 43
penile squamous cell carcinoma, 261
pergolide, for Cushing's disease, 271
periosteum, damage exploration, 211–12, **211**
permethrin, 48
pH, and wound healing, 208
phaeohyphomycosis, 115–16, **116**
phagocytosis, in inflammatory response, 5
photodermatitis, in dermatophilosis, 102, 105, 106
photographs of skin disease, 18
photosensitization, 183–5, **184**
phycomycosis, 117–19, **118**
pigmentation
alterations, 80, **81**
hypo-/hyperpigmentation definition, 10
'pin firing', 218, 219
pin worm infestation, 143, **143**
pinky syndrome, 150, **150**
pinnal papilloma, 95, **95**
'pitting-on-pressure' test, 157
plants
poisoning, 185–6, **186**
seleniferous, 186
plaque, definition, 8
podophyllin, 51
for sarcoids, 251
poisoning
arsenic, 187
iodine, 189–90, **190**
mercury, 187–8, **187**

poisoning (*cont.*)
plant, 185–6, **186**
selenium, 186–7, **186**
potassium iodide antifungal, 44
potassium monopersulphate, 45
poultry red mite infestation, 128–9, **129**
povidone-iodine, 36, 37, 46
for folliculitis control, 100
lavage fluid, 212
pox *see* viral diseases
prednisolone, 48, 49
for immune-mediated vasculitis, 165
for insect hypersensitivity, 173
for pemphigus foliaceus, 163
topical, as antimitotic, 51–2
for urticaria, 160
see also corticosteroids
pressure necrosis, 220–1, **220**, **221**
prostaglandins, in inflammation, 5–6
proteinases, in inflammatory response, 6–7
protozoa, nodular syndromes, 74, 75
protozoal disorders, 121–2, **121**, **122**
proud flesh, 214–15, **214**, 217–18, **217**
provocation tests, 32
pruritus, 18, 66
in alopecia classification, 69
classification of causes, **67**
Pseudoallescheria boydii, in mycetoma, 114
pseudoglanders, 117, **117**
Pseudomonas, antiseptic control, 36
Pseudomonas mallei, in glanders, 108
Psoroptes equi, 124, **125**
Psoroptes hippotis, 124
psoroptic mange, 124–6, **125**
purpura haemorrhagica, 180–1, **181**
after abscess, 98
pustule, definition, 8
pyrethrins, 45
pyrethroids, synthetic, 48
pythiosis, 69, 117–19, **118**

quarter cracks, 228, **229**
treatment, 230
Queensland itch, 171–3, **172**
quittor, 236–7, **237**

radioallergosorbent test (RAST), 33–4
in urticaria, 160
radiofrequency hyperthermia, 55
of sarcoids, 250
radiology, in tumour diagnosis, 243
radiotherapy, 60–2, **61**
of sarcoid, 251–2
of squamous cell carcinoma, 60–1, **61**, 265
restriction tests, 32
Rhodococcus equi, 97
ringworm
antifungal therapy, 44–5
identification, 24
microsporosis, 113–14, **114**
trichophytosis, 111–13, **111**, **112**
rotenone, 45

'saddle rash', **106**
saline, as lavage fluid, 212
sarcoid, 244–52
aetiology, 244
clinical aspects, 244
of foot, 238–9
treatment, 248–52
benign neglect, 249
chemotherapy, 252
choice, factors in, 249
immunological, 58–9, 251
limitations, 249
radiation, 252
surgical, 53, 249–51
topical cytotoxic/antimitotic, 51, 251
types
fibroblastic, 246–7, **246**, **247**
malevolent, 247–8, **248**
mixed, 247, **247**
nodular, 245–6, **246**
occult, 244–5, **244**, **245**
verrucous, 245, **245**
at wound site, 208
sarcoidosis, 169–70, **170**
Sarcoptes scabei, 126, **126**
identification, 24
sarcoptic mange, 126, **126**
scalding
diarrhoea/urine, 224–5, **224**, **225**
thermal, 219
scales, definition, 9
scaling/crusting syndrome, classification, 76, **77**
scar, definition, 9–10
scarring, after traumatic injury, 221–3, **221**, **222**, **223**
see also exuberant granulation tissue
screw-worm larval infestation, 136
scrub-itch, 127–8, **128**
mite identification, 24
sebaceous gland tumour, 266
seborrhoea, 179–80, **180**
sedation *see* tranquillization
see also anaesthesia
seedy toe, 237–8
selenium poisoning, 186–7, **186**
selenium sulphide, 48
sensitivity reactions, 4, **6**, 7–8, **7**, **8**, **9**
septic arthritis, wound complication, 210
shampoos
antiparasitic, for psoroptic mange, 126
for folliculitis control, 100
fungicidal, for ringworm, 113
selenium sulphide, 48
shoeing, and thin walls, 228
Simulium, bites, 133–4, **134**
smears *see* impression smears
sodium iodide antifungal, 44
soles
bruising/haematoma, 234
cracks, 229, **229**
treatment, 230
fibroma, 267, **267**
genetic defects, 228
puncture wounds, 232–3, **232**
spider bites, 135, **135**
Sporothrix schenckii, antifungal therapy, 44
sporotrichosis, 116–17, **116**
squamous cell carcinoma, 261–6, **263**, **264**
clinical signs, 263–4, **263**, **264**
diagnosis, 264
prevention, 266
prognosis, 265–6
tabulated summary of, 262
treatment, 264–6
immunotherapy, BCG, 58, 60
radiotherapy, 60–1, **61**
surgical excision, 53
types, 261–3
stable fly, 131
bites, 133, **133**
staphylococcal infections
folliculitis, 99
pastern, 100
pseudomycetoma, 101–2, **101**

skin, 106–7, **106**
steatitis, 176
stickfast fleas, 129–30
stings, insect, 133–6, **133**, **134**, **135**
stomatitis, vesicular, 92
Stomoxys calcitrans see stable fly
strangles, 97, 107
streptococci
antibiotic sensitivity, 41
infections, 97, 99, 107–8, **107**
abscess, *S. equi*, 97
Strongyloides, identification, 24
sulphonamides, 43
potentiated, for besnoitiosis, 122
sunburn, 183, 184, **184**
surgery
indications for, 53
methods, 54–7, **54**, **56**
principles, 53–7
for pythiosis, 119
scarring, 221, **221**, **222**
tumour excision *see by individual tumours*
suturing, 213, 215–16
swabs for culture, 25–6
swamp cancer, 117–19, **118**
sweat gland tumour, 266–7, **267**
sweating, 3
in Cushing's disease, 269, **269**
sweet itch, 171–3, **172**
systemic lupus erythematosus (SLE), diagnosis, 32
systemic lupus erythematosus-like syndrome, 166–8, **166**, **167**

Tabanus, 131, 133
tail dystrophy, 147–8, **148**
teeth *see* dentigerous cyst
teleradiotherapy, 61–2
of sarcoid, 251–2
of squamous cell carcinoma, 265
tendons, damage exploration, 211, **211**
tertiary amine disinfectants, 37–8
tests, diagnostic/investigative, 20, 21–34
allergy, 32–4, **33**
antinuclear antibody, 32
immunofluorescence, 32
practice laboratory equipment, 21, 22
restriction/provocation, 32
samples for, 21–32
acetate tape, 26–7
biopsy, 27–32
groomings, 22, **22**
hair, 22
scrapings, 24–5
swabs, 25–6
tetracyclines, 43
thermocautery, 54–5
thrush, hoof, 236, **236**
tick infestation, 135
and pruritus, 67
toe cracks, 228, **228**
togavirus infection, arteritis, 93
toxic dermatoses *see* chemical/toxic dermatoses
toxicity, of parasiticides, 45
toxins, in alopecia, 69
tranquillization
for biopsy, 28
for intradermal allergy testing, 32
see also anaesthesia
traumatic injury
bursitis, 225–6, **226**
chemical, 223–4, **223**, **224**
hoof
coronary band, 230–2, **231**
foot disorder syndrome, 86
sole puncture, 232–3, **232**
nodules in, 73
pressure necrosis, 220–1, **220**, **221**
scalding (diarrhoea/urine), 224–5, **224**, **225**
scarring, 221–3, **221**, **222**, **223**
thermal burns, 218–20
see also wounds
triamcinolone, and laminitis, 49
Trichophyton, antifungal therapy, 44–5
trichopytosis, 111–13, **111**, **112**
see also ringworm
tripelennamine hydrochloride, 52
trombiculid mites, identification, 24
trombiculidiasis, 127–8, **128**
Trypanosoma equiperdum, in dourine, 122
tumour, definition, 9
see also neoplasms

Uasin Gishu disease, 93–4
ulcerative lymphangitis, 109, **109**
ulcers
decubitus, 220–1, **220**, **221**
definition, 10
oral, in Cushing's disease, 269, **270**
ultrasonography, in tumour diagnosis, 243
ultraviolet exposure, actinic dermatoses, 183–5, **184**
unilateral papular dermatosis, 198–9, **199**
urine scalding, 224, 225, **225**
urticaria, 156–60, **157**, **158**, **159**

vaccination, 57
for papillomatosis, 95
for pythiosis, 119
in sarcoid treatment, 251
see also immunomodulation
vasculitis
immune-mediated, 164–5, **164**, 180–1, **181**
leukocytoclastic, pastern/cannon, 165–6, **165**
venereal diseases
dourine, 122, **122**
exanthema, 95–6, **96**
verrucous nodules, 73
see also warty sarcoid
vesicle, definition, 8
vesicular stomatitis, 92
viral diseases, 91–6
arteritis, 93
coital exanthema, 95–6, **96**
horse pox, 91–2, **91**
molluscum contagiosum, 92, **92**
papillomatosis, 94–5, **94**, **95**
congenital, 94, **94**
papular dermatitis, 93–4, **93**
vesicular stomatitis, 92
see also antiviral agents
viral infections
alopecia in, 69, 70
nodular syndromes in, 75
scaling/crusting, 77
weeping/seeping, 79
viruses, swabs for detection, 25
vitamin deficiencies, 192, **192**, **193**
and wound healing, 208
vitiligo, 195–6, **195**, **196**
acquired, 196–7, **196**
vulval carcinoma, 262, 263
treatment, 264–5

wall
break-back, 234, **234**
rings, 234–5, **235**
warble fly infestation, 132, **132**

warts, neonatal, 94, **94**
  see also 'grass warts'; papillomatosis
warty sarcoid, 245, **245**
  mixed, 247, **247**
wasp stings, 134, **135**
weeping/seeping syndrome, 78, **79**,
wet dermatoses, 78, **79**
wheals
  definition, 9
  in urticaria, 157–8, **157**, **158**
white line disease, 237–8
wire injuries, 231, **231**
withdrawal syndromes, corticosteroid, 50
withers bursa, 226, **226**
wounds
  clinical signs, 216
  exuberant granulation tissue, 214–15, **214**, 217–18, **217**
  healing, 205–8
    factors affecting, 207–8
    summary principles, **206**, 207
  preliminary approach, 208–12
    diagnosis, 216
    history, 208–9
    preparation/exploration, 209–12
    restraint/anaesthesia, 209
  sole puncture, 232–3, **232**
  treatment, 217
    closure, 215–16
    debridement, 213–14
    lavage, 212–13
  see also traumatic injury

zinc deficiency, 191, **192**
  and wound healing, 208